MW01196752

Karen Kirkness has written a highly individual and intensely interesting book. If you have not been exposed to the "new" anatomy, Karen will definitely expand your concepts about our unfolding life-long dance between stability and mobility.
Thomas W. Myers, Author of *Anatomy Trains*

I really enjoyed reading this book. It offers unique images to support very well-researched views, presented in a conversational tone that I know readers in fascia will not want to miss. Well done!
Prof. Dr. Andry Vleeming World Congress on low back and pelvic girdle pain

Karen approaches the interweaving of gross and subtle in a captivating way, highlighting the connections between ideas with such curiosity and openness. It has and will continue to change the way I look at movement.
Yashodha Govindaraju Yoga practitioner

This book builds a bridge between the outdated classical biomechanical anatomy and the concept of human posture and movement as a holistic manifestation of a self-organizing and shaping organism. The subtitle of this book rightly speaks of a new anatomy, a trans-anatomically oriented architectural anatomy, an "integrated anatomy." With that, the book is not only an enrichment for yoga-oriented people but is warmly recommended for anyone who really wants to delve into what moves us. And that is spirit.
Jaap van der Wal Phenomenologist, Morphologist and Embryologist

In a clear, precise and conversational way, Karen guides us on a journey into our spiraling selves, shining a light on why this is of the utmost importance for any movement modality.
Rachel Tudor tudorpilates.com

Karen's dynamic teachings are imbued with intelligence, humor, experience, and an infectious energy that I adore. She's extraordinary!
Karyn Stillwell www.stillwellyogaonline.com

I recommend this book for serious yoga educators and practitioners, and all who want an in-depth illustrated manual of how the embryo becomes a living, spiraling manifested mystery.
Carol M. Davis DPT, EdD, MS, FAPTA, Professor Emerita, University of Miami School of Medicine; Myofascial Release Physical Therapist and Teacher; Author and Editor: Integrated Therapies in *Rehabilitation/Evidence of Efficacy in Therapy, Prevention and Wellness*

There is no other book like this out there, it takes you from the beginning, and it will forever change the way you look at your own movement and how you help your clients. Absolutely stunning work!
Olivia Kampe Pilates teacher https:∥kinuum.com

I am blown away by Karen's gifted use of language and story-telling as she guides readers through the embryonic roots of spiral movement, leaving you in awe of the human form, where there are no individual parts, only a magnificent, ever spiralling and pulsing whole.
Eija Tervonen Yoga teacher, Somatics practitioner, Spiral Stabilisation trainer

Karen Kirkness has created a trailblazing paradigm of human anatomy that explains why yoga has such a profound impact on body, mind and spirit. She provides a brilliant new model of anatomy that will transform how you experience and view yourself. Reading this book will absolutely elevate your yoga practice.

Mercedes (Didi) von Deck MD Orthopaedic surgeon, Fellow of the American Academy of Orthopaedic Surgery; Ashtanga Yoga Teacher (Director of Down Under Yoga Mysore Ashtanga Program); Guild Certified Feldenkrais Practitioner

This is not just a yoga book but a clearly referenced anatomical journal of movement, which has now become my go-to book for all things fascia, embryology and their spiral connection. In simple terms ... After 30 years of involvement in exercise and movement anatomy ... This book answers questions that I didn't know had to be asked!

Mark Flannigan Neuromuscular therapist, Exercise scientist

The value of Karen's work to our yoga teaching community shines an important light on how we can enliven the beautiful matrix within us through subtlety. Her depth of knowledge of the subject matter and her creative approach to bring this to life makes it an important book for our times.

Hayley Winter MSc, BWY Dip, E-RYT 500, YACEP Founder of the Institute of Yoga Sports Science®

Karen is one of a rare breed of exceptional teachers who takes complex topics and delivers them in a simple, fun and enticing manner that leaves you craving more. Like all Karen's teachings, this is a MUST HAVE book for all yoga teachers and practitioners.

Bruce Mackay Director, Yoga Alliance Professionals

Karen's real skill, along with her incredible depth of knowledge and enthusiasm on all things anatomy and yoga-related, is her ability to communicate that knowledge and enthusiasm at all levels.

Joanne Merritt, Former Team GB cyclist, Yoga & Pilates practitioner

Spiral Bound will produce a better understanding of functional anatomy for everyone involved with the human form. The book is written in a colloquial language that pulls you in and explains complicated concepts in bite sized pieces.

Janet Philp Anatomy Fundamentals @anatomyfoundations

This book will be valued by all somatic practitioners. It expands the understanding of the human form, from its embryological foundations to how these inform our movement. For yoga practitioners, Karen's detailed exploration of the Five Filaments supports the interconnection and continuity of a yoga practice reflecting yoga philosophy and Dhatu Siddhanta from Ayurveda.

Caroline Phipps-Urch Vice Chair, Yoga Scotland

Karen is a phenomenal anatomy and yoga teacher. Her work is particularly suited for anyone interested in putting the nuances of anatomy into motion thus enabling them to weave her teachings into their practice. Highly recommended!

Aimee Alexandra Schmidt Cranio-sacral therapist, Pilates practitioner & Yoga teacher

This book will shake you to the core. It is about anatomy and yoga but not in the way we usually think about them. This is no fusty list of time-honoured descriptions and impossible poses but a deep insight into the living body and how it moves the way it does.

Graham Scarr Author of Biotensegrity: The Structural Basis of Life

The discussion of the Five Filaments movement rubric in its simple, elegant form is perfection – the way it is broken down into simple, practical language is so useful. A gift for yoga teachers and movement therapists to cue rotation in movement for every level of experience.

Nadine Watton Co-director of Meadowlark Yoga YTT programme

Sensitively written, with an admirable understanding of movement and body. This book provides clarity, it is insightful and engaging. Well done Karen!
Ana Outsubo MPT São Paulo, Brazil

Understanding the concept of spirality has been nothing short of a game changer both for my practice and for my teaching.
Kate Towers www.katetowersyoga.com

Human anatomy is often presented as mechanical and gross; Karen shows us that its essence is subtlety and interconnection. A tour de force of creativity and intellectual brilliance to reimagine anatomy in a way that is holistic and deeply embodied.
Paul Fox Yoga in Healthcare Alliance | Promoting Yoga in the UK & Internationally

This text offers a groundbreaking look at understanding around anatomy and beyond that is softer and more connected than the sometimes reductionist, linear traditional approach to the subject. This approach is mirrored in yoga culture as conversations around power dynamics, lineage and new ways of working evolve and it is therefore a relevant and timely addition to the field.
Lorraine Close Outreach director, Edinburgh Community Yoga, MSc, RYT TCTSY-F

I met Karen some years ago when I traveled to Edinburgh to interview her. I knew immediately that my meager anatomy brain was outmatched as Karen managed to paint detailed muscle interconnections on my body while at the same time fielding questions with insight and wit on the not so straightforward topics of Fascia and Biotensegrity.
Stu Girling Loveyogaanatomy.com, Author of Illustrated Yoga Anatomy

Karen's approach to anatomy has been transformative for both myself and my students; she has been a real inspiration and I can't wait to continue learning from her.
Fern Ross Yoga teacher and Journalist www.fernrossyoga.co.uk

This book is an adventure, both fun and exhilarating, a paradigm shift in our understanding of biological systems, and a huge bonus for all curious yoginis and yogis.
Brian Cooper PhD, Yoga Alliance Professionals www.yogaallianceprofessionals.org

Karen's book provides an updated approach to understanding anatomy as it applies to yoga through the lens of biotensegrity and holistic human movement. It creates the groundwork for using rotation and spiraling movements within your yoga teaching and practice and moves beyond linear asana. Spiral Bound is a must read for all yoga teachers!
Trina Altman, BA, NCPT, E-RYT 500, YACEP Author of Yoga Deconstructed®: Movement science principles for teaching

Karen's work is the missing link in the way anatomy is traditionally taught, and her book is an absolute must for anyone working within the world of holistic movement.
Sally Parkes BSc SYT Pregnancy & Yoga teacher trainer

This book transcends the status quo for yogis. It takes the fabric of traditional yoga and delicately weaves the latest research and techniques into its seam. A must-read for the next generation yogi.
Joe Robinson Director, Mana Fitness Byron Bay & Byron Bay Fitness Retreats

Karen's book brings a focus to the natural constraints of the human body and how we can use movement to support, rather than disrupt, these rotational patterns. I would highly recommend Spiral Bound to anyone in the pregnancy and postpartum community as a big picture anatomy reference for their professional practice.
Dr. Sarah Ellis Duvall PT, DPT, CPT, CNC

The integrated approach to anatomy that Karen brings to us, in her workshops and book, is the missing link we have not only in movement but also in physical and manual therapy education.
Ângela Elias Fernandes Physical therapist

Karen brings a refreshing account of living anatomy that is rooted in the embryo, informed by biotensegrity and shaped for practical applications of movement and exercise.
Niall Galloway MD, Author of *Seeking Symmetry*

Spiral Bound is not a mere translation of ancient ayurvedic concepts into modern anatomical terminology, but a pioneering exploration of the relationship between subtle and gross that makes for essential reading by anatomists, ayurvedic practitioners and yoga teachers alike.
Elise Hill Ayurvedic counsellor

Not going to beat around the bush, traditional anatomy isn't accessible and to be fair can be boring. Karen goes about it in a completely different way, she shows us how it all works in the most innovative way using tactile props and imagery that grab your imagination and bring anatomy to life and when she gets you moving, oh boy, you learn all about what you haven't been using.
Jodie Reynolds www.yogijodie.com

Karen has a natural, inclusive and encouraging ability to make anatomy and movement theory interesting and accessible no matter your starting point or approaching perspective (within yoga or a general interest in the subject).
Alasdair Bruce Yoga practitioner, 200 Hr YTT grad

Karen's book is a practical and eye-opening approach to the complexity of anatomy and body movement in yoga.
Benji Pérez Salinas http://www.instagram.com/benji_yoga/

Karen is an extraordinary trainer who blends her anatomical insight into all of her teachings. Spiral Bound is a wonderful piece of work which will assist the reader to spiral under their own skin.
Janet Richards E-RYT 200, YACEP, Founder, The Yoga Studio Carlisle, Owner and Director of Carlisle Yoga School

Spiral Bound has challenged, humbled and inspired my understanding of anatomy and embryology, as it serves a cause beyond its progressive scope and [spoiler alert] is a revolution in its own right.
Mihai Bob MD PhD Lecturer of Human Anatomy and Embryology at the "Iuliu Hatieganu" University of Medicine and Pharmacy Cluj Napoca, Romania .

Karen's approach to the study of anatomy for yoga is an unforgettable experience! This is absolutely a very modern, integral approach to teach yoga.
Kostyantyn Yaremenko Costa Yoga

Explanations of Andragogy and the interrelatedness of muscle function and fascia and much more are lessons that have a direct impact on my approach with elite athletes, enhancing my views across the entire psychosocial biological spectrum of coaching practise.
David Tilbury-Davis Elite athletics coach

Spiral Bound

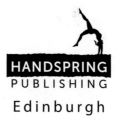

HANDSPRING
PUBLISHING

Edinburgh

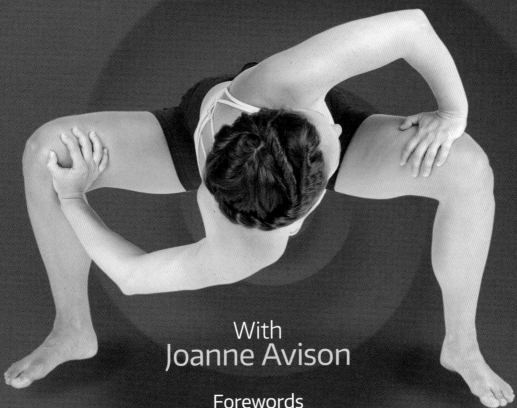

Spiral Bound

INTEGRATED ANATOMY FOR YOGA

Karen Kirkness

With
Joanne Avison

Forewords
Corrie Ananda ◆ Tiffany Cruikshank
David Keil ◆ John Sharkey

HANDSPRING PUBLISHING LIMITED
The Old Manse, Fountainhall,
Pencaitland, East Lothian
EH34 5EY, United Kingdom
Tel: +44 1875 341 859
Website: www.handspringpublishing.com

First published 2021 in the United Kingdom by Handspring Publishing

Copyright ©Handspring Publishing Limited 2021
Photographs and drawings copyright ©2021

All rights reserved. No parts of this publication may be reproduced or transmitted in any form or by any means, electronic or mechanical, including photocopying, recording, or any information storage and retrieval system, without either the prior written permission of the authors and publisher or a license permitting restricted copying in the United Kingdom issued by the Copyright Licensing Agency Ltd, Saffron House, 6-10 Kirby Street, London EC1N 8TS.

The right of Karen Kirkness to be identified as the Author of this text has been asserted in accordance with the Copyright, Designs and Patents Acts 1988

ISBN 978-1-912085-03-3
ISBN (Kindle eBook) 978-1-912085-04-0

British Library Cataloguing in Publication Data
A catalogue record for this book is available from the British Library

Library of Congress Cataloguing in Publication Data
A catalog record for this book is available from the Library of Congress

Notice
Neither the Publisher nor the Author assumes any responsibility for any loss or injury and/or damage to persons or property arising out of or relating to any use of the material contained in this book. It is the responsibility of the treating practitioner, relying on independent expertise and knowledge of the patient, to determine the best treatment and method of application for the patient.

All reasonable efforts have been made to obtain copyright clearance for illustrations in the book for which the authors or publishers do not own the rights. If you believe that one of your illustrations has been used without such clearance please contact the publishers and we will ensure that appropriate credit is given in the next reprint.

Commissioning Editor Sarena Wolfaard
Project Manager Morven Dean
Copy Editor Susan Stuart
Cover and Design Direction by Bruce Hogarth
Typesetter Ditech, India
Printer Replika, India
Book printed in Minion Pro Regular 11/13 pt

The
Publisher's
policy is to use
paper manufactured
from sustainable forests

CONTENTS

Forewords   xiii
About the Author   xix
About Joanne Avison   xx
Contributors   xxi
Acknowledgments   xxii
Preface   xxiv
Glossary   xxx
Introduction   xxxvii
Anatomy of this book   xlii

Chapter One   Across anatomy   2
    1.1 In the beginning   4
    1.2 Embryology   6
    1.3 The meso story   9
    1.4 Mighty somites   12
    1.5 Out on a limb   16
    1.6 Legacy of limb symmetry   23
    1.7 A more useful neutral   28

Chapter Two   The Five Filaments   36
    2.1 Into the round: mapping movement   38
    2.2 Kinematics of coupling   43
    2.3 Rotational redux   51
    2.4 Spiral motion in yoga   56
    2.5 The Five Filaments rubric   58
    2.6 From coupled to throupled   73
    2.7 The spirals as patterns of movement   78
    2.8 Guiding the glide   82

CONTENTS *continued*

Chapter Three   Srotas-kinematics (tubular movement)   **90**

3.1   Steady and comfortable   92

3.2   A hole in the middle   93

3.3   Gross and subtle   96

3.4   Gastronomical   101

3.5   The mystery   103

3.6   Prana   105

3.7   Srotamsi: many rivers   107

3.8   Akasha by Kate O'Donnell   110

3.9   Srotas: subtle kinematics   111

3.10 Weaving the threads   115

3.11 Subtle body, spiral bound   118

3.12 Vayu   120

3.13 Integration   125

Chapter Four   Kinematics come to life   **134**

4.1 Simplicity emerging   135

4.2 Aims and objectives   143

4.3 Samasthitih   144

4.4 Statement of constraints   147

4.5 The Five Filaments in postural yoga: one example   148

- One: Shoulder Filament – the scapulohumeral rhythm (A, B)   148
- Two: Hand Filament – supination/pronation (A, B)   150
- Three: Hip Filament – the pelvifemoral rhythm (A, B)   152
- Four: Foot Filament – supination/pronation (A, B)   154
- Five: Axial Matrix Filament – twist/lateral flexion (A, B)   156

Chapter Five	Acoustics of self	160
	5.1 Self-directed transformation	162
	5.2 Dvandva	163
	5.3 Breath	166
	5.4 Bandha: de facto structure	172
	5.5 Dṛṣṭi	178
	5.6 Seated in spirals	179
	5.7 Resources for teachers	183

Appendix A	Yoga's missing link	186
	A.1 Modeling movement	188
	A.2 Tensegrity	189
	A.3 On the value of models by Susan Lowell de Solórzano	190
	A.4 The tensegrity icosahedron (T-icosa)	192
	A.5 In the wild	192
	A.6 Biotensegrity	195
	A.7 Heterarchy: simultaneity and circularity	195
	A.8 Modularity	200
	A.9 Expansion and contraction: outward push and inward pull	202
	A.10 The body: a home for configurations	203
	A.11 Biotensegrity in yoga practice by Chris Clancy	211

CONTENTS *continued*

Appendix B   **Nonlinear teaching**   **216**

     B.1 Nonlinear pedagogy   218

     B.2 Non-proportionality   219

     B.3 Fluxtability   221

     B.4 Noise   223

     B.5 Creativity and empowerment: the rewards   224

Online Chapter   **Reflection and growth: spiral shareera**

This chapter, Reflection and growth, contains an overview of spirality, sacred geometry, why spirals are so integral to life and more about how spirality shows up in human tissue. Simply scan this QR to access the online chapter free of charge.

Permissions   231

Index   237

FOREWORDS

The dedicated yoga practitioner spends hours on their mat each day exploring and expressing their inner life through movement, breath, and stillness, day after day, year after year, through health, sickness, injury, births, and deaths. Over time they awaken to and understand not just the innate intelligence of the tissue that they live in, but its interconnectedness to thoughts, emotions, and life events.

In my earlier years as a yoga student and teacher, anatomy books were mostly a dry and theoretical list of isolated parts to memorise. Little about them felt relevant to a lived experience as a breather and mover and none of them helped me understand my hypermobile body and its constant injuries. I sought out specialists in different movement modalities and compiled my understanding of the physical prerequisites needed for the safe practice of physical postures. Had I had a resource such as *Spiral Bound*, I would have visited it again and again as it reveals the full ecosystem of our anatomy and the interweaving elements that give rise to the whole. The aim for the yoga practitioner is to come into a stronger connection and understanding of their unique organism to experience how the microcosm relates to the macrocosm. Karen's book is the ideal companion to this explorative journey.

In my role as a teacher of guided self-practice Ashtanga yoga, I see up to 70 students each morning, from committed practitioners and teachers, to new students and casual practitioners; bodies come through the door *demonstrating* different abilities, ages, sizes, and shapes – emotions are high, low, calm, irritated – minds are fast, slow, filled with predetermined expectations, or open and keen to absorb. As a teacher facilitating someone's practice, I have to be able to "read" the person before me, not just their physical capability but where they are psychologically, emotionally, and energetically – in short – their whole organism. Resources such as *Spiral Bound* provide the discerning teacher and practitioner a shared language to draw from during the collaborative process of cultivating a personal yoga practice under guidance.

The instructional language I choose when teaching students is specific and inclusive. I often refer to the "spirals" of certain movements and guide practitioners to "draw up the tissue of the thighs," for example, rather than "engage your quadriceps." The latter is not inclusive to a new practitioner and can overwhelm them with too much information, it is also separatist, singling out one muscle rather than the collective use of the mass of tissue that works together as the thigh. Karen's book clearly explains integrational anatomy, it is thorough and profound, yet practical and accessible. *Spiral Bound* uses familiar yoga postures to demonstrate complex structures, bringing them to life. The use of spirals in my teaching comes from the visual patterning of the body's tendency toward spiralling in movement; Karen's research goes way beyond this to the core of the spiral, its construct, and how it inspires and informs our anatomy.

As a Doctoral student of existential psychotherapy, I *am interested in western psychology and the philosophical concepts* of freedom, choices, and suffering and their parallels to the ancient Indian wisdom traditions. The mind lives in the body and the body lives in the mind, there is no separation.

FOREWORDS *continued*

Karen's work affirms the interconnectedness of the organism, tracing it back to its embryonical creation (as far as conception!), taking us on an intricate journey of the interconnectivity of the gross and subtle aspects that bring about the whole. It is a complete and holistic approach that naturally lends itself to the yogic philosophy of the Vedic corpus which Karen draws upon linking Eastern thought with Western science in a way that is both comforting and reassuring.

Spiral Bound brings together cutting-edge, progressive anatomical ideas around biotensegrity and fascia amongst others, it is important information that any mover can benefit from, an ideal reference point for yoga practitioners, teachers, seekers, experimentalists, and anatomy geeks. I have come across many people who have a good understanding of anatomical theory but their connection to it is unconvincing; theirs is a knowledge that is cerebral, not kinesthetic.

Whilst Karen's research comes to us from the academic study of anatomy and medical science it also comes from the experience of a long-term dedicated yoga practitioner, someone who has spent years observing, experiencing, and inquiring into her own psycho/emotional/physical organism. This book has heart and wisdom, it is a unique contribution to the field of yoga and movement. It is one of those books that you will want to refer to again and again.

Corrie runs one of the leading Mysore programs in London. Corrie teaches asana and yoga philosophy to practitioners of all levels and trains and mentors teachers. Her teaching is progressive, inclusive and from the heart.

Corrie Ananda
PG Cert. Psychotherapy and Counselling
MA Traditions of Yoga and Meditation
Yoga Alliance Senior Teacher
Authorised Level II Ashtanga Yoga Teacher
Certified mobility specialist (FRC)
London, UK
March 2021

We live in the age of yoga and, with that, comes a responsibility and a code of duty. As teachers, it is our duty to convey a message to our students that empowers and educates them. As a teacher trainer, I have to train my teachers to do their best to support their students and be compassionate guides through an understanding of the body and the practice. The root of this understanding leads us to appreciate what Karen brings to light at the heart of *Spiral Bound*: the body's intrinsic constraints.

With more and more research and information about the biochemistry and biomechanics of yoga being published daily, it is our job as teachers and students of this practice to continue to learn, to incorporate this new information, and to expand our awareness. We need to stay open to how the research, so elegantly expressed in the story of this book with all its scholarly references, can further inform our practice to be a powerful modality of complete health and wellness. And at the core of this work, as Karen reminds us throughout, is always our own practice, history, and what we bring to the mat every day.

The development of Yoga Medicine was inspired by just this intersection of science and personal experience, which is why Karen asked me to write a foreword for her. I started out practicing Ashtanga and had achieved advanced asana, but I hit the limits of a purely physical progression in my practice when an unexpected injury forced me to rethink my entire approach. That devastating injury became one of life's greatest gifts, broadening my perspective and giving me a reason to learn much more about myself (and my anatomy) than I would have otherwise.

At that moment, I was inspired to look more deeply into my training in Traditional Chinese Medicine, sports medicine & orthopedics, and it was here that I developed a unifying vision of yoga that embraced the idea of anatomy and meridians as well. I brought that perspective back into my practice. I created Yoga Medicine, a program that has given me a vehicle to teach students, yoga teachers, and medical practitioners the philosophy and practice of yoga as a legitimate medical therapy. I became a devoted advocate for the study of anatomy as a means of unleashing a deeper understanding of yoga and holistic health.

Since then, I have realized that this story of stepping into power and developing it as a creative practice is a narrative that I share with many others. As teacher trainers, our job isn't merely to pass on information about anatomy and practice, but to inspire others to find their power and live to their greatest creative potential. This common ground is one that I know Karen brings to life in this book and her points about learning anatomy in order to transcend the limitations of nomenclature are close to my own aims as an educator.

A comprehensive understanding of anatomy enables us to more easily access a sense of the subtle body being an interconnected web, what Karen explains as closed kinematic chains, a key theme of this work. Doing this work has always afforded me a daily, intimate understanding of the primary role of fascia and connective tissue. Recent research on fascia has only further validated the interdisciplinary approach – and what is fascia but an extremely interdisciplinary tissue in the body!

The field of connective tissue is a quickly expanding area of study with so much to teach us. As we embrace an understanding of the more concrete anatomical information, books like Karen's provide a gateway to interpreting the subtler information systems of the body and the interconnected web of the fascial matrix and meridians as coupled systems.

We must learn to embrace this deeper study of anatomy, kinesiology, and new research for a complete understanding of yoga and holistic health, both to serve our own needs as well as the needs of our community. This rethinking of anatomy can lead all of us to a rethinking of our entire practice—and as Karen reminds us in this book, ultimately to a sense of connectedness with all.

Tiffany Cruikshank LAc, MAOM
Founder of Yoga Medicine® E-RYT 500
Seattle, Washington, USA
February 2021

Whenever an author takes the time to both educate and propel our understanding of a subject forward, we should celebrate. Karen has done just that with *Spiral Bound*.

This book represents a new arc of understanding from the perspective of spirals. These spirals start in the structure of our DNA, move through our embryological development, and ultimately express themselves in the way in which we move both in everyday life and in the practice of yoga asana.

Ultimately, yoga asana practice is about us understanding the felt sense experience in our body as a way of knowing ourselves. Karen's work will help us become more aware of and attuned to what has been there all along. It has just been waiting for us to recognize it.

The East and West have been cross-pollinating for some time now. Most people don't even remember the first Western academics to travel East and explore the arts and sciences of meditation, yoga, and Traditional Chinese Medicine. People like John Kabat-Zinn and Dr David Eisenberg were some of the more famous ones. Between the internet and advances in travel, this is happening through all of us!

We are now in the midst of the largest experiment of these practices. There have never been more people doing these yogic practices at once. Books like *Spiral Bound* help us to bridge the gap between East and West and make meaningful connections.

As humans, we desire to make meaning and understand how everything is connected. We want to understand how we, as humans, start as a single cell and then evolve into all of the complexity that we are. Karen has done a fantastic job of reminding us that we are not parts and pieces (that's just a perspective). No, we are unfolding beings that have been unfolding (in spirals) from the very beginning.

Karen reminds us that it's not East versus West, it's East and West describing the same thing in different ways. Mostly, it's the West catching up and pushing our own science to expand and encompass what has already been known in the East. As we expand our understanding, we still include old Cartesian thinking (parts and pieces) and then expand it so that we may have a more full experience of the whole.

Karen's work will help us recognize, become more aware of, and then feel and experience these spirals in our own bodies. Through this, we may find a more integrated experience of our bodies. Without a doubt, this will inform our understanding of how we do asana practice.

Finally, I remember meeting Karen almost 20 years ago on a teacher training. I was the anatomy teacher and was on my own journey to make anatomy simple and understandable to the yoga community. Nothing makes me happier than to see students grasp the subject of anatomy and take it on in a way that enriches their personal experience of practicing yoga.

The pinnacle is to see one of these students (in this case Karen) take on the subject academically and write a book that takes the subject forward. Not that it is my place, but I am so proud of what Karen has achieved with this book. She has explored the current depth of a subject that has always fascinated me, anatomy, and more specifically, fascia. She has managed to spiral it together with the experience and science of yoga.

I am sure you will find valuable and practical information in the pages that follow.

David Keil LMT, NMT
Author of Functional Anatomy of Yoga and
Founder of Yoganatomy.com
Miami, Florida, USA
March 2021

Congratulations to you, the reader, for investing in your own continuing education. I believe this book will prove to be a rare find having spiraled and folded within its pages the potential to transform yoga, in fact, all movement disciplines. Having received an invitation, from anatomist and senior yoga teacher Karen Kirkness, to pen the forward for this truly exceptional academic, educational tome, *Spiral Bound*, I was truly honored. Karen's observant and informed writing style is supported by the nurturing encouragement and guidance of fellow yoga expert Joanne Avison. Karen has delivered a book that has academic rigor and impressive anatomical accuracy and yet avoids being "too dry", and will, I am confident, prove accessible to the widest possible audience. Karen's writing style provokes a voice that talks with a quietly spoken wisdom from within the pages, a voice that exudes a welcome to you to explore new frontiers in yoga, movement, anatomy, and language.

Containing anatomical and biomotional detail, chronicled in a factual, entertaining, yet detailed manner, this carefully crafted book has been informed by, and reflects, nature's sagacity. Straight lines are a fallacy in living anatomy, human or otherwise. Karen Kirkness brings style and substance to support her supposition. Karen describes the process of embryogenesis in a manner that is a joy to read while empowering the reader with the confidence needed to move away from lines and to move towards an omnidirectional, model-dependent reality. A reality that resonates with natures twists, writhes, coiling, and uncoiling.

Embryogenesis is informed by the tensional and compressive forces of a fluidic world void of gravity. Informed also by Coriolis forces and the forces within that nurture and support appropriate cellular expression. Such forces combine with genetically informed proteins supported by fabric stiffening fats, sugars, and inorganic molecular phosphates (e.g., metals) resulting in emerging spiral bound, curved anatomy, helical proteins, collagens, and DNA. The talented anatomist, Karen Kirkness, twists and folds this story of a new anatomy for yoga, into anatomy fit for the 21st century. All the while providing the reader with a riveting read.

As a wordsmith, Karen Kirkness tackles the issue of anatomical language, *"the dogged adherence to tenets of anatomical nomenclature"* (Preface). The issue of anatomical nomenclature is not restricted to what the language of anatomy does not tell us but calls our attention to what it does tell us. For example, much of anatomy's descriptive language has, historically, relegated women as inferior to men. Exemplified in the use of the word "Pudendum" (n); Human external genital organ, especially of a woman. From Latin pudēre; to be ashamed (1). This is not acceptable in the 21st century. Neither should the use of reductionist, linear, outdated "origin and insertion" terminology currently used to describe what is truly "origin-less and insertion-less" (2). This book packs a powerful pedagogical message that, while focusing on anatomy and yoga, will resonate within a wider conversation promoting connectedness and continuity within our local and global communities.

Yoga and movement modalities are not exclusive to the elite. By elite I mean amazing individuals who perhaps can curl one foot behind their head or persons who can do box-splits and touch the floor with their chest. If you lack such capacity you, too, are amazing. As pointed out in Chapter 4, a practitioner develops their body wisdom with time-bound care, appropriateness and guidance for the sake of learning.

Movement should be nutritious and this book highlights the need to invest the time and seek professional guidance to ensure safe, effective, and appropriate practice parameters.

The Five Filaments model is one that will resonate with anyone who grew themself. Rather than fighting against an outdated anatomy of point to point postulates and straight lines, the Five Filaments approach invites and encourages us to better understand and extend the development of our anatomical foundations. I urge the reader to pay special attention to Chapter 5 with a focus on breath, acoustics of self, and how *"tuning into the breath"* can result in a recalibration of oneness.

I am delighted that I share things in common with Karen Kirkness. We are both formally trained anatomists. We both studied in Scotland and have been influenced by topics including platonic solids, geometric shapes, and the work of D'Arcy Wentworth Thompson. We both see anatomy through the lens of the integrative model of Levin's biotensegrity, *"the model that binds"*. We also share a love and respect for our fellow human beings with the wish that perhaps we can have a lasting, positive impact on the lives of others; after all, we are all spiral bound.

John Sharkey MSc
Anatomical Society (Full Member)
Clinical Anatomist (BACA)
Exercise Physiologist (BASES)
Biotensegrity Interest Group (Founding Member)
Dry Needle Trigger Point Specialist
Senior Lecturer and Programme Leader MSc NMT
University of Chester
Dublin, Ireland
March 2021

References

1. Draper A. The history of the term pudendum: Opening the discussion on anatomical sex inequality. Clinical Anatomy. 2021-03-30 DOI: 10.1002/ca.23659

2. Sharkey J. Tensegrity informed observations in human cadaveric studies - a clinical anatomist's perspective. Integrative Journal of Medical Sciences (online). 2020;7. Available at: https://mbmj.org/index.php/ijms/article/view/260

ABOUT THE AUTHOR

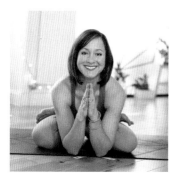 **Karen Kirkness**, MFA & MSc Human Anatomy from the University of Edinburgh, is a yoga practitioner with broad and branching roots. Originally an Ashtangi, Karen has been practising since the late 1990s. She is the creator of **Anatomy Inspired**, an online course for creative movers to practice innovative anatomy teaching and learning techniques. She contributes as guest faculty on training courses internationally.

Always adapting, Karen's style now incorporates unconventional movement exploration and fascination with helical patterns found throughout nature. Her teaching is informed by early influences of endurance sports and, more recently, motherhood. Karen is a Pregnancy & Postpartum Corrective Exercise Specialist (PCES) and weaves threads of theory, creativity, and healing into her functionally fun and fascia-aware approach to yoga.

Karen is an E-RYT 500, YACEP and Senior Yoga Teacher with the Yoga Alliance Professionals, and PhD candidate with research in Medical Sciences and Anatomy Education at Hull York Medical School. She founded her Edinburgh-based studio, Meadowlark Yoga, in the early 2000s and since then has embraced an inter-lineage approach to yoga. She seeks to foster community and facilitate a constraints-led journey toward self-care and personal growth for all levels. Karen presents creatively in both art and science festivals and is a member of the Anatomical Society and the International Symposium of Clinical and Applied Anatomists (ISCAA). She lives with her husband Simon and their two toddlers in the Scottish Borders.

Get in touch with Karen's work through her website http://karenkirkness.com/.

ABOUT JOANNE AVISON

Joanne Avison, mother, artist, author, advanced Yoga Teacher and Yoga Therapist (C-IAYT), is also a manual practitioner/teacher in Structural Integration; her Masters' Degree is in Spiritual Sciences (MSS). Author of *YOGA: Fascia, Anatomy and Movement* (Handspring Publishing 2015, 2nd edition 2021), Joanne presents structural anatomy of fascia and biotensegrity to movement and manual therapists. Her unique presentations distinguish our innate "biomotional intelligence". Honouring new fascia research and the ancient wisdom of sacred geometry, Joanne shows how body, mind and being remain entirely unique and interconnected, inside and out. From considerable experience in the anatomy dissection laboratory, with Clinical Anatomist, John Sharkey, Joanne is able to make sense, for movement teachers and manual practitioners, of how our own bodies are unique instruments, resonance fields that we can tune and optimise, to present ourselves in our own archetypal ways. Our patterns matter! As a graduate of the CMED institute,

Joanne asks, "We are the architects who self-assembled the architecture, through which to express the architect. How can knowing that transform our ability to move congruently in harmony with our own archetypal nature and movement patterns?" Joanne was delighted to work with Karen Kirkness on *Spiral Bound*, encouraging her deeply to foster her own unique style in presenting "double-dead anatomy" through her unique vision of human motion. Karen understands how the innate chirality of the human forming motif, expresses as Spiral Bound movements. "With her genius for language and creative expression of anatomy art, Karen's work is a golden resource."

Joanne Avison MSS, CMED
Advanced Yoga Teacher (E-RYT500) Certified Yoga Therapist (C-IAYT)
Structural Integration Manual Practitioner/Teacher
Brighton, UK

CONTRIBUTORS

Chris Clancy

Chris Morita Clancy is a retired Vijnana yoga teacher and teacher trainer. She is the creator of Embodied Biotensegrity, a training course for yoga teachers. As a leader within the community, Chris now serves as a board member of the Stephen M. Levin Biotensegrity Archive, a founding member of Pacific Northwest Biotensegrity Interest Group (PNWBIG), and co-host of the BiotensegriTea Party. https://www.embodiedbiotensegrity.ca

Susan Lowell de Solórzano

Susan C. Lowell de Solórzano is co-founder of the Stephen M. Levin Biotensegrity Archive. She holds an MA, Human Development & Education with a focus on kinesthetic learning, is a certified Level III T'ai Chi instructor, co-author of *The Soft Answer: Verbal T'ai Chi for sociable self defense*, and is also a certified FlexAware teacher. Susan co-hosts the popular online BiotensegriTea Party and is the author of *Everything Moves: How biotensegrity informs human movement*.

Sam Moor

Sam began exploring Mind/Body modalities when he was 16 years old and settled onto the path of Internal Martial Arts a few years later. For the last 25 years he has trained extensively in China, Europe and the UK, taught internationally and written widely on the subject. As a teacher he specializes in facilitating the cultivation of whole-body perception and movement via direct-experience.

Kate O'Donnell

Kate O'Donnell is the author of three books on Ayurveda, including bestselling *The Everyday Ayurveda Cookbook*. She is an Ayurvedic Practitioner, senior yoga teacher, and international presenter, as well as the founder of the Ayurvedic Living Institute, an online resource for Ayurvedic education and lifestyle. She continues to travel annually to India for study.
www.kateodonnell.yoga

Contributing demonstrators

Sarah Durney Hatcher – find Sarah teaching Mysore style Ashtanga Yoga through her website, https://www.sarahhatcheryoga.com/.

Amy Hughes – Amy offers a range of yoga-based classes, workshops, and trainings via https://amyhughesyoga.com/.

Emma Isokivi – Emma is Programme Director of Ashtanga Yoga Edinburgh, find out more on http://www.emmashtanga.com/.

Fadzai "Fudge" Mwakutuya – Fudge is a visual artist and life model sharing creative practice via https://fadzaimwakutuya.co.uk/.

ACKNOWLEDGMENTS

Dakshina – gratitude

My teachers, students, and friends in yoga have all contributed to this book in no small way. Collective movement and the endless negotiations of a collaborative workspace inform my understanding of yoga more than any other means of study. Evolving in movement within my community is a constant inspiration, providing the source material and stamina both needed for finishing this book.

How can I possibly thank the wise and generous mentors, including Joanne Avison, who have made it possible for me to upgrade my curiosity to a level of clarity suitable for bringing this book to market? Thank you, Graham Scarr, for your guidance and for making the excellent book, *Biotensegrity: The Structural Basis of Life*[1] that lit the way for my biotensegrity journey, and your continued publications that inspire us all.[2–4]

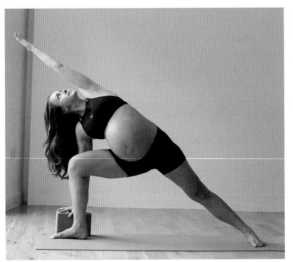

The author at 40 weeks pregnant

Danièle-Claude Martin opened my eyes to the inherent confidence we can feel by tuning into what she calls "comfort self-stress"[5] and what I have explored in yoga through bandha as "intrinsic comfort." Her collaboration with Dr Stephen Levin is advancing the movement community with their insight into the geodesic nature of body fabric as soft matter.[6] Thanks to Professor of Exercise Physiology, Natàlia Balagué, whose work on nested constraints in sports has informed my suggestions for where we go next in yoga pedagogy.[7] David Muehsam, experienced yoga practitioner and biophysicist, provided enormously helpful critical input where my understanding of oscillating biorhythms needed tuning.[8]

Through the influence of a handful of mentors combined with research and personal practice, I started to see the pattern revealing itself. My teaching colleagues Sarah Hatcher, Nadine Watton, Emma Isokivi and Amy Hughes, pictured in this book, embody that ultra-fine line of honed/softened intensity. David Keil has been another source of practical insights that help me bring sensible, critical thinking about anatomy into the Mysore room (a place that, as history is revealing, could do with a lot more of such sensibility).

Thanks to Fadzai Mwakutuya for your artistic and conceptual collaboration over the last four years, and for modeling the spirals. Thanks to friend and yogi colleague Amy Hughes for parsing the spirals with me to endlessly geeky details for all the asanas. Joanna Darlington, thank you for getting it and endlessly giving of your profound understanding in the visual stages. Enormous thanks to photographers Anna Henly and Charlene Lim. Big shout out to Professor Gabrielle Finn, my friend and PhD supervisor.

To Dena Kingsberg, thank you for your inspiring and supportive teachings. Thanks to John Sharkey for your encouragement, for pioneering the fluid matrix of anatomy at the highest level and for the use of your cadaveric photos. Kate O'Donnell, thank you for your Ayurvedic expertise and collaborative spirit in the central themes of this book. Thanks to Olga and Stephen Levin for opening your home to me and sharing your hospitality.

A heartfelt thanks to Sarena Wolfaard for your confidence in my ability to take this project through two pregnancies and emerge with the goods on the other side. The process of deploying humans, experiencing their gestation and two very different births, then watching them develop from babies into toddlers has been the most exceptional education of my life. Without the grace of our two kids, who chose us to be their parents, the fundamental sense of this book would not have materialized in the same way.

To my endlessly supportive husband: thank you, Simon.

Karen Kirkness
Edinburgh, UK
February 2021

References

1. Scarr G. Biotensegrity: The Structural Basis of Life. Handspring Publishing; 2014.

2. Scarr G. A consideration of the elbow as a tensegrity structure. International Journal of Osteopathic Medicine. 2012;15(2):53–65.

3. Scarr G. Health and Disease: what is the difference? In: Pilat, A., (ed.), Fascia: scientific advances, Proceedings of the 28th Jornadas de Fisioterapia Conference, March 1–3, Madrid: Escuela Universitaria de Fisioterapia de la Once; 2018:219–225.

4. Scarr G. Biotensegrity: What is the big deal? Journal of Bodywork and Movement Therapies. 2020;24(1):134–7.

5. Martin DC. Living Biotensegrity: Interplay of Tension and Compression in the Body. Kiener Verlag; 2016.

6. Levin SM, Martin D-C. Biotensegrity: The Mechanics of Fascia. In: Schleip R, et al, editors. Fascia: The Tensional Network of the Human Body. Elsevier Ltd; 2012. p. 138–55.

7. Balagué N, Pol R, Torrents C, Ric Á, Hristovski R. On the relatedness and nestedness of constraints. Sports Medicine - Open. 2019;5(1):6

8. Muehsam D, Ventura C. Life rhythm as a symphony of oscillatory patterns: electromagnetic energy and sound vibration modulates gene expression for biological signaling and healing. Global Advances in Health Medicine. 2014;3(2):40–55.

PREFACE

What makes the study of anatomy distinct from the study of yoga? Across movement disciplines, practitioners yearn for greater understanding, not only of the anatomy but how it *moves*. Why? I can think of two reasons nestled into one overarching theme. First of all, from where I am standing, it looks like we are all really tired of suffering. Since moving in harmony with the lay of the land feels good, it follows that the literature base is building a core of new structural ideas for how and why our bodies might move the way they do.[1-3]

Can it be that simple? To me, feeling good in yoga simply means being empowered and sustainably pain-free. Conversely, measured discomfort (not simply "pushing through pain") can also yield considerable dividends toward feeling good over time. How can the study of anatomy help us sort out one from the other? Calibrating such parameters of physical experience represents a life's work, an effort that takes different forms for different people.

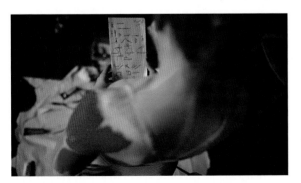

Professor Gabrielle Finn, Professor of Medical Education and PhD Supervisor to the author, here painting the physicist-Iyengar-yoga-teacher Louise Belshaw ahead of the yoga anatomy session co-taught at the Northern Ireland Science Festival, 2019.

Broadly speaking, I see a kind of polarity that effectively separates those who explore the parameters of physical practice kinesthetically, and those whose research lives in the academic shades of the spectrum. A passionate investigation of anatomy on both fronts has helped me unlock the source of confidence I needed to make informed decisions about how I practice and teach yoga. My aim in this book is to help you discover and reinforce your own.

Secure, comfortable, and *connected*

As my practice of yoga matures, my appetite for asana changes. Instead of a ravenous hunger for achieving kudos, I am hungry for ease. I can *feel* that things are a whole lot more comfortable in my body when I practice and teach within my body's natural constraints. As I have learned and hope to share with you in this book, these constraints are spiral bound, and drinking deeply of their wisdom might represent our best chance of optimized longevity.

Constraints offer rhythm, balance, and... space. These qualities come from the body's tendency to rotate in spiral patterns that appear in a chicken-and-egg kind of story. From the tiniest particles of organic chemistry and during processes that precipitate embryonic development, all the way through the narrative showing up in our present adult tissues, anatomy *curls*.

At its heart, this book is all about how to let your own body be the teacher. Once we get to grips with the embryology and the structure of collagen, the spiral motif is so fundamental that a spiral-bound approach is the obvious one. This approach is first a lens for studying anatomy and then a method of curating movement that harmonizes with the story of our tissues. Our bodies are indeed repositories of wisdom that may continue to reveal itself as part of a lifelong tango if we are lucky. By lucky, I mean fortunate enough to inherit favorable genes with sufficient privilege.

That brings me to the second reason why I think the world yearns for a greater understanding of the body: *connectedness.* Human anatomy is broadly the same across gender and ethnicity, but that underlying sameness is not enough. We have proof and can intuit that our tissues are not only *alike* but also *connected.* I suggest that this desire to be more broadly connected to each other requires more aptitude than classical systems of nomenclature allow. Globally, the paradigm is shifting toward the wisdom of empathy and interconnectedness.

How do we coax out this inner wisdom? It *can* be as simple and innate as breathing. The innovative forms of vinyasa have given us cues centered on drawing in, expanding out, rotating internally or externally. These cues do not just make for an excellent yoga class; they form the language of biology.

It took me a long time to learn to trust this language and let it take the helm of my movement. When I did, this connecting pattern of breath-centered, in-and-out movement conjoined with a sense of spiraling, offered natural kinesthetic confidence that I could experience in my own body. Latterly, I have come to see that "coupling" in this sense is more accurately described as a kind of "throupling," as the laws of coupled motion co-create a thirdness.

Joanne Avison, my collaborator, dear friend and mentor, talks about this as the "law of tripled motion" in the latest edition of her book[4] and it is a major theme of this text as well. Before I had a name for the phenomena I was experiencing in practice, I nevertheless knew the feeling was real. A deep curiosity about its structure led me to a phenomenological study of anatomy.

Reflexivity

Most of us start with the gross, and my story is undoubtedly rooted in that. So, who am I? I'm a cisgender, white progressive American ex-pat mother of two young children living in Scotland, currently experiencing the accelerating erosion of what little edge I once had. I remember spontaneously acknowledging this privilege in my twenties, begrudgingly, despite having worked tooth and nail for everything I had.

Then I realized, of course, that privilege resides in the opportunity to have work in the first instance, and the space to carry it out without the constant threat of bodily harm. Indeed, the nature of most bodily harm I have experienced has been self-inflicted. Speaking of which, I am also a self-diagnosed recovering practitioner of Ashtanga yoga trying to make sense of yoga in a post-MeToo and post-lineage, quite possibly post-yoga, yoga world.

OK. But this is a book about anatomy? Yes! It is. My ongoing research resides in art and anatomy. At heart, I am a yogi. My background and personality color my worldview, line of questioning, methods, approach, and synthesis. It is only fair to acknowledge my personal bias and not get hung up on the pretense of objectivity, which is an impossible point of view in anatomy for yoga. My bias is not that I see spirals everywhere (although I do)[5–8] or that I still think physical adjustments in yoga can heal (although I do); it is that I am increasingly dubious about dogged adherence to certain tenets of anatomical nomenclature.

As much as I love words and am seriously invested in anatomical terms, I am afraid that the reductionism fails us where the living anatomy of yoga is concerned.

You will see my nomenclature aversion as a theme throughout this book, a book that I started writing in 2017. The manuscript was due for completion in the winter of 2018, and, two babies later, it is now 2021 as I write this. Living through #MeToo, a pandemic, and the intensification of the social justice movement as part of a global **paradigm shift** that has everything to do with anatomy for yoga, I am immensely grateful that I did not finish this book on time.

The yoga system is visibly feeling the shift. We are experiencing a pivotal moment for yoga practitioners everywhere, and now there is truly no way to put your head in the sand and "just talk about anatomy". So many members of the physical culture community have stepped forward to share stories of shocking abuse rooted in reductionist views of previous generations bent on performance, from USA gymnastics to the lineages of yoga and beyond. My own truth is finding its wave, and I hope to add volume to the collective tidal shift.

Pre-2020, I was struggling to contextualize what I wanted to say in this anatomy for yoga book, which is at its heart about the body as a resonant meta continuum. Anatomy is continuous not only structurally, but also in spatiotemporal and behavioral ways that interconnect all living things at various levels. Biologic tissue is liquid crystalline[9,10] communication. Granularity can be modular, modularity can be collective, and all oscillating amongst states in time with a diffusion of information, appearing to flow like a murmuration of starlings darting hither and yon.[11–14]

Nomenclature in anatomy, born out of the need to reduce in order to understand, is ill equipped for naming the behavior of starlings or whitebait or our limbs in space.[15] Nomenclature keeps us steeped in the linearism and lineages of a narrowed, purely hierarchical perspective, blinding the seeker to the nonlinear balance of forces that *is* any organism. This disconnect with lived experience not only sets the stage and sanctions the kind of abuse we still see as a society, it further allows communities to ignore, subvert, and even excuse behavior that is inconvenient or professionally dangerous for it to address. How can we evolve collectively when the suffering of others remains closed into discrete systems and cut off from informing the whole?

This paradigm shift is a move away from lineages to networks and from the anatomical planes to the vector space of dandelions and resonance with nature. As per the worldview of **organicism**, which has influenced embryology since Kant,[16] our view looks at the embryo as a whole that gives rise to themes influencing our continuing experience as mature organisms.[17,18] This view reckons anatomy is resonant with a collective universal rhythm.

Anatomy is far from a dead -ology only to be memorized and then regurgitated as parts, locked in perpetual self-conflict, confusion, and competition. Instead, it is a living science that has the potential for the same kind of updating that we are demanding of our behavioral systems as a society. In the yoga world, we are revising our power structures to define consent and scope of practice to improve student–teacher relationships.[19] We are upgrading our pedagogical (andragogical, to be more accurate) standards in training courses and developing tools for addressing

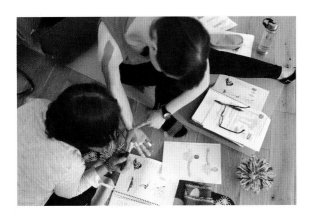

Embryology informing the yoga anatomy curriculum by way of body painting the dermatomes; 2019 workshop at Meadowlark Yoga.

cultural misappropriation and recognizing the effects of dopamine traps.[20,21]

Is it time to revise what we mean by "anatomy"?

In a word: yes. Bearing in mind that organisms of our complexity are all almost entirely composed of atomic space, bound water, a trillion-count smattering of micro-organisms, and a relatively infinitesimal sprinkle of minerals, traditional anatomical nomenclature is way out-gunned when it comes to naming the essential ingredients. If linear language cannot get a handle on the ingredients list, then how could it possibly offer the recipe for anatomy that we are interested in as yogis? After all, yoga is unifying by definition.

Our bodies are made up of mini-systems, intra- and interconnected to other bodies through oscillatory subtle architecture. Catches in the cloth anywhere in our shared system, at any time in its history, leave lasting and continuous effects that come to bear on outcomes everywhere else in our shared reality and, by extension, our shared anatomy. As we get our heads around this murmuration of morphology, we can genuinely unblinder ourselves to the structuralized, congenital suffering that has, thus far, been endemic to the human condition.

Once the view opens, it might even be possible to contain outbreaks of abuse, to heal, and finally harness some valuable tools in overcoming future suffering as a people.

Seeking subtlety in the open source

Before embarking on this writing journey, I looked at meridian systems, reviewed ancient and modern yogic texts, dissected cadavers, studied anatomical atlases, drew from life, made sculptures, and painted on the body. I broke many bones and underwent several surgeries from orthopedic to obstetric. As fascinating as it all was, studying gross anatomy left me feeling like something was missing. Could that missing ingredient be related to the so-called *subtle body*?

My approach to rounding up sources came out of an increasing fascination with what lies beneath and what patterns might be held in the tissues of all living things. I could see the spiral unfolding all around me in the natural world. All in, I intended to craft a book that weaves these threads together for a conversational, yogi-friendly, and most importantly, *practical* perspective on anatomy. That lasting intention is folded into the pages of this book.

I want to let you know from the outset that this book does what it says on the cover: *integration*. I am suggesting something that is virtual witchcraft to the anatomy establishment. Here goes: just because you can't dissect it out with the tools we have inherited from the post-classical period, doesn't mean that it isn't there. In my twenty years of teaching and practice, I have heard from yoga students and colleagues echoing my intuition that there must be something more than the nuts and bolts of codified anatomy screwed down by its own nomenclature.

In the yoga conversation, this idea of integration goes beyond the nomenclature of developed parts to encompass embryonic development in looking for that "something more." The whole yoga project resides in the connection of subtle and gross, which in the old paradigm is problematic, as mainstream anatomy is only now just recognizing the interstitium as a named system.[22] As fascia researchers explore new ways of codifying structure, we are seeing the rise of more -egrities and -ologies branching from the myofascial chain theories of previous generations.

As much as I welcome innovation, the multiplying array of semantics is dizzying and threatens to alienate those with genuine interest. I wonder if the increasingly trademarked ideas and attendant camps and committees keep us mired in terminology? As far as the establishment goes, the hallowed halls of anatomy are still a long way from updating the books to include anything subtler than fascia,[23,24] and even the fascia as a system is still on thin ice in mainstream anatomical nomenclature.[24] For an anatomist to suggest that there is something more than the material (or that the material itself is multi-dimensional) is radical, but to offer a possible *means* of connection within the realm of "the imaginary" is practically rebellion. Witchy, antipatriarchal, and *nerdy* rebellion at that. Welcome to my world, deeply informed by all of the above.

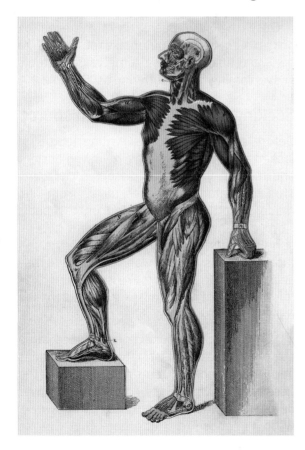

Engraving from 1872 featuring the muscles of the human body.

(www.thegraphicsfairy.com)

Karen Kirkness
Edinburgh, UK
February 2021

References

1 Bordoni B, Myers T. A Review of the Theoretical Fascial Models: Biotensegrity, Fascintegrity, and Myofascial Chains. Cureus. 2020;12(2):e7092-e.

2 Yang L, Carrington LJ, Erdogan B, et al. Biomechanics of cell reorientation in a three-dimensional matrix under compression. Experimental Cell Research. 2017;350(1):253–66.

3 Epstein M. The Elements of Continuum Biomechanics. Wiley; 2012.

4 Avison JS. Yoga: Fascia, Anatomy and Movement. 2nd Edition. Handspring Publishing; 2021.

5 Paul SP. The golden spiral flap: a new flap design that allows for closure of larger wounds under reduced tension – how studying nature's own design led to the development of a new surgical technique. Frontiers in Surgery. 2016;3:63.

6 Cartwright JHE, Checa AG, Escribano B, Sainz-Díaz CI. Spiral and target patterns in bivalve nacre manifest a natural excitable medium from layer growth of a biological liquid crystal. Proceedings of the National Academy of Sciences. 2009;106(26):10499–504.

7 Okabe T, Ishida A, Yoshimura J. The unified rule of phyllotaxis explaining both spiral and non-spiral arrangements. Journal of the Royal Society – Interface. 2019;16:20180850.

8 Martín-Durán JM, Vellutini BC, Hejnol A. Embryonic chirality and the evolution of spiralian left–right asymmetries. Philosophical Transactions of the Royal Society B: Biological Sciences. 2016;371(1710):20150411.

9 Hirst LS, Charras G. Biological physics: Liquid crystals in living tissue. Nature. 2017;544(7649):164–5.

10 Hyde ST. Crystals: animal, vegetable or mineral? Interface Focus. 2015;5(4).

11 Lin S-Z, Li Y, Ji J, Li B, Feng X-Q. Collective dynamics of coherent motile cells on curved surfaces. Soft Matter. 2020;16(12):2941–52.

12 Kim SE, Kim WS, Kim BG, et al. Spatiotemporal dynamics and functional correlates of evoked neural oscillations with different spectral powers in human visual cortex. Clinical Neurophysiology. 2013;124(11):2248–56.

13 Cao Y, Lopatkin A, You L. Elements of biological oscillations in time and space. Nature Structural & Molecular Biology. 2016;23:1030.

14 Rossi F, Ristori S, Rustici M, et al. Dynamics of pattern formation in biomimetic systems. Journal of Theoretical Biology. 2008;255(4):404–12.

15 Goodenough AE, Little N, Carpenter WS, Hart AG. Birds of a feather flock together: Insights into starling murmuration behaviour revealed using citizen science. PloS One. 2017;12(6):e0179277.

16 Gilbert S, Sarkar S. Embracing complexity: organicism for the 21st century. Developmental Dynamics. 2000;219:1–9.

17 Jones E, Ruse M. Human Evolution: From Fossils to Molecules, Reductionism to Holism. In: Rethinking Biology. World Scientific; 2019. p. 117–39.

18 Beach P. The contractile fields: A new model of human movement. Journal of Bodywork and Movement Therapies. 2007;11(4):308–17.

19 Farhi D. Teaching Yoga: Exploring the Teacher–Student Relationship. Shambhala; 2016.

20 Remski M, Rooney S, Dissette J. Practice and All Is Coming: Abuse, Cult Dynamics, and Healing in Yoga and Beyond. Embodied Wisdom Publishing; 2019.

21 Miller L, Balodis IM, McClintock CH, et al. Neural correlates of personalized spiritual experiences. Cerebral Cortex. 2019;29(6):2331–8.

22 Long R. The Key Muscles of Yoga. BookBaby; 2010.

23 Benias PC, Wells RG, Sackey-Aboagye B, et al. Structure and distribution of an unrecognized interstitium in human tissues. Scientific Reports. 2018;8(1):4947.

24 Allen WE. Terminologia Anatomica: International Anatomical Terminology and Terminologia Histologica: International Terms for Human Cytology and Histology. Journal of Anatomy. 2009;215(2):221.

GLOSSARY

Acharya

An ancient physician in Ayurvedic practice.

Agni

Fire; in Ayurveda, agni is the catalyst for digestion and tissue genesis.

Amorphous

Not regularly organized.

Anatomical position (AP)

Standing erect, facing forward, arms at the sides, palms forward.

Andragogy

Methods for teaching adults.

Apana

Outward push; apana vayu is the downward and outward movement wind.

Architecture

The architecture of the body is the histological continuum of fascia, elements arising out of the embryological mesoderm.

Ashtanga Vinyasa Yoga

Influential system of dynamic yoga developed in the 20th century in Mysore, India, by the late Pattabhi Jois with the guidance of his guru, Krishnamacharya.

Auxetic

The quality of having a negative Poissin's ratio, which means auxetic materials don't get thinner when they are stretched. Auxetic materials expand when stretched.

Ayurveda

"Science of life" from the Vedas; "yoga's sister science".

Bandha

Lock, bond, area of tensioned in-drawing (see Chapter 2).

Basal tension

The resting tonus of living tissue; the extent to which tissue draws inwards without us making any effort to do so.

Biomotion

Term coined by Joanne Avison for how organisms move in the round, as opposed to lever system actions in a single plane.

Biopolymer

A polymer (Greek *poly-*, many + *-mer*, parts), or large molecule composed of many repeating subunits, that occurs in nature; e.g., protein, DNA, cellulose.

Biotensegrity

A living system; new paradigm for considering balance of forces in biologic structure.

Blastopore

The hole where gastrulation begins in the developing embryo.

Bound water

Water molecules in body tissues which are bound to macromolecules or organelles as part of their structure.

Chakras

Energetic "wheels" or centers of converging energy within subtle body anatomy (see Neuroendocrine system)

Chirality

From the Greek for handedness, chirality describes something that has a left or right-hand bend; it can be thought of as the characteristic of necessitating a mate.

Chondrocyte

A mature cartilage cell.

Chordata

The phylum of animal, including vertebrates, that is classified according to the presence of a notochord during some stage of their development.

Chronotype

A person's unique profile of circadian rhythms.

Circadian rhythms

Daily 24-hr chronocycle of neurobiologic cascades; *circa*, about + *diem,* a day.

Circulatory

The comprehensive organ system of interconnected, circuitous vessels related to the circulation of blood and lymph.

Closed kinematic chain

"Closed-chain kinematics" in biology, including human anatomy, is the coupling of multiple parts into continuous mechanical loops allowing the structure to self-regulate complex movements at all scales.

Compression

A force that presses or pushes together.

Collagen

Most abundant (up to 30% of total protein mass) fibrous protein in the ECM of animals; resists tensile forces, secreted as procollagen by fibroblasts.

Complementarity

Principle from quantum physics that two sets of seemingly opposite views/systems can hold true simultaneously; wave/particle duality/simultaneity.

Constraints

Guiding limitations; in a human movement context, constraints guide how we move as a species.

Continuum

A coherent whole defined by the gradual spread of interconnected differences.

Cosmogony

Study of the origin and early evolution of the universe.

Cosmology

Study of the continuing evolution of the universe

Cytoskeleton (CSK)

Present in all domains of life, the CSK of a cell consists of interconnected microtubules, actin filaments, and intermediate filaments (proteins) distributed throughout the cytoplasm, giving unit shape and interfacing within the collective dynamics of tissue.

Dhātu

Sanskrit word for the tissue principle of Ayurvedic anatomy.

Deep fascia

Dense layers of connective tissue which surround individual muscles and groups of muscles to form fascial compartments. Two kinds: aponeurotic and epimysial fasciae.

Dermatome

A sort of "map" derived from the embryonic ectoderm from which the skin and subcutaneous tissues also develop and become the areas of skin innervated by a single dorsal root ganglia.

Deuterostomes

Of the Bilateria; the blastopore of these organisms will develop first into the anus.

Dorsiflex

Action of drawing the dorsal surface of the foot (top) toward the shin.

Dorsolateral

Pertaining to the back and the side.

Doshas

The Tri-dosha theory of Ayurveda includes three physiological qualities: Vata, Pitta, Kapha. These arise from the interplay of the panchamahabhutas; their relative imbalance dictates states of health and disease.

Dṛṣti

"Looking place" associated with turning the senses inward (pratyahara) and concentrating (dharana) during yoga practice.

Duhkha

Lack of space; discomfort.

Dvandva

Sanskrit for "pair of opposites".

Elasticity

The tendency of a material to "bounce back" to its original shape after a deformation.

Electromagnetic field (EMF)

Spectrum of waves within which different frequencies give rise to various properties; i.e., the light spectrum of color visible to the human eye.

Embryogenesis

The formation of an embryo.

Embryology

The study of an organism's early development.

Embryological mesoderm

The region of the trilaminar disc (one of three layers of the early embryo) that gives rise to "middle" tissues: the myofascial system.

Enantiomorphic pair

Enantiomers are chiral molecules that are mirror images of one another.

Epi -

On, above, or over.

Epistructural pathways

Routes of force/communication that flow over or above anatomical structure.

Extracellular matrix (ECM)

The matrix of support materials secreted by cells, extending from the molecular level to the macro level.

External/lateral rotation

Joint action moving away from the center relative to classical AP.

Fascia

Matrix of fibers secreted by cells that encompasses cellular structure.

Fibonacci sequence

Starting with 0 and 1, the sequence is: 0, 1, 1, 2, 3, 5, 8, 13, 21, 34..., where each number in the sequence appears by adding up the previous two numbers (the Golden ratio). This sequence holds virtually endless cultural, biological, astronomical, mathematical, and cosmological discussion.

Fiber

The rope-like components of ECM classed in three types: collagen, elastin and fibronectin. Gives tissues their tensile strength, or resistance to stretch.

Fibronectin

A non-collagenous fibrous connective protein that helps cells to adhere to the ECM.

Force

An effort or exertion of power.

Garbha shareera

Ayurvedic embryology, "embryo body".

Gastrulation

In humans, the process by which an embryo goes from blastula stage to the gastrula stage during which further differentiation happens.

Gheranda Samhita

One of the three classic texts of hatha yoga (the *Hatha Yoga Pradipika* and the *Shiva Samhita* being the other two); meaning "Gheranda's collection".

Golden ratio, φ

A so-called irrational number (phi) that describes the relationship between two quantities or lengths in which their ratio is the same as the relationship of their sum to the larger of the two quantities (Fibonacci sequence).

Golden spiral

A logarithmic spiral whose growth factor is φ, a geometric expression of the Fibonacci sequence, the golden ratio, a pattern of growth and form observed in nature.

Ground reaction force

Force exerted by the ground on a body in contact with it.

Ground substance

The amorphous, thixotropic, negatively charged, hydrophilic constituent of ECM, consisting of large GAG molecules linked to form larger molecules (PGs), excellent at resisting compressive forces.

Guru-shishya

Traditional teacher-disciple format for the transmission of yoga practice; lineage (parampara).

Hasta Bandha

Tensional in-drawing of the palmar arches through activation of the fingers in conjunction with upper limb spirality.

Hatha Yoga Pradipika

Ancient Sanskrit text on Hatha Yoga by Swami Swatmarama.

Helix

A three-dimensional spiral.

Heterarchy

A flexible system of organization in which the unranked elements form a network of distributed influence.

Hierarchy

An organizational system where elements are arranged in a graded order.

Histology

The study of biologic tissue.

Hoberman sphere

A spherical structure composed of closed kinematic chains often used in movement culture to illustrate breathing (and thus also known as the "breathing ball"), described as "isokinetic" by its patent-holder, Chuck Hoberman.

Hydrophilic

Material with an affinity for water.

icosahedron

One of the Platonic solids; frequently used to model shapes of the natural world due to its geometric properties of triangulation and closest packing.

Ida nadi

In yogic anatomy, the major left-side pranic current coiling around sushumna carrying "feminine force".

Inchoate

Not yet clearly or completely formed or organized; rudimentary.

Intermediate filaments (IFs)

Tensional elements of CSK.

Internal/medial rotation

Joint action moving toward the center relative to classical AP.

Intrinsic stress/tension

Prestress, basal tonus, intrinsic tension, "drawing in," prana vayu.

Isometric

Unchanging length.

Isotonic

Tension without contraction.

Jalandhāra Bandha

"Chin lock".

Kha/khe

Space, ether.

Koshas

Five "sheaths" of the subtle body, arranged from gross to subtle.

Krishnamacharya

Guru of both Pattabhi Jois and B.K.S. Iyengar; progenitor of Vinyasa.

Kumbhaka

Breath retention.

Kundalini

Branch of yoga interested in activating kundalini shakti; the potential feminine energy said to rest dormant like a coiled snake at muladhara chakra.

Lever model

The mechanistic idea of the body as a collection of levers and pulleys operating in a uniplanar, binary, linear hierarchy (a.k.a. the "old" paradigm).

Linear

Linear behavior follows the stress/strain curve of classical mechanics and is typical of Newtonian materials; see nonlinear.

Liquid crystal

A mesophase of matter exhibiting both the properties of flow characteristic of a liquid and the properties of particle orderliness normally found in solids.

Lymphatic

Relating to the lymph (Latin *limpa*, water), the interstitial fluid that collects through lymph capillaries as part of the circulatory system.

Mamsa vaha srotas

The srotas system of myofascial region, relates to the embryological mesoderm.

Mechanotransduction

The responsive process by which cells convert mechanical stimuli into biological signals.

Menisci

Greek *meniskos*, "crescent"-shaped fibrous cartilages or "discs" that partially line a joint cavity, e.g., the knee meniscus, wrist, acromioclavicular, sternoclavicular, discs, and TMJ.

Meridians

Lines on a body drawn for the purpose of navigation, understanding, and manipulation.

Mesenchyme

Mesodermal embryonic tissue.

Mesoderm (meso)

"Middle" layer of the embryological trilaminar disc giving rise to fascia and related tissues.

Mesokinetic

Martin and Levin's term for the biologic CKCs in an organism.

Mesophase

Middle phase of matter, somewhere between its liquid and solid form, i.e., liquid crystal.

Metameric

Relating to or consisting of several similar segments or somites; from somitomeres.

Microfilaments

Actin microfilaments generate cellular tension and, together with the microtubules and intermediate filaments (IF), comprise the filamentous components of the CSK.

Microtubules

Hollow tubes that act as compression-bearing elements in the CSK.

Microvacuoles

A term coined by Guimberteau to describe the volumetric routes he observed in the interstitium using endoscopy.

Minimal-energy

The most energy efficient strategy always used in natural processes.

Modularity

The characteristic of a system to be organized in compartments, often in patterns at different scales.

Morphology

The study of shape; morphogenic, the embryonic process by which differentiation of cells and tissues gives rise to consequential shape in the adult.

Morphological constraints

Shapers of experience as generated in the shape of one's actual form.

Mudra

Seal; energetic fastening especially through positions of the hands and feet.

Mūla bandha (mūlabandha)

"Root lock".

Multipotent

Cells which are able to differentiate along several lines.

Multistability

Multiple performance effects brought about in a nonlinear system.

Myofascia

Myo, muscle; fascia, connective tissue. The myofascial system incorporates all structures of the musculoskeletal system, factoring bones and blood into the fascia.

Myotomes

Embyronic meso giving rise to skeletal muscle; in the developed body, it is a specific region of muscle innervated by a single nerve.

Nadis

Subtle energy srotamsi (tubes, channels) transporting prana.

Nagadi vayus

Pranic currents of the outer body.

Neuroendocrine system

Together, the nervous system (instant communication using impulses) and the endocrine system (longer-term communications using hormones) form feedback loops linked to the chakras of the subtle body.

Neurulation

Formation of the embryonic neural tube.

Nonlinear

Nonlinear behavior is not proportional and is characteristic of living organisms such as humans.

Non-proportionality

The characteristic of nonlinear systems that makes them impossible to reverse engineer; complexity of interconnected variables not linked proportionately.

Notochord

An axial structure that develops in the early embryo during gastrulation.

Organismic constraints

Factors built into a person's organism, including personality factors (e.g., risk-taking behavior), personal fitness, mental skills such as concentration and emotional control, individual anthropometrics (height, weight, and limb lengths), as well as perceptual and decision-making skills.

Oscillation

Periodic fluctuation, swing, vibration.

Pada bandha

Tensional in-drawing of the metatarsal arches through activation of the toes in conjunction with ankle spirality.

Panchamahabhutas

The five elements that come together to form an embryo in Ayurvedic embryology (Garbha shareera).

Parametric controls

Changing the parameters of a nonlinear system will affect its behavior; see Tristana.

Pedagogy

Methods for teaching.

Phi, φ

1.6180339887498948482… The golden ratio, Fibonacci sequence.

Pingala nadi

In yogic anatomy, the major right-side pranic current coiling around sushumna carrying "masculine force".

Prāṇa

Life energy, breath (in yoga philosophy).

Prāṇāpāna

The balanced pairing of prana with apana, representing balance, breath, and complementarity.

Prana vayu

Inward pull.

Pranayama

Yogic technique of manipulating breath flow.

Prestress

Pre-tension, basal tonus, intrinsic tension, "drawing in," prana, intrinsic stress/tension: the state of being materially reinforced.

Pronation

Anatomical term for rotating the distal aspects of limbs so the palmar/plantar surface presents inferiorly; medial rotation.

Protein

From Late Greek *prōteios*, of the first quality; Greek *prōtos*, first; a biopolymer, the "building materials of life" made of long chains of amino acids (as compared to carbohydrate).

Protostomes

Of the Bilateria; the blastopore of these organisms will develop first into the mouth.

Pulmonary ventilation

Mechanical action of breathing.

Quantum biology

Inspired by the paradigm shift in physics, the hard and soft sciences are adopting complementarity to account for the unaccountable in nature.

Raja Yoga

The "royal" path of yoga techniques going directly to Samadhi.

Resonance

The effect when an oscillation is "pumped up" with the well-timed addition of another oscillation of equal frequency.

Resting tonus

The basal tension of living tissue; the extent to which tissue draws inwards without us making any effort to do so.

Samadhi

Final stage of yoga; union with Brahman.

Saṃskāra (sankhara, samskara)

Sanskrit term for generalised patterns (impressions, or residues) that make up personal psychosomatic conditioning.

Sattva guna

The middle path, balance.

Sarcomere

Contractile areas of myofascial system where actomyosin motors operate.

Scapulohumeral rhythm

Biomotion of the shoulder describing the movement of the scapula in time with the humerus.

Sclerotomes

Embryonic meso giving rise to the axial skeleton.

Sharira/shareera

The human body.

Soft matter

The branch of physics studying all things squishy, including biologic tissues.

Somites

Transient, embryonic structures that give rise to vertebrae, ribs, dermis of the dorsum, and body fabric of the limbs.

Somitomere

Gives rise to somites; a partially segmented whorl of mesenchymal cells embryologically derived of the paraxial mesoderm.

Spiral

The spiral is a line curving continuously away from a central point. There are many types of spirals (including but not limited to the Golden spiral found ubiquitously in nature).

Spirality

The condition of being formed of spiral components and behaving as such.

Sravanam

Listing, hearing, and experiencing: receiving truth.

Srotamsi shareera

Body matrix of tubules.

Srotas (srotamsi, pl.)

Tube or tissue construct in Ayurvedic anatomy.

Srotas-kinematics

A new term for the theory of interconnected movement on every level in the tubular body from gross to subtle anatomy.

Sthiram

Steadiness; Sthira-sukham, steadiness and comfort, Patanjali's definition of asana.

Subtle body

Energy-based yoga anatomy as derived from the cosmology of Sā khya philosophy and Tantra yoga.

Sukha

Sanskrit for space, comfort, pleasure, ease.

Supination

Anatomical term for rotating the distal aspects of limbs so the palmar/plantar surface presents superiorly; lateral rotation.

Sushumna nadi

In yogic anatomy, the central channel of space flowing from seat to crown.

Syndetome/fasciatome

Embyronic meso giving rise to fasciae; in the somite this is classically known as a region of "tendon progenitor cells".

Synergic/synergistic

The combining of two or more forces so that the result is more than the sum of the original two.

T-icosa

Tensegrity icosahedron and 24 tensile vectors.

Talar mortise

The talocrural joint of the ankle.

Tantra

The interwoven hatha yoga techniques relating to purification of nadis and awakening of shakti.

Tensegrity

Tension + integrity, a term coined by Buckminster Fuller to describe the concept of floating compression previously proposed by Kenneth Snelson.

Tension

A force of pulling apart, stretch.

Therapeutic modalities

Received therapies such as massage, physiotherapy, myofascial release, chiropractic adjustments, etc.

Thixotropy

Greek *thixis*, touch + *tropy*, turn. The property of some gels that are ordinarily viscous (thick) but become thinner (less viscous) when agitated, shaken, or stirred (like ketchup, and synovial fluid). After a period, these gels return to their original state.

Tissue

Specialized regions of cellular organization between the level of the cell and the organ.

Torus

A donut-shaped piece of topology with celebrity status in sacred geometry.

Transanatomical architecture

Van der Wal's term for tissues beyond borders.

Tristana

Breath, bandha, and drsti: an important set of parametric controls in Ashtanga Vinyasa Yoga.

Uddīyāna bandha

"Upward flying lock".

Vayu

Movement "airs" or "winds" that carry certain directionalities of Prana; there are five main vayus (with many more sub-vayus): prana, apana, samana, udana, vyana.

Vector

A line that has magnitude and direction.

Vector space

Each element in a vector space is a list of objects, or vectors, that has a specific length.

Ventromedial

Pertaining to the front and to the middle.

Vesalius

Known as the "Father of modern anatomy," 16th century Flemish anatomist, author of *De humani corporis fabrica*.

Vestibular

Parts of the inner ear that control balance.

Vinyasa

Movement–breath coordination in yoga practice; derived from the Sanskrit *nyasa*, "to place," and the prefix *vi*, "in a special way."

INTRODUCTION

Welcome, reader

Whatever kind of movement you are into, you're welcome here. This book is for anyone with a curiosity about anatomy, with any level of yoga experience. Any insight I have to offer comes from failing very obviously at learning anatomy and embryology the "normal" way; I had to build ten models of everything in order to understand it (and always with the cheapest materials around). If I could learn it, *anyone* can, and we can all benefit from making models. I will say that this is not a technical manual for learning about fascia, nor is it a textbook for anatomy in the usual sense. There are plenty of reference books out there you can look to for beautiful illustrations of anatomy for yoga.[1,2]

This book is about morphology, or how we got to be shaped the way we are and how this shape influences movement. I point to the umbrella of coupled functions in biology, the means by which every system is affected by every other system. I am also exploring the underlying mechanism (closed kinematic chains, or CKCs) that describes how the bits of anatomy could join up and dance. I talk about CKCs to highlight interconnectedness in the yoga body, a body I see as filamentous.

This book is not about stretch science or classical biomechanics, although you will see that these related studies inform my view. My interest in the shape of things is couched in my broader epistemological framework: hermeneutic phenomenology.[3] In a simplified sense, this research framework interprets the felt experience of individuals as source material for the kind of knowledge-gathering that can link us together.[4–6]

The following are valuable assets for the reader:

- Familiarity with the subtle body.
- Some experience of yoga.
- Basic anatomy background.
- General curiosity about the interconnected-ness of patterns in nature.

Even if you are a complete anatomy novice, each chapter offers information panels and Key concepts, with accompanying images to explain details. This book integrates threads from several selected disciplines, so the range of vocabulary is referenced in the Glossary (spot the colored words in the text).

As a semi-academic work, I have referenced the evidence base and provided a bibliography at the end of each chapter to facilitate smooth coordination between the text and references. I chose the Vancouver style to leave the numbered citations as breadcrumbs that you can take or leave.

My message is rooted in an empirical study of rotational movement applicable to any style of moving. As such, it is very much a creative work built around visuals to animate the felt sense of anatomy. The concepts are often best visualized with models, toys, and shapes easily made and/or observed around us all in nature. The underlying message is that what we learn at a high-school level in the basic sciences of biology, chemistry, geometry, and physics have so much to offer in the consideration of integrated anatomy.

The ideas and spirit in these chapters owe much to the work of Joanne Avison, who remains a key mentor of mine and whose comments appear throughout this book. Joanne allowed yogis to recalibrate the way we think about biomechanics in her use of the term "biomotional" in her influential book, *Yoga: Fascia, Anatomy and Movement.*[7] When I sometimes I use the pronoun "we", I am referring to Jo's influence throughout the book.

As a long-term yoga practitioner and teacher, and through her extensive experience in the fascia revolution that is flourishing in the field of manual therapy, Joanne established a groundbreaking interdisciplinary link. As a key contributor/protagonist to the BIG (Biotensegrity Interest Group), Jo's mentorship has emboldened my exploration of yoga anatomy in conversation with geometry (she still blows my mind into wordless smithereens, an amusing side effect of her superpowers).

For me, yoga is about personal experience and without talking personally about my journey, this narrative would be not only dull but also false. Joanne has encouraged me to keep the tone of a conversation, rather than a dissertation, throughout the work. That is to make it accessible, despite the research behind it. So, regardless of your background: please stay with me for the story as it is intended to inspire yours.

My story

Finding yoga in my late teens was nothing short of life saving. Yoga first taught me to discipline myself with its arm-balances and early wake-ups. It grew into something spiritual that offered a broad and profound model of lineage with ancient texts and deep insights from the philosophical aspects. Latterly, the importance of discernment over blind discipline has become key to my practice. I learned, through trial and much error, how to honor and care for my body, mind, and voice through practice. More recently, I have been moved by the importance of cultivating the same qualities within my community.

I first became interested in geometry as an art student working with ideas about space and nature after picking up Daud Sutton's beautifully bijou *Platonic and Archimedean Solids.*[8] Platonic solids became influential in my work at the Edinburgh College of Art, where I also first encountered the work of D'Arcy Wentworth Thompson[9] and other naturalists fascinated with patterns in nature.[10] Living in Scotland and working as an artist and a yoga teacher, my figurative work became physical in a literal sense, as I got involved with the body as a medium.

I worked solo and in collaboration with other artists on performance and time-based works rooted in body culture. On top of that, extreme cycling and Ashtanga yoga led me to some intensive physical circumstances in which I was pushing my tissues until they showed the limits of their compliance. I broke bones and tore myself up every which way on the bike and used yoga as a kind of first aid. When naïve addiction to intensity took hold of yoga practice, injuries appeared there too. That is when I first turned to anatomy, out of a visceral need to know more about the limitations of trying to achieve the impossible mixed with a deep and reverential curiosity about how the body works.

I spent a year studying classical human anatomy through cadaveric dissection, and my life was forever changed. Taking the body to bits was as humbling as it was inspiring. It became increasingly apparent that the only distinctions amongst all the parts were the ones *we made* as we dissected out "areas of interest" and threw all the fat and fascia into the bins.

I knew, from having read the second edition of *Anatomy Trains*,[11] that this was the way mainstream anatomy worked. However, until then I did not fully realize the extent to which, just as a hammer sees everything as a nail, the scalpel sees everything as needing to be separated and cut into pieces, sections and parts. After looking inside the body, I could see that all parts are artefacts of dissection.

It is not just the muscles that we have carved out of context, but the anatomically described, discrete units of fascia too. There are no nuts and bolts. Everything in the body is part of an interconnected mesh made whole through the dance of life. That interconnectedness was something I could *feel* in my body, as a living experience. I could also see it in the cadaver, before cutting, most notably in certain types of cadaveric preservation.

Yes, it does very much matter how the cadaver is prepared. Most mainstream institutions use a process of embalming with formalin to preserve cadaveric material. The Thiel method is an alternative "soft-fix" embalming technique that is best known for retaining the look and feel of a living body. Formalin-embalmed cadavers can last decades, but this "hard" process of preserving vital structures inherently dries and discolors the specimen. In comparison to formalin-embalmed cadavers, research shows that the Thiel soft-fix method fosters a more realistic learning experience.[12]

As I grappled with core concepts of dissection artefacts in my Master's course work, I considered undertaking a comparison study of Thiel and formalin prepared cadavers for my dissertation.[13,14] Around that time, circa 2013, I became familiar with the Centre for Anatomy and Human Identification's work on soft-fix cadavers at the University of Dundee. Soon after, I discovered the Biotensegrity Interest Group. The BIG group seemed to be dealing with the same issue I was facing: that there was indeed a basis of natural architecture that plays an *essential* role in understanding living anatomy. *So why bother studying tissue that is doubly dead?*

Around this time, clinical anatomist and BIG protagonist John Sharkey was paving the way for independent study of the soft-fix cadavers. Through his enthusiastic efforts toward opening the closed doors of the dissection lab, people like me with a genuine interest in anatomy could gain access to soft-fix cadavers in his Biotensegrity Dissection seminars. Studying classical anatomy showed me how to take everything apart for a close examination of segments, whereas the work of BIG visionaries like John now helps me put it all back together again to make sense of the whole in motion.

When I first encountered the BIG, I had that sick, helpless feeling you get when something outrageously beautiful that defies categorization totally grips your soul. It was not long after I met Susan Lowell de Solórzano on social media that she opened the door to the inner sanctum of the biotensegrity community and invited me to my first BIG meeting. There I had the pleasure of meeting Dr Stephen Levin MD, and since then my art–science dreams have come to life in a big way.

The wild and cerebral journey of coming to reconcile structural anatomy with what I was experiencing on the mat in my actual body was only possible by maintaining a daily yoga practice. In the years researching and writing this book, I realized that all the seemingly disparate views on anatomy converge into one self-centric personal experience; they have to. The reductionist limitations of words and the resulting confusion (and even hostility) that words can foster are all part and parcel of the intellectual realm in which it is possible to be very accurate about *naming parts*.

In the simple act of using yoga to quell the raging mind and move the curious body in which it resides, I have enjoyed many hours of clarity. For me, the real experience of *being* **spiral** and listening to the reverb of breath leaves all other methods of study behind. Without that kinesthetic experience, there can be no grounding or fundament for real understanding. I hope this book offers you some rope bridges across the divide that it attempts to weave together.

Shravanam: listening through doing

You may ask what happened to my addiction to intensity? Did I stop hurting myself? Over the years, I realized that it *is* possible to channel intensity in a non-harming (*ahimsa*) mode by observing natural patterns. Studying the nature of tissue gave me the confidence to wriggle free of the "need to achieve" trap. Gradually, my understanding of natural constraints redefined my core understanding of achievement. I brought this approach to my studio and found that the fundamental nature of tissue was something others were interested in exploring as well.

That emerging pattern forms the basis of this book and the scaffolding of the *Five Filaments*. The Five Filaments rubric is an approach to postural anatomy that shifts from the guru culture to cultivate the exploration of yoga from a place of personal empowerment rather than subservience. I would love to share it (and the profound value of listening to your inner voice) with you, from my heart, especially if it can assist you in discovering how to feel good in your body and teach from a wellspring of confidence.

On a practical level, the Five Filaments will best serve the practitioner interested in safely progressing and perhaps redefining their practice, whatever that may be. Of course, transformation calls for embracing the journey. Wherever I am now, I have reached this point through riffing on, responding to, rebelling against, and ultimately reframing the Ashtanga method for over two decades.

Far from doomsaying, the abuse revelations are a call to action, and reform is happening through acknowledgment, empowerment, and innovation. As we continue listening to victims who have survived abuse within the lineages of yoga, it is a time to look at our teaching tools. I feel inspired to share the ideas in this book as a unique contribution to the anatomy for yoga conversation, intended to spotlight common ground.

Furthermore, it is high time for healing. The yoga-as-lineage community at large has faced reckoning upon reckoning in recent years, reflecting the spirit of the times. The conversation around ethics and scope of practice has been a long time coming, and it is also informing how we talk about tissue. The paradigm shift in biology is indeed so profound and so interconnected that it cannot but include a transformation in how we treat ourselves, each other, and maybe even the planet (or so we can hope).

References

1   Kumka M, Bonar J. Fascia: a morphological description and classification system based on a literature review. The Journal of the Canadian Chiropractic Association. 2012;56(3):179–91.

2   Long R. The Key Muscles of Yoga. BookBaby; 2010.

3   Babich B, Ginev D. The Multidimensionality of Hermeneutic Phenomenology. Springer International Publishing; 2014.

4   Rudebeck CE. Grasping the Existential Anatomy: The Role of Bodily Empathy in Clinical Communication. In: Toombs SK, editor. Handbook of Phenomenology and Medicine. Dordrecht: Springer Netherlands; 2001. pp. 297–316.

5   Leder D. The Absent Body. University of Chicago Press; 1990.

6   Laverty SM. Hermeneutic Phenomenology and Phenomenology: A Comparison of Historical and Methodological Considerations. International Journal of Qualitative Methods. 2003;2(3):21–35.

7   Avison JS. Yoga: Fascia, Anatomy and Movement. Handspring Publishing; 2015. p. 376.

8   Sutton D. Platonic and Archimedean Solids. Wales: Wooden Books Ltd; 2002.

9   Thompson D'AW. On Growth and Form. Cambridge University Press; 1945.

10   Cook TA. The Curves of Life. London: Constable; 1914.

11   Myers TW. Anatomy Trains: Myofascial Meridians for Manual and Movement Therapists. Elsevier; 2009.

12   Kennel L, Martin DMA, Shaw H, Wilkinson T. Learning anatomy through Thiel- vs. formalin-embalmed cadavers: student perceptions of embalming methods and effect on functional anatomy knowledge. Anatomical Sciences Education. 2018;11(2):166–74.

13   Eisma R, Mahendran S, Majumdar S, et al. A comparison of Thiel and formalin embalmed cadavers for thyroid surgery training. The Surgeon. 2011;9(3):142–6.

14   Eisma R, Lamb C, Soames RW. From formalin to Thiel embalming: What changes? One anatomy department's experiences. Clinical Anatomy (New York, NY). 2013;26(5):564–71.

ANATOMY OF THIS BOOK

I wrote this book in the spirit of discovering anatomy for a progressive understanding of yoga. It is not about individual anatomical parts, although learning about classical anatomy is undoubtedly a worthwhile pursuit in itself. In the *Spiral Bound* approach, fascia and all the structures arising from the early embryonic *meso* (and the analogous *mamsa vaha srotas* of Ayurvedic anatomy) form the key anatomical instrument.

In the interest of integration, we will start our investigation of anatomy in **Chapter 1** as a continuum of embryology. **Chapter 2** follows with a closer look at how the rotational patterns established in the embryo continue to shape our grown-up anatomy through the biologic coupling of closed kinematic chains (CKCs), introducing what we call the **Five Filaments**.

With a foundation in structure giving us channels of space, the narrative flows through **Chapter 3** as our investigation of tubular anatomy continues in a way that works more congruently with a flow of Prana in the subtle body. This chapter offers the crux of the book: *srotas-kinematics*, "tube movement" – the mechanism of integrating the Inside and Outside, within the Self and as well as in collective behavior.

In **Chapter 4**, I apply the spiral-bound yoga approach to teaching and practice with a series of large full-color images featuring the Five Filaments (5F) , a constraints-led rubric applied to a range of asanas with suggested micromovement to support working toward each asana presented. **Chapter 5** progresses with subtle body concepts of coupled oscillatory systems into a discussion of how breath and bandha bear the gift of vinyasa.

This sets the stage for looking in more detail at the key sitting positions and leaving the reader in a neutral position ready for taking next steps in real life.

Like our human limbs, the appendices of this book are more than just add-ons. As we focus on the commonalities amongst styles, **Appendix A** explores biotensegrity, ushering us deeper into the interconnected, sensory web that brings postures to life through the building of models that explore tension and compression. **Appendix B** examines the teaching space in yoga anatomy, and we get our heads around nonlinearity with Chow's Four Points of nonlinear learning in skill acquisition as applied to andragogy of anatomy for yoga.

Online resource

The online chapter, **Reflection and growth,** riffs on the *Spiral Bound* message, weaves all the threads together, and suggests lines of further enquiry for the keen student of integrated anatomy.

https://www.karenkirkness.com/offers/oy66hJdW

Who will get this book?

I wrote this book for yoga practitioners and movement professionals as well as anyone curious about how gross and subtle body anatomy can come together practically. It presents a selection of anatomical concepts through learning, research and years of personal yoga study. In my experience, the most potent way to interpret anatomical theory is through direct experience, relating abstract academic concepts to what we feel in the body on a personal level.

Central to my approach to this learning of "living anatomy" is the kinesthetic experience of making models, making shapes, and playing. I hope to show clearly that functional anatomy for yoga is seated in voluminous spirals, or helices, that integrate to form rotations through the trunk and limbs. No matter the style, asana practice works most safely and efficiently when the instruction includes recognition of these spirals, and there is no surer way to know this than to feel it for yourself.

Instructing asana in spiral form is not a new approach.[1-3] We are coming to realize our duty of care as teachers and finally considering how tissue responds to load, and that *is* new. Jules Mitchell, in particular, has forged a brave and evidence-based enquiry into biomechanics as she elegantly explains key research findings that inform her views in *Yoga Biomechanics: Stretching Redefined*.[4] Although Jules does not particularly point to spirality, she does lead her readership to question critically both the limits of quantitative measurements and the usual script in yoga cueing.

My contribution in this book is to explore the andragogical (adult learning) space of anatomy for yoga, suggesting a curriculum built around rotation on a practical level and the value of personal experience in the broad sense. I intend to simplify the material into something accessible to yoga practitioners in the language of yoga. I am looking at the evidence of spiral movement in the body, reminding us that all structures are part of an interconnected web of tissue.

Key ideas include:

- All elements of the body materials arising from the embryo (including, but not limited to, fascia) influence movement, as movement influences them.

- The foundational pattern of these movement influences, our "organismic constraints", is spiral.

- These spiral movement patterns are the same for all humans and similarly color the morphology of all vertebrates.

- These spiral movement patterns are composed of closed kinematic chains (CKCs) throughout the living form.

- These CKCs are distinct from classical biomechanical levers. Instead, they model the "throupled" arrangement of unlimited interconnectivity at all size scales (from subtle to gross).

- This throupledness appears in biological coupling within and amongst individual bodies, subtle to gross.

Looking at the body in this way, as a unified whole rather than the sum of parts, represents a paradigm shift in anatomy. What seems revolutionary for some is perhaps an acknowledgment of what yogis feel every time they get on the mat. The yoga world is feeling the same kind of shift, as we reframe patriarchy into something more like a network of peers. We are embracing a constraints-led curriculum with a nonlinear approach[5] to skill acquisition across disciplines of physical culture.[6,7]

It only makes sense that it is also time for us to reframe our approach to anatomy, to better understand and manipulate breath-centered movement. In the chapters that follow, you will find a straightforward presentation of spiral-bound anatomy that relates specifically to the practice of yoga, presented alongside classical and contemporary movement concepts for an integrated approach.

Building models, being models

In its presentation of biotensegrity, Appendix A offers further exploration of the links introduced in the earlier practical chapters. From there, you could spiral back into earlier chapters and continue the exploration in your practice. Words and even pictures are not an ideal way of presenting ideas about movement! You have to feel it for yourself. Although any codification has its limitations, what I love about biotensegrity is how it makes us think about the dimensionality of tissue. It gives us tools for holding ideas in our hands.

Most yogis learn through their bodies, so when things get more abstract, it is worth making a model of tensegrity and effectively feeling the geometry. You can source DIY options on the web or check out my online course, Anatomy Inspired, for bespoke instructions in the context of anatomy, https://www.karenkirkness.com/anatomyinspired. Working in real-time with *push* and *pull* gives rise to a practical understanding of the body fabric we inhabit. In yoga, we do this at every level, starting with the most straightforward aspect of pranayama: the retraction and expansion of every breath. The model-play will nourish your felt sense of these first principles.

Of course, as living beings, we have the condition of built-in subtlety. This situation gives rise to a conundrum. You *are* biomotion making a model of biomotion to learn about biomotion! It is like the snake eating its own tail – the *ouroboros* at the heart of sacred geometry. Whether you are a person or a panda, if you are alive, then you are a mystery, and that mystery is spiral bound.

As such, I encourage readers to build the models and to *be* your own model of mystery on the mat. You can consciously incorporate these ideas into your actual practice. I believe that rotation-based movement can make asana safer and more effective in teaching and personal practice.

Vedic Gayatri Mantra of the Pāñcajanya Shaṅkha (conch)

पाञ्चजन्याय

Oṁ
Panchajanyaya vidmahe
Padma garbhaya dheemahi
tanno Shankha prachodayaat
Oṁ Shāntiḥ, Shāntiḥ, Shāntiḥ

Translation:

Let us contemplate Pañcajanya,
He/she who is installed in a lotus,
May that Shankha (sound of Shankha: Om)
inspire us and awaken our Consciousness.

References

1   Friend J. Anusara Yoga Teacher Training Manual. Anusara Press; 2009.

2   Borg-Olivier S, Machliss B. Yoga Synergy: Applied Anatomy Physiology Yoga Book (illustrated edition). Yoga Synergy Pty Limited; 2005.

3   Scaravelli V. Awakening the Spine: The Stress-Free New Yoga that Restores Health, Vitality and Energy. Aquarian; 1991.

4   Mitchell J. Yoga Biomechanics: Stretching Redefined. Handspring Publishing Limited; 2018.

5   Chow JY. Nonlinear learning underpinning pedagogy: evidence, challenges, and implications. Quest. 2013;65(4):469–84.

6   Button C, Seifert L, Chow JY, et al. Dynamics of Skill Acquisition: An Ecological Dynamics Approach. Human Kinetics, Inc; 2020.

7   Balagué N, Pol R, Torrents C, et al. On the relatedness and nestedness of constraints. Sports Medicine – Open. 2019;5(1).

1.1 In the beginning 4

1.2 Embryology 6

1.3 The meso story 9

1.4 Gastronomical 12

1.5 Mighty somites 16

1.6 Legacy of limb symmetry 23

1.7 A more useful neutral 28

Across anatomy

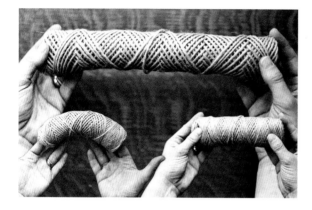

FIGURE 1.1

(Photo by Charlene Lim)

Like the caterpillar that takes the thread from its own mouth and builds its cocoon and at last finds itself caught inside the cocoon, we have bound ourselves by our own actions, we have thrown the network of our actions around ourselves.

Vivekananda[1]

Key concepts

1   To study embryology in the broader context of evolution is to appreciate how things come to be the way they are in the developed anatomical configuration we experience in adulthood.

2   Van der Wal's term "transanatomical" refers to structure that is trans, or across anatomical structure.

3   The notochord offers an attachment site or guiding central theme to developing tissues and a role in our development beyond the embryo.

4   Meso is the middle tissue that relentlessly orchestrates, connects, supports, and defines the bodily structure.

5   Thinking of the embryo in terms of distinct germ layers with definitive fates hides some of the more enlightening plot twists in the story of our spiral-bound tissues.

6   Dermatomes show us how our surfaces arrived as a result of early tissue wrapping around a central axis (notochord). The innervation patterns of these surfaces reveal how branches of the nervous system hitched a ride on these tissues during embryological development.

7   Even though we use the term layers for convenience, bear in mind, as we traverse the basics of classical embryology, that this transanatomical architecture isn't separate anywhere, ever.

8   Embryology shows how the limbs rotate out of their original limb buds into their recognizable forms as arms and legs, emerging from the tissue and in continuity with it.

9   Between weeks five and eight, the limb buds elongate and spiral into the positions characteristic the newborn.

CHAPTER ONE

10 Prestress, or pre-tension, is the quality by which our bodies draw into themselves through the spiralling filamentous development of cellular architecture.

11 Working with the limbs and their rotational origins in yoga is easier when you consider their embryological journey.

12 Limbs emerge from the trunk; the trunk is an interconnection, or continuum of the limbs.

13 Hands and feet can be platforms for standing; fingers and toes are structurally similar.

14 Limb structures broadly reflect one another.

15 For a positional basis of yoga anatomy, we often need something that is less preferential regarding which end is up.

1.1 In the beginning

I first picked up the *Hatha [Yoga] Pradipika*[2] (HYP) back in the 1990s (widely regarded as the oldest surviving text on Hatha Yoga, compiled by Swami Swatmarama somewhere between the 16th and 15th centuries CE). There was no chance of me taking it seriously – how could a middle-class sophomore raised in 1980s suburban Florida possibly relate to the self-application of a paste made from ash and semen (verse 98)? I was in college when I got the reading list for my 200 Hour YTT. Would I be fashioning a rectal syphon as part of my morning ablutions? What could this possibly have to do with nailing a handstand? One has to laugh, imagining these scenes as the cliché of a yoga-mad generation.

Looking at this juxtaposition of cultures on a grand scale, we find tropes of absurd incongruities as present populations encounter ancient cultural texts filtered through the blogosphere. Yoga's explosion in popularity is impossible to ignore. As ancient yogic practices find their way into the Millennial mindset, cultural appropriation highlights ironies and interpretations from hilarious to hurtful. I wonder what the next generation of young yogis will make of the classical works of yoga such as the HYP and the *Gheranda Samhita*?[3]

As a teacher, I'm now sitting on the other side of the pedagogical table. I have to laugh (that inward smile of recognition) whenever we start a new 200-hour training at my studio, as I observe keen beginners getting their first glimpse of the *kriyas*. When we turn to the HYP pages, a collective cringe settles over the room: it is easy to understand why. The mood is in stark contrast to the determined focus of the anatomy class – and the divide between them is a chasm, a gap that can perhaps be bridged.

Talking point

 Being honest, how many of us "anatomy people" rate the yogic "subtle body" as anything but esoteric oddities of another time and place? Chakras, prana, vayu? Seventy-two thousand rivers of shakti flowing through my nadis. *Hmmm*. Dropping the pretense, those of us that come to yoga as purely physical movement cringe at the concept of the subtle body. Likewise, those whose interest revolves around the subtle body might write off the idea that physical postures are much more than posing. Is there a middle ground?

Across anatomy

What do I mean by subtle body? That is the critical question that usually knocks back methods of empirical research. However, I will offer suggestions based on my journey so far, with a surprising conclusion at the end of Chapter 3. Elements of the subtle body from yogic literature contribute to the telling picture of what is also happening on the level of the gross anatomical structure. It took me a long time to see those distinctions between subtle and gross are just a matter of perspective.

Seeking subtlety, and with the benefit of further experience, I rediscovered the ancient yogic texts, and explored more modern ones. I reviewed a range of Ayurvedic literature,[4–8] inadvertently crashing into fields of soft matter physics, symmetry breaking, architecture, music theory, sacred geometry, and Turing mechanisms. Tubes and spirals seemed to bind it all together. Was there some simplicity here after all?

Somewhat to my surprise, studying Western biomedical anatomy and embryology brought me closer to an appreciation of ancient ideas about the nature of living tissue. What at first seemed to me like super weird (and potentially dangerous) superstitious rites represent what I now see as legitimately insightful human attempts at understanding our place in nature, with due respect for its mysteries.

Through the lens of holism, everything in the natural world is a living microcosm, reflections of the greater cosmic whole. However, conventional anatomical nomenclature reduces our personhood to a box of levers and pulleys installed in an isolated fleshy framework of linear relationships. As if our tissues were organized on the inside by a stack of bones – something of an internal scaffold tethering it to uprightness.

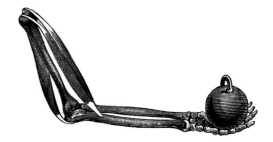

FIGURE 1.2

Levers and loads. Drawing from an 1872 physiology textbook demonstrating traditional anatomical lever mechanics: the rigid lever (radius and ulna) pivots about a fulcrum (elbow joint).

(thegraphicsfairy.com)

We are not stacked, literally or symbolically: we remain connected inside and out by webs of different densities, physically and metaphysically. That we still accept the principles of lever mechanics as the basis of all movement – indeed, adhere to them wholesale as facts – to me seems incompatible with the experience of physiological movement. If levers don't define gross anatomy, how could they possibly coordinate the energy-based context of yoga's cosmological anatomy? (Stay with me – we'll come back to the subtle body in Chapter 3).

In this chapter, we unpack the title of this work and explore a selection of body ideas in support of seeing innate anatomical patterns of spirality. These pervade our physiological (and psychosomatic) lives during embryogenesis (formation of the embryo after conception – the pre-embryonic stage) and embryonic development (up to eight weeks after fertilization).

CHAPTER ONE

 Spiral or helical: what's the difference?

Let's boil it down to basics. The term spiral can be a noun or a verb, and either way it is key to any readership interested in movement. A **helix** is a three-dimensional spiral, often seen in counter-spiraling pairs that form tubes, which are relevant to gross and subtle anatomy. Something that has the shape of the helix is *helical*, or *helicoid*. I use both terms throughout the book, depending on the context.

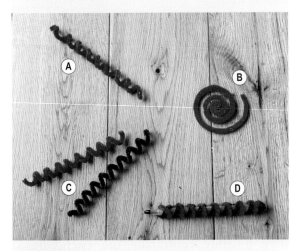

FIGURE 1.3

Spiral and helicoid pipe cleaner models: (A) helix in 3D; (B) 2D spiral; (C) two separate helices of opposite handedness (chiral); (D) a tube formed by pairing chiral helices of opposite handedness.

Here, we will take a closer look at the spiraling embryonic arrival of our limbs into their common configurations to see how our adult movement in yoga plays off these earliest patterns. All threads weave into the fundamental idea that there is value in incorporating spiral anatomy principles into personal and professional practice. Later, we'll see that these spiral principles aren't just the stuff of the gross anatomy: they live at the core of the subtle body anatomy as well.

Key concept 1

To study embryology in the broader context of evolution is to appreciate how things come to be the way they are in the developed anatomical configuration we experience in adulthood.

1.2 Embryology

Embryology is the study of an organism's development in the womb up to the eighth week after conception. The related disciplines of embryology and **histology** (the study of cells and tissues) are usually clustered together in the anatomy department, often in the context of developmental biology. It was only after several years of puzzling over how things got to be arranged as they are in the cadaver that I understood why.

Jaap Van der Wal PhD, MD is a medical doctor (emeritus associate professor) from the Department of Anatomy and Embryology at the University of Maastricht, The Netherlands. He is known as a phenomenological embryologist whose dedication to wholeness in describing the development of the embryo shifts the traditional way in which this subject is generally taught. Van der Wal suggests that the unicellular organism (the living zygote), continuously shape-changes *as a whole*, deploying its self-assembly as an embryo. An author, philosopher, and inspiring presenter, Van der Wal introduced the notion of *transanatomical architecture* into the literature with his tissue-sparing dissection of the human elbow; done in the opposite way to traditional anatomical dissection.[9]

Across anatomy

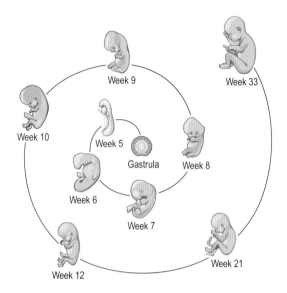

FIGURE 1.4

Human embryo in development.

(apokusay at www.vectorstock.com, with modifications by the author.)

Studying embryology, particularly in this expanding perspective, gives yoga practitioners exceptional insight into functional, postural, living anatomy in asana. Looking at the earliest developmental stages of our bodies means seeing ourselves as stories-in-process-of-unfolding, rather than as a collection of parts that can or can't do specific asanas. With such a big-picture view, we become *trans-asana*. We can thus see our ever-emerging, transanatomical selves as we practice the possibilities of our shape, our unique morphologies, in all their wholeness.

But how do we start and where do we begin? The bursting forth of a limbed creature from a spherical ball of cells is a sophisticated, complex, multidimensional process.[10–14] Studying it involves so much preloaded expertise that the mere prospect of considering embryonic development can be daunting. Take heart; it is well worth persevering with, at the very least, an overview that includes the spiral-bound nature of our formation.

Key concept 2

Van der Wal's term "transanatomical" refers to structure that is trans, or across anatomical structure.

Jaap van der Wal, through the careful and experienced understanding of anatomical dissection and embryological development, offers what many consider to be a maverick view of the human form. His understanding (of both evolutionary history and developmental histology) invites us to find the unique shapes (morphologies) of living bodies, as whole in themselves, at every stage of development.

Joanne Avison

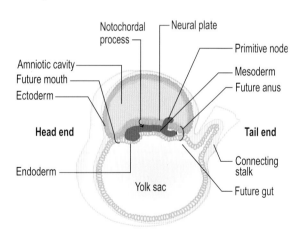

FIGURE 1.5

Gastrulation: sagittal view of the trilaminar embyronic disc around 16 days after fertilization.

CHAPTER ONE

One way for beginners to approach the intimidatingly complex story of embryology is to use an analogy. Reckoning with our roundness means visualizing voluminous shapes that are continually in-folding and unfolding themselves. This spiraling pattern, inherent to our forming process, has certain similarities with ribbons winding around a maypole.

The blue whale, the three-toed sloth, and your grandmother, all share the distinction as members of the classification in biology called phylum Chordata. That means, at this level, we are defined (among other fundamental features) by the embryonic presence of a notochord, a polarized axial structure (meaning one that provides axis) that develops during gastrulation (see Fig. 1.5). The notochord becomes the flexible longitudinal axis of this developing pre-embryonic circus.

Gastrulation (after gastro, belly-forming) is the invagination (folding into itself) of the fertilized egg (conceptus, or blastula) into what is classically described as three aspects, known as germ "layers."

The presence of this axis, in turn, induces the formation of what will become the neural tube in a process called neurulation (see Fig. 1.7). *This* tube eventually becomes the central nervous system. In a process something like structuring a maypole, the notochord provides a kind of mast during embryological development. It generates the metameric array of vertebrae, around which other tissue elements self-organize in species-specific ways, waves, and whorls. Whether water-bound, earth-bound or upright, the tissue ribbons all dance around the notochordal guide-pole.

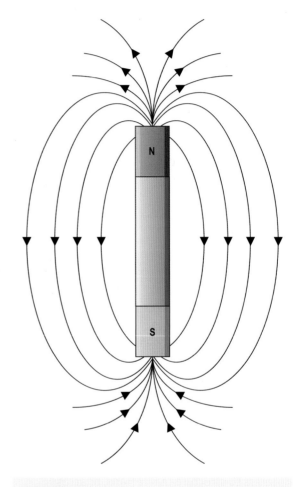

FIGURE 1.6

Vertebrate eggs are polar structures like the example shown here of north and south. In the embryo, the two opposite poles are differentiated as animal pole and vegetal pole. Polarity is an electromagnetic phenomenon, and it is the basis for the earliest orientations of the embryo that determine everything that comes next in development. The axis passing through the embryo is known as the animal-vegetal axis. Polarity is normally expressed in the egg as a gradient in the ratio of cytoplasm and yolk from animal to vegetal pole.

The notochord later becomes a somewhat different player in the developmental dance. After serving as the central theme around which the *whole spine* dances into being, the notochord becomes the nucleus pulposus (NP, inner gel substance) of the individual, intervertebral discs. Traces of the notochord persist into early adolescence, and there is enquiry around pathogenesis related to replacement of the notochordal remnants with chondrocytes in the maturing child.[15,16]

Suffice to say, nothing is redundant, and it is worth considering from a shaping/balancing body point of view, that the more global embryonic notochord (a so-called transient structure of the embryo) becomes a local notochordal echo in each disc. Together, the discs act as spacers; organizing the spine *as a tube* of sorts. Each disc retains an NP, and our movements could be said to join the dots when we integrate spinal motion well, at the gross level of asana practice.

Joanne Avison

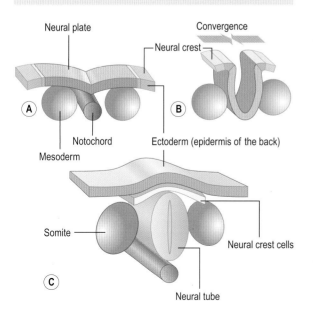

Neural plate

Convergence

Neural crest

(A)

(B)

Notochord

Ectoderm (epidermis of the back)

Mesoderm

Somite

Neural crest cells

(C)

Neural tube

Key concept 3

The notochord offers an attachment site or guiding central theme to developing tissues and a role in our development beyond the embryo.

1.3 The meso story

Soon after you embedded yourself into the uterine wall of your mother, you went through this most important transition of your life: gastrulation. Forget adolescence, university, marriage, children: by far the most significant moment of your life was when you became a trilaminar disc. Sometime after compaction of your first cells, but before you grew limb buds, you transformed yourself from a hollow ball of cells into a double bubble. One bubble became a cavity containing amniotic fluid (the amniotic sac), your personal ocean that you instinctively wrapped around yourself. The other bubble was to be your yolk sac (this process of gastrulation is hungry work; you instinctively enveloped your yolk sac too).

FIGURE 1.7

Neurulation: the folding "burrito". (A) Coronal view of the notochord in situ; (B) notochord signals induce tubification of ectoderm at the neural plate as shown through Day 18; (C) the ends of the neural plate fuse to form the autonomous neural tube with neural crest cells visible by Day 23.

The two surfaces of the joined bubbles are then known as a two-layered oval, or the bilaminar disc, in classical terminology. Amid some jostling between the upper and lower

CHAPTER ONE

floors, there suddenly appeared an in-between, composed of eager cells that migrated from the ground floor into the basement down a spiral staircase between them. They poured downstairs as a crowd, in response to different growth rates and patterns. These highly responsive cells found themselves forming this 'tween tissue, a kind of mezzanine, known classically as the **mesoderm**, or middle layer. This now *tri*-laminar disc whorls, folds and enfolds itself into nested tubes, and from here a whole new level of tubular partying exudes from this early patterning.

is not a "derm", bearing little or no resemblance to a layer),[17] is comprised of a primitive field of fluid and **protein**. This field is an embryological juice called **mesenchyme**, a soupy spectrum of loose fibers suspended within a mucous **ground substance**. This juice is worth the squeeze; from it, we derive the tissues of locomotion and circulation. The urogenital systems also arise from within (and around) this juicy milieu. They appear according to the species-specific plan that orchestrates the chrono-structural origami of your unique architecture.

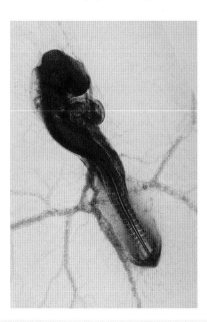

FIGURE 1.8

Brightfield photomicrograph of chick (*Gallus gallus domesticus*) embryo development at 60 hours; 29–32 somites.

(Scenics & Science/Alamy Stock Photo)

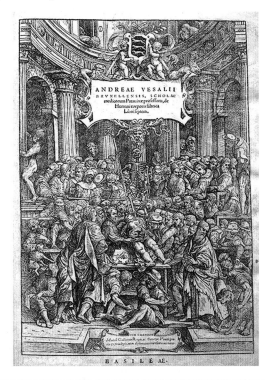

FIGURE 1.9

Frontispiece of Vesalius' *De Humani Corporis Fabrica* (1543).

This so-called mesoderm (that Van der Wal calls the *meso:* he emphatically demonstrates it

From this same soft start, the **lymphatic** and **circulatory systems** emerged, which (along with the nerves) were later intimately woven around the maypole of your body plan. The tirelessly winding somites led this part of the dance, bent on rotating to become the fabric of your torso, arms, and legs. These rapidly differentiated on their journey towards their more familiar final configurations.[18]

In an average anatomy lesson since the time of Vesalius (see Fig. 1.9), one would likely learn that this preceded the fully developed human body: ultimately composed of approximately 206 bones and 640 muscles. Unlike your average anatomy lesson, in this chapter we will stop seeing the developed body as a parts list of separate structures and separable layers. Here, rotation and invagination never come to a definitive end.

Key concept 4

Meso is the middle tissue that relentlessly orchestrates, connects, supports, and defines the bodily structure.

Instead, we will start from the embryological soup and decline to separate it into three layers. Since all the membranes are swimming in their respective sub-soups, they contain and are contained by the fluid body that continuously emerges through itself. The body is relentlessly subtle. It is composed of a continuous, collagenous, spiraling, semi-conducting liquid-crystal arrangement of tubular structures arising from a primitive stew (gelled in bound water like a gelatin dessert).

Memorizing all the detailed embryological strata presents the same trap as memorizing the yet-to-become 206 bones and 640 muscles designated to the developed human body. I'm inviting us to reframe yoga anatomy to allow for the notion that the in-between spaces (which are not empty) incorporate something much more usefully considered as the fluid-fascial matrix we all embody.[19] In real life (and living motion) the mesenchymal milieu of the embryo doesn't really disappear, despite what labels we assign to its final structures.

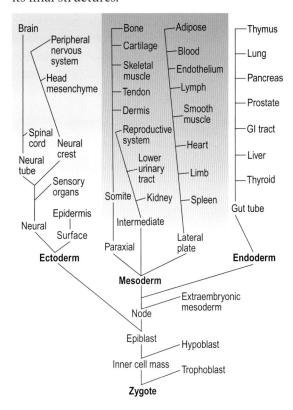

FIGURE 1.10

Fields of development: ontological tree showing the gist of the germs/derms. In embryology infographics, the usual color code is as shown: blue is ectoderm, yellow is endoderm, and red is mesoderm.

Classically, post-neonate, the cell and that which surrounds it factor separately. That is, what surrounds the cell is more generally referred to as the extracellular matrix (ECM), meaning "outside" the cells. Recent research is following the same pathway to wholeness we all seek (at least philosophically). Pathologists Neil Theise and Rebecca Wells (and colleagues)[20] have suggested the term *interstitium*, to encompass the nature and structure of the internal tissues.

This tissue field comprises a continuum, containing virtual spaces and fluidity classed as fascia in the literature,[21] and always expressing as filamentous variations on a soft-matter theme. As such, the body is a spectrum of thicknesses, folding, unfolding and in-folding, imbuing and self-organizing to form its own pockets and tubes within pouches and pipes, to become itself. Howsoever you cut it – it begins and remains one piece.

Key concept 5

Thinking of the embryo in terms of distinct germ layers with definitive fates hides some of the more enlightening plot twists in the story of our spiral-bound tissues.

 Meso and the layerless cake

This inner world of the *meso* derives from the embryological region between the ectoderm (upper or outer layer) and endoderm (innermost layer). Classically known as the mesoderm, or middle layer, this inner-middle world generates fields of muscular tissue that develop into what is generally referred to as the musculoskeletal system and its attendant fasciae.[9]

This layer, or derm, is not a layer in the strict sense. Instead, it is a specialization of cells that I'll refer to here as meso, and later as the *mamsa* (the Ayurvedic anatomical equivalent that is also all-encompassing). Factor in the multipotent neural crest cells (NCC) that feature in peripheral innovation and contribute to the locomotor system as well, and it becomes clear that pinning down the development of these tissues to any one term is just not congruent with what happens in real life. (See "Head, shoulders, knees and toes" below for more on neural crest cells.)

In her book, Avison introduces another applicable term, alongside the classical specialization that refers to the differentiation of these structures. Tissue formation is a process of instinctively knowing what to become and becoming – this is what Avison calls the "pre-formance", and van der Wal calls the "performance" of creating ourselves as living volumes.[22] Whatever you call it, development cannot be entirely explained by genetic, chemical interactions: we push and pull ourselves into being[23,24] as mechanical forces (tension and compression) act in continuity.[25–27] It is a self-perpetuating process.

Donald Ingber was among the first to use the term mechanotransduction as the structural/action-based foundation of tensegrity and gene expression.[28] Closely reflecting a key component in the study of yoga, Avison describes the process of *spacialization* that the meso, notochord and somites undergo as the kinetic organization of the form. Genetic signaling, polarity, impulses, fluids, and fabric folds prompt that process – as they, in turn, sculpt the very same flows and folds they call into placement.

1.4 Mighty somites

During the earliest stages of embryological development, the neural tube wraps itself up like the folding of a burrito. As this innermost inner-tube forms (in response to the notochord), it zips itself up to create a tube that induces the formation of still more tubes. Much tubification occurs in parallel with the notochord, animating pairs of cells that run along the length of the forming neural tube, from head to tail end. These pairs give rise to polarized somites (from *soma*, or body), and their path is a bit like the ribbons weaving around the maypole, from the top down.

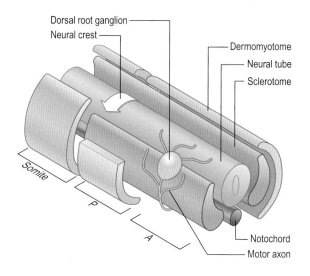

FIGURE 1.11

This diagram of the anatomy of spinal nerve segmentation shows the early elements of the developing peripheral nervous system including the migrating neural crest cells and outgrowing motor and sensory axons. These are shown with reference to the somite derivatives (dermomyotome and sclerotome). Most of the dermomyotome has been peeled back from the somite on the left, revealing the sclerotome as subdivided into anterior (A) and posterior (P) aspects.

(Redrawn from Kelly Kuan CY, Tannahill D, Cook GMW, Keynes RJ. Somite polarity and segmental patterning of the peripheral nervous system. Mechanisms of Development. 2004;121(9):1055–68.)

The "little bodies" of these somites arise as spheres from the mesenchymal paraxial mesoderm in a regular, rhythmical sequence. They migrate along the head to tail axis (anterior-posterior, cranio-caudal axis) as pairs of epithelial balls, forming the body-tube of the whole torso (see Fig. 1.7). Somitogenesis, the origin of somites, is driven by a clock and wavefront mechanism[29] that transforms the somites, one on each side of the developing neural tube, into sets of more differentiated tissues.

The spheres further subdivide as the animating structures of potential muscle, bone and connective tissues (termed **dermomyotomes**, **sclerotomes** and **syndetome/fasciatomes**),[30] placed and spaced by polarity[31] toward their transforming position. The **ventromedial** portion of the somite becomes mesenchymal sclerotome (together with the midline notochord) which, with increasing maturity, differentiates into the ribs and spine. The spine is destined to encase the neural tube (early central nervous system), a tube-within-a-tube around which the tubular torso is simultaneously choreographing a burrito ballet of its own.

Key concept 6

Dermatomes show us how our surfaces arrived as a result of early tissue wrapping around a central axis (notochord). The innervation patterns of these surfaces reveal how branches of the nervous system hitched a ride on these tissues during embryological development.

The **dorsolateral** (front/back) portion of the somite becomes the dermomyotome, fated to become the axial dermis from the dermatome portion, and skeletal muscles from the myotome aspect.[32] A further subdivision emerges between

CHAPTER ONE

 Dermatomes

Dermatomes are perhaps the most famous of the somitic subdivisions as they track the story of development. The somites form whorls that abseil around (like ribbons dancing around the maypole from top to bottom), taking with them the nascent neural tissue expressed into the dermatomes as seen in Fig. 1.12. Dermatomes derive from the embryonic outer layer (ectoderm) from which the skin and subcutaneous tissues also develop. These become the areas of skin supplied by the branches of a deeper aspect of the central nervous system (known classically as single dorsal root ganglia). Essentially, they give us a map that illustrates the journey of the inside becoming the outside.

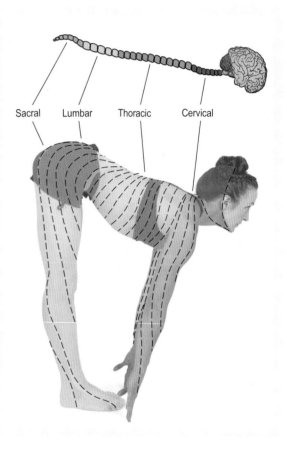

FIGURE 1.12

Dermatomes: the nerves originating from the neural plate take a circuitous route, hitching a ride along with the myotomes and sclerotomes to reach their final destinations as shown.

the myotomes and sclerotomes; this, the *syndetome*, is destined to become the tendinous tissues of the segmental muscles attaching to the vertebral array.

Although this is metaphorical and the somites don't literally go on to wrap repeatedly around the notochord, the tissue streams they initiate *do* weave around the trunk, arms and legs. It is illustrative of the spiraling nature of embryonic development. Once the axis establishes itself, our proto-tissues wrap around the longitudinal tubes ventrally and dorsally. Somites are the whorled organizers of the body plan.[33] They define the spine to create another set of tubes: the belly cavity ventrally and the cavity for the central nervous system along the inner dorsal contour.

Appreciating the transformative wrapping, it becomes easier to see how our compartments wind and twirl around the inner tubes. These, with use and time (and under the influence of differential growth rates and force transmission through the body), will eventually become articulated bones. Even the bony arrangements are evidence of this deep, spiral strategy. How our limbs rotate into position embryologically is a crucial feature of this chapter, setting the stage for a focus on the rotational nature of the limb patterns as they develop.

Across anatomy

Head, shoulders, knees and toes

As far as Earthlings go, to say that the vertebrates are evidence of a successful strategy would be a monumental understatement. To develop the predatory lifestyle needed to carry out world domination, organisms required a head. It turns out that having a head is structurally and functionally critical. So complex was the task of generating head structures that an extraordinary type of vertebrate cell population emerged to carry out the process: thus evolved the neural crest cells (NCC) (see Fig. 1.7).

Often regarded as the fourth germ layer, the NCC form in the neural primordium of vertebrate embryos.[34] This structure arises in conjunction with the other architectural derms and contributes to nearly all tissues and organ systems throughout the body.[35] The craniofacial skeleton (referring to the head and face – not the fascia as such), the peripheral nervous system, and pigment cells are among the many tissues that arise from NCC.[36]

The NCC not only give rise to our skin color (i.e. pigment-producing cells called melanocytes), peripheral nerves and their ganglia, but also to a variety of connective tissues, bones and cartilages of the head, known as mesenchymal derivatives. In other regions of the body, these tissues are described as mesoderm-derived, meaning they arise from between the ectoderm and endoderm (i.e. from the meso according to van der Wal).

In reality, however, the so-called derms are not distinct, or separate or layered. The literature tells the story of what makes vertebrates truly unique embryonically, and of course, it scales up to our adult configurations.[37] It is well-accepted that NCC persist into adulthood and form a reservoir of stem cells with therapeutic potential.[38] It transpires that NCC aren't just multipotent and pervasive, they also yield surprising interconnectivity throughout the entire body from the earliest stages.

Key concept 7

Even though we use the term layers for convenience, bear in mind, as we traverse the basics of classical embryology, that this transanatomical architecture isn't separate anywhere, ever.

What all that means in plain English is: these highly potent, original cells of the embryo form our color on the outside, our gut, nerves and connective tissue system on the inside (which are unpigmented; we are all the same on the inside), and they give rise to a great deal of what connects them in between. This suggests that separating the body into classical classifications (just as separating humans beings based on color) is missing a very significant point. Essentially, this points to a layerless, in-the-round reality in which the derms are NOT as distinct as we might wish them to be in advance of an embryology exam.[39,40] Keep this in mind as we traverse the layered terrain of basic embryology.

Talking point

Yoga is rapidly expanding as a transnational, trans lineage practice. Do we need to expand our ideas of anatomy for yoga to encompass the bigger picture and consider the transanatomical nature of our living architecture?

CHAPTER ONE

1.5 Out on a limb

The activity of living things is primarily dictated by which element they navigate with their limbs, be it the sky with wings, the land on legs, or swimming in the water with fins. Vertebrates, in general, tend to be characterized by their limbs: they fly in the sky, knuckle-drag, pronk, paddle, prance, pose, and run marathons. In humans, the trunk contains the organs responsible for immediate survival, but it is our limbs that define us as bipedal quadrupeds (from a structural point of view).

> These definitions arise from the forces those limbs negotiate in motion, which also generate the patterns of this soft matter we each self-assemble. The pattern of matter is the essence of this species-specific, environment-dependent, space-time configuration we call form or structure, which, in turn, defines the species and the forces it can negotiate. Every maypole begins in 360 degrees of whatever it calls home (earth, air or water). This matters, as we understand the relentlessly spiral patterns in which our soft matter architecture is bound.
>
> **Joanne Avison**

Dr Stephen Levin, originator of the term "bio-tensegrity" – a blend of biology and tensegrity, describes the spine as a tensegrity truss system[41] (we will come back to Dr Levin and biotensegrity in Appendix A). The truss model necessarily includes the whole body; extending it to the limbs, we can incorporate it to understand the body *as a whole*. These trusses are modular body segments that have an aspect of chirality, or handedness, with constraints that we pair in both flow and opposition in asana.

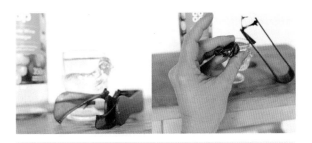

FIGURE 1.13

The body is entirely composed of soft matter, even the bones. In this simple learning activity, you can soak a bone in vinegar for some time and feel for yourself how the bone crystals dissolve, leaving the bendy fascia behind. Living in the countryside, we often find a bony specimen while out walking. I took the opportunity to use a pair of rabbit scapulae for this demonstration.

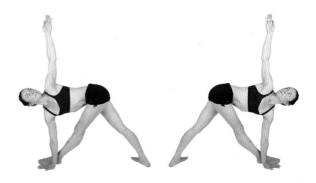

FIGURE 1.14

Yoga postures are often chiral, as pictured here in Parivrtta Trikonasana

(Demonstrated by Sarah Hatcher)

Chirality leads body elements to twist in a particular direction. Arms rotate inwardly when we ground them downwards and unfold externally when we reach out into the world. Legs have a similar rhythm, literally configured in rotation. In truth, the appendages are not appended to the trunk at all. Instead, you can think of them emerging from the axial body compartment as extensions of the spiral (helical) tracks of the trunk.

(i)

Chirality refers to mirror-image pairs of objects that cannot be superimposed onto one another. To find a great example, just look down. Your two feet are identical and opposing shapes. Chiral things tend to appear as a complete pair with a function greater than the sum of the individual parts. Together they facilitate our gait motion through rotational correspondence. This is a fundamental clue to understanding non-linear biologic forms and the keystone of this book.

Limbs unfurling

It is hard to imagine that we all begin life as a single (if charmed) cell, a fertilized egg made up of both its mother's and father's genetic material, uniting their respective DNA. As Avison points out, "acorns don't go to acorn school to learn how to become oak trees." We have all that we require to become us baked into the ingredients at the outset. The being precedes the body, so-to-speak, and once that loaf is baked, it cannot be unbaked or reduced to parts.

That unicellular sphere soon becomes multicellular (the one becomes the many). They go on to differentiate (specialize and spatialize), enfolding and curling eventually into a flexible and flexed trunk. Our limbs come later to the party: only after four weeks, relatively late in

the process after the foundational body plan has formed, do our limb buds appear.

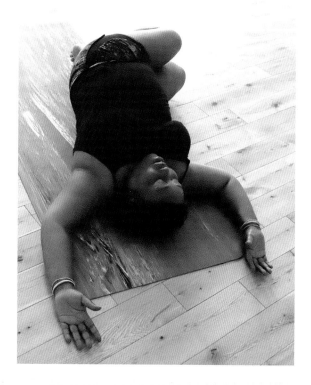

FIGURE 1.15

A supine twist is formed as gravity stabilises the opposing pairs of limb trusses.

(Demonstrated by Fadzai Mwakutuya)

Exquisitely intricate molecular choreography regulates limb development in vertebrates like us. The chemistry of the limb dance is much the same across species and, as it turns out, the recipe for baking limbs is also very similar across species.[42,43] Limbs develop as outpouchings of mesenchymal cells. These pouches of goo undergo tremendous shape changes (or morphological transformation), that give rise to

CHAPTER ONE

different thicknesses of the tissues in different places, such as the cartilage "condensations".[42,44,45] Such condensations are the fundamental cellular beginnings of our manifesting morphology.[46]

What we now experience as our bones are such cartilaginous (fascial) elements, pimped out with bone-forming minerals that we pinched from maternal reserves (typical). These we reorganized as we self-assembled and found our forms ever-informed by the original recipe of our blueprint, and reinforced by the particular ways our species interacts with earthly constraints. Bone formation occurs much later in development and continues post-neonate; however, the pathways are writ large in these embryonic condensations.

Key concept 8

Embryology shows how the limbs rotated out of their original limb buds into their recognizable forms as arms and legs, emerging from the tissue and in continuity with it.

The sophistication of this process genetically stands outside the scope of this book. For understanding how movement patterns appear in the limbs, it is enough to know that limb development begins as the tiny buds emerge through the body wall. The complexity of the somite choreography initiates a longer axis in each. These arise as condensed inner-tube tissues that trigger the dance into formation.[47] The various tissues have different growth rates, which (besides the complexities of a heart-led patterning for the circulation with which to grow) keeps our maypole theme, continuous within each limb.

The central pole is analogous with the core cartilage that bolts, piston-like, through the middle. The ribbons are the other limb tissues, wrapping around the pole – but pulled under tension into form by the inner-tube, as they grow at a slower rate and get pulled into their pre-tensioned architecture. As these limb sproutings continue, their journey takes them inevitably along a gently twisting path into recognizable arms and legs.

The far (distal) ends of the limb buds, most distant from the spine, spread out to form handplates and footplates before they differentiate into fingers and toes by about week six. The finger-forming process involves as much editing as it does the production of a new structure, another layer of the morphology process that reminds us of the importance of negative space.

 Limb development

- Upper limb buds are visible by days 26–27.

- Lower limb buds are visible by days 28–29.

- Upper limb buds develop along the lower neck (inferior cervical) segments.

- Lower limb buds develop along the lower torso (inferior lumbar) and upper tail (superior sacral) segments.

- Each bud forms a specialized ridge that guides the growth and development of that limb.

- Each pair of limbs rotates around the body axis.

Across anatomy

- Each pair of limbs experiences differential growth rates that cause them to curl around their axis.
- Around week six, the handplates and footplates begin to differentiate by spatializing the digits.
- Limbs are structurally established by the eighth week of development, by which time they have digits (fingers and toes).

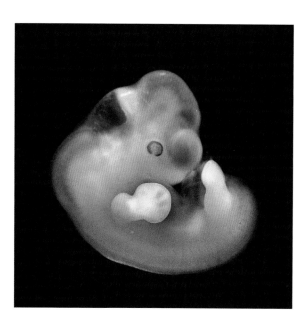

FIGURE 1.16

Human embryo, six weeks. The black circle is the edge of the fundus of the eye. Visible here is the umbilical cord, a strand of tissue containing the two spiraling arteries that carry blood to the placenta (the organ embedded in the uterine wall that interfaces maternal and fetal circulations) plus one vein with return supply to the fetus.

(Lennart Nilsson, TT/Science Photo Library)

 Out of the flatness of fishes

Evolutionarily speaking, our limb patterns come from those of primitive fishes.[48,49] As the planet's atmosphere changed, life took to the land, and gravity was experienced very differently by those creatures that emerged from the buoyancy of saltwater. Limbs, initially flat fins, evolved rotatory shoulder and pelvic joints as a direct result of navigating over slippery muddy flats and mounds, and the need to lift the head to see the emerging view. Imagine the change in perspective as the once-uniplanar perspective scaled up and around into 360 degrees!

It was imperative to develop the ability to look up (push up from the ground) and see around to where the body could go, all while navigating slithery surfaces to push upon, pulling along the rest of the gravity-bound body. This evo-devo (evolutionary development) dance was led by the instinct to move forward and, later, to look up. Further rotation at the elbows would follow, as part of this ongoing evolutionary process toward *orthograde* (walking upright with limbs swinging independently) posture. Given what we have developed into, this was essential.

The legs of land-walking bipeds eventually needed some kind of jointing at the knees to organize the seeing, moving body relative to the earth. Further, they needed to move even more efficiently over land while navigating with agility around who or what might be in their way. We, humans, continue to experience changes in our strategy, particularly noticeable in how the elbows and knees bend in opposite directions. In humans, the arm buds develop earlier than the leg buds emerge and continue their advantage throughout gestation.

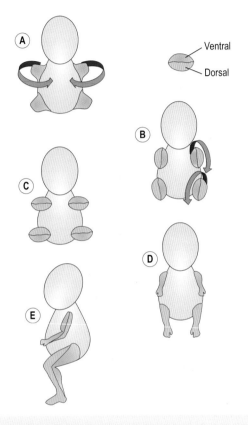

FIGURE 1.17

Ventral-dorsal rotation.

A We start out as a belly-up turtle with our four limb buds directed laterally

B Rotation of the limbs around to the front of the body brings the limbs out of the coronal and into to the parasagittal plane (to the front)

C The limbs continue to spiral around their long axis: upper limb externally, lower limb internally. The dorsal surfaces of the limbs are then facing each other as the limb buds continue to develop.

D As the limbs mature into their adult position, the tissue that started out in the ventral is now anterior in the upper limb, but posterior in the lower limb.

E Looking at the adult from the side, with bent knees and elbows, the ventral surfaces are the flexors.

During the seventh week of gestation, we see the limbs spiraling into place. The arms slide down from the neck as they emerge from the sides as limb buds emerge and rotate ventrally. Their ventral surfaces rotate upwardly (laterally/externally), offering the medial arm and palmar surface of the hand upward, evident in the carrying angle of the elbow. The legs rotate inwardly (medially/internally), taking the medial aspect of the limb bud into a dorsal position distally (what was the ventral lower limb, becomes the back of the lower legs and soles of the feet). These leg rotations lay the tracks for future knees and their so-called screw-home mechanism.

These significant turnings take tissue along for the ride, bringing the body elements of the arms and legs into a future readiness for the anatomical position (see Section 1.7). In this position, the elbows point toward the back (dorsally) and thumbs seek a lateral home (pointing out to the sides). Likewise, we see the knees take their place on the front surface of the body (ventrally), and the big toes coming together into their position we know so well from looking down at our feet on the mat.

At the eighth week of development, the embryo is approximately 23 mm long. By this time, the hands stretch through the inchoate arms and continue to reach through, as an echo of something you might feel when pulling on a latex glove. The cartilaginous precursor of the yet-to-be bone grows many times faster than the surrounding tissues, spiraling into form.[50]

Across anatomy

Elbows and knees arise as the different bands of tissue grow at different rates, like pea tendrils wrapping around their trellis, or ribbons around the maypole of their yet-to-become bony inner-tubes. The process is spatiotemporal sculpture.[51] The self-sculpting tissues of the embryo require both fluid-like and solid-like states to deploy themselves into wholeness.[52]

Key concept 9

Between weeks five and eight, the limb buds elongate and spiral into and out of the positions characteristic of the newborn.

From these somewhat undignified-looking beginnings, with our developing limbs poking out furtively from the still-tailed body wall, the buds spiral their way into a more advantageous position and differentiate to allow us a reasonable means of interacting with the world. The action happens through the balance of chirality (the counter-spiraling essence of our forming formula). The limbs extend from the trunk and converge through the trunk. In yoga, it becomes increasingly apparent that the limbs connect us to the earth, the sky, each other, and into ourselves, hugging these original patterns to us, to transcribe forces of the dance into form.

Tuned into tension

At this point in the story, we need to recognize that we are prestressed from the outset. Let's expand on what **prestress**, or pre-tension, means. When you put a tent pole into a tent, it has to be ever so slightly longer than the pocket housing it. This relationship allows the canvas to be held open and upright (between the tent poles of the whole structure). Thus, it contains a volume, essentially tensioned by the compressive forces of the rods (which are compressed by the tensional forces of the tent fabric). It is the reciprocal balance between these two forces that creates and maintains the shape or volume of the structure. The third force is the result of the particular combination of the other two.

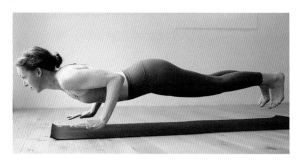

FIGURE 1.18

Nakrāsana (Crocodile pose). Cellular prestress (self-stress) in the structural matrix is what gives our bodies the stiffness and elasticity to bounce high after greeting the ground.

(Demonstrated by Emma Isokivi)

Unlike us, a tent has to be tethered to the ground to find its shape. Nevertheless, it is classed as a tension-compression based architecture, and the canvas or fabric has to be under tension to hold its shape. We are born with that pre-tension (or prestress) in place as a result of our bones growing faster than the surrounding tissues, within the limb tubes. In other words, our muscles and tendons and nerves and tissues are all pulled into shape embryonically. Some evidence of this is that we naturally curl into the fetal position, our hands and feet rest in slightly arched shapes, and our undone posture default is curved and folded.

Think child's pose. That is our prestressed pattern, dyed in the wool before the forces of life bring our bones into the more adult expression. Our bones become something like the tent poles in the example of the tent, even though in the embryo, they are not yet fully formed. The bony precursors, however, prestress the architecture in differential growth patterns as closed couplings formed in concert with the surrounding tissues.

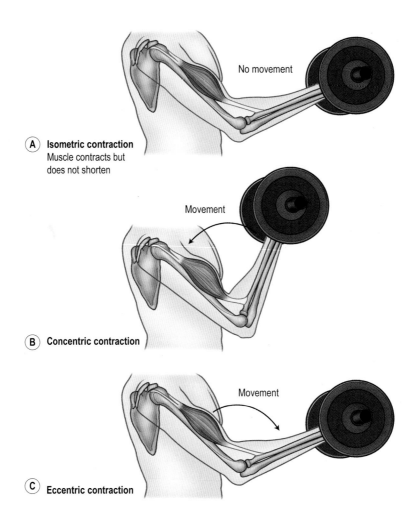

No movement

(A) **Isometric contraction**
Muscle contracts but
does not shorten

Movement

(B) **Concentric contraction**

Movement

(C) **Eccentric contraction**

FIGURE 1.19

The classical explanation of musculoskeletal movement is based on a model of simple levers in which a discrete muscle acts on a joint to pull one bone toward another in a single plane.

Across anatomy

Key concept 10

Prestress, or pre-tension, is the quality by which our bodies draw into themselves through the spiral development of cellular architecture.

Biologists have shown that not only is the prestress reinforcement strategy found in the cell, but it is also a global feature of all organisms[53] (explored further in the online chapter, Reflection and growth – see p. xii for access details). Danièle-Claude Martin describes one influence of prestress in functional movement in her book when she refers to the phenomenon as "comfort self-stress."[54] It is "self-stress" in the sense that no outside forces are doing it to us. As such, the structure of the organism itself provides the internal pattern of couplings, which is reflected in the weave of the prestressed architecture.

An invitation

For a lively conversation between anatomy and yoga, let's consider the entire organism. Not just as it is now, but as it has been since conception, as it may have been evolutionary eons ago, and where this trajectory is likely taking us into the future. As yogis, we are genuinely interested in the body regarding its entire timeline, not just the isolated components of a reductionist or mechanistic view. That view is the box we have inherited and the one into which we are trying to cram our understanding. Because it doesn't fit as such is why we benefit from unboxing anatomy to see it integrated with the bigger picture.

I invite you to consider a new way of envisaging those adult human arms and legs, as we have become used to calling them. We draw them as sticks on a stick figure; work them out on a quad press in the gym and talk about "flexing the knee" and "extending the elbow" as if they ever do that at right-angles. Consider now that their journey, entirely emerging through a process of fluidic, pretensioned rotation, cannot make sense if we attempt to attribute their motion entirely to a lever model and bending moments at the joints.

Key concept 11

Working with the limbs and their rotational origins in yoga is easier when you consider their embryological journey.

Moreover, how could a lever model (see Fig. 1.19), that by definition can only move in one plane, describe the motion we experience? How does it make sense that one muscle could move independently and to the exclusion of others, when we know from the lightest consideration of the embryology that the entire process is orchestrated as a whole, at once, by the time the whole body is the size of a walnut? Let's take a more in-depth look at how these limbs relate to the trunk invariably in *continuities* that are *always* influencing the rest of the system from which they emerge.

1.6 Legacy of limb symmetry

The limbs take root posteriorly in the torso tube, or the thoracolumbar region (see Figs 1.20 and 2.36). They emerge from and converge into a dynamic cross-ply that weaves into deep fibers and sheaths around what will become the abdomen, diaphragm and pelvis; all made of fascial pockets, self-assembling from the folding and unfolding process we have described. That includes the internal sheath of the diaphragm and the fascia that wraps and encompasses the posterior abdominal wall, forming the structures known as the endopelvic fasciae en route.

This is another challenge of continuity, connectivity and chirality. Everything arises from this unicellular beginning; using the connective (and connecting) tissue template, from which it self-assembles and forms. There is only one continuum: nothing is added or bolted on that doesn't emerge from the original structure. This entirely undermines the most basic notion of levers (open two-bar chains – what is open?) and goes further to suggest that the fascia is the fabric of the unicellular architecture that becomes the multicellular architecture that there is only ever one of! You are one, containing the all as a continuum. Even the cells are made of it; so that the torso tube is part of the whole weave. The ONE wholeness; the one fascia – in all its paradoxical variations.

Joanne Avison

Discrete limb boundaries do not exist in a seamless model. The smaller bones and joints integrate as part of the continuum of tissue, deploying even before they have had sufficient forces put through them to become bony as such.[41] Research in limb disparity (long legs, short arms) in

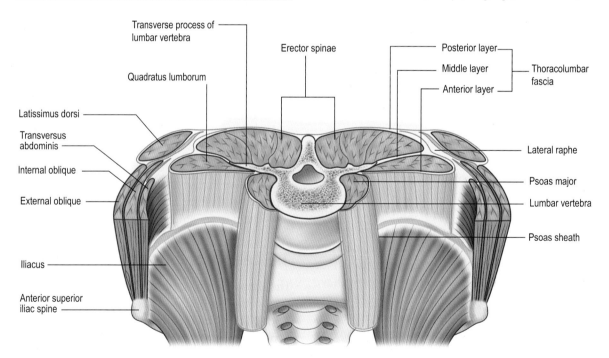

FIGURE 1.20

The thoracolumbar fascia includes the deep fascial compartments of the limb trusses woven through the X of the lumbosacrum from superficial to deep, extending to contain the psoas in continuity with the diaphragm and peritoneal cavity within.

Across anatomy

Table 1.1 Comparison of a basic selection of anatomically allied parts in the upper and lower limbs		
	Upper limb	**Lower limb**
Soft tissue	Pectorals	Hip flexors
	Latissimus dorsi	Tensor fasciae latae/gluteals
	Deltoids	Gluteals
	Rotator cuff	Deep 6
	Biceps brachii	Biceps femoris
	Triceps	Quadriceps
	Anterior compartment of forearm	Posterior compartment of lower leg
	Palmar surface of the hand	Plantar surface of the foot
Skeletal elements	Scapula	Hip bone
	Humerus	Femur
	Olecranon	Patella
	Radius/ulna	Tibia/fibula
	Thumb (pollex)	Great toe (hallux)

humans, when compared to other primates, shows that development continues to shape evolutionary change.[55] We point to the whole story, not just a retrospective view of development, but also a full picture including that of potential future scenarios.

Key concept 12

Limbs emerge from the trunk; the trunk is an interconnection, or continuum, of the limbs.

We are similarly invited to consider the relationships between the upper and lower limbs. Even though our arms and legs have evolved to manage different loads and maneuvers, it is useful to reflect on their equivalence, certainly from a postural point of view. David Keil writes about his observations of the upper and lower limbs in comparison to one another, likening the deltoids to the gluteals.[56] In a practical sense, we explore and compare the upper and lower limbs, in that they can both do some of what the other can.

Although we are moving away from parts-list thinking, it can be handy to see how some of the classically named bits of anatomy mirror one another not only bilaterally, but also as pairs of limbs. In arm balances, for instance, the arms can behave as the lower limbs and take on functionality similar to the legs in the anatomical position. When the forearms are in grounding mode, or pronation, the hands can become more like the feet. Rotational patterns of the arms in handstand echo what happens with the legs in a footstand (i.e. what we think of as ordinary standing). This approach to anatomy is rooted in the Five Filaments, the constraints-based movement rubric proposed in this book.

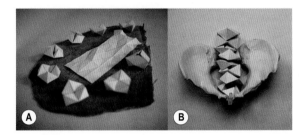

FIGURE 1.21

Constraints: 3D flexagon (you can make one yourself to get a feel for morphological constraints. (A) In the centre, the paper shows the creases that guide how the shape comes together and continues to move. (B) The particular features of the flexagon make it an interesting model for tissue. (Find another example of this topology in Chapter 3, and another relating to spirality in the Reflection and Growth chapter available online.)

Origami is an excellent example of how constraints shape movement.[57–59] You can fold and crease paper to direct its deployment into shapes. Extra creases will impose new constraints on a piece of origami, making it move differently. When I first started folding flexagons (see Fig. 1.21), I noticed that any extra creases would make the structure floppy, compromising the shape's integrity. Constraints shape a structure, and we can manage the

movement of that structure to reinforce those constraints. We'll come back to variations on the flexagon throughout this book.

 Foot fingers

We yogis could talk all day about the hands, feet, and their tendrils, the phalanges: fingers and toes. All five toes, or foot digits, have developed as grippers of the earth. As such, they all have a likeness in the pattern of their form and function. Fingers, on the other hand (lol), have a fully developed oppositional arrangement as hand digits. Sticking out from the five fingers is the ornery pollex (Latin for "the strong one"), referring to the thumb.

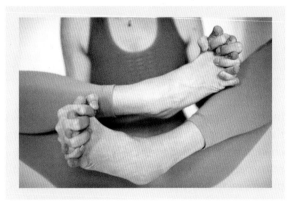

FIGURE 1.22

Foot fingers and hand toes: the autopods can get a grip on each other.

Thumb-like structures appear in a vast range of species. However, the ability to oppose the *little* fingers and thumb is unique to primates. (To consider the evolving feature of thumbs check out the *alula*, or bastard wing, of a bird in flight). In humans, the thumb can move at various angles to the other hand digits and permits the delicacy of fine motor skills of which we are capable. The thumb gives us more than a grasp on our world; it allows us a vast range of creative detail and subtlety of motion unique among organisms.

Key concept 13

Hands and feet can be platforms for standing; fingers and toes are structurally similar.

Since the toes all flex in apparent uniformity, they are classically grouped in anatomy as a set of five, with no special designation given to the great toe apart from its comparison to the thumb in the nomenclature. In the Arabic language, for example, toes don't even get a special designation, they're known only as "foot fingers." In Latin, the medical terms are *pollex pedis* (meaning "foot thumb") or *hallux*.

If we consider the hallux as the thumb of the foot (in each case the attaching muscles have been given distinctive anatomical names:

"pollicis" to the pollex and "hallucis" to the hallux), we can make a useful comparison. As man evolved from quadruped, the upper limbs developed increasing dexterity as a survival adaptation. Standing on tiptoe, for example, to reach up and pick small berries (and put them quickly into the mouth) would require a specific grounding through the foot and hallux, while delicately opposing thumb and fingers to select the fruit (and an organization such as the arm and hand, to eat them). Such ideas are where the understanding arises that the upper limbs have evolved to be used differently from the gravity-bound basis of the lower limbs.

In yoga, we regularly and intuitively ground through the big toe mounds. In handstands, we learn to harness the roots of the thumb and forefinger similarly. This action works through the pre-tensioned endpoints of the limbs; predisposed to have a hollowing ability in the palmar and plantar surfaces of each. In yoga, we call this amplification *hasta* and *pada bandha*. Like a sprung floor, the hollowed surfaces are pre-stiffened structures and can become springier.

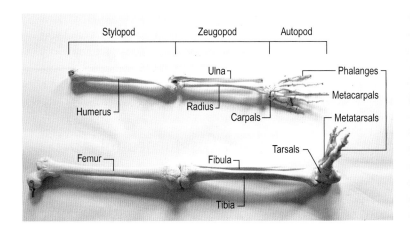

FIGURE 1.23

Stylopod, zeugopod, autopod in the upper and lower limbs.

This springy hollowing provides the body with a suitable standing apparatus by allowing that spring to extend when weight-bearing and navigating ground reaction force (GRF), either way up (see the windlass mechanism in Chapter 2). We can evoke and intensify this pre-stiffening to consciously deploy the hands into the behavior of a second set of feet, so that a handstand is functionally comparable to a footstand. In this sense, if the toes are foot fingers, then similarly, we can see the hands as the feet of the arms.

Key concept 14

Limb structures broadly reflect one another.

We explore this in yoga. However, there are biological limits that honor the innate structure of each. Interestingly, the overall pattern of one proximal bone, two distal, three then four to shape the wrist and ankle bones respectively and then the pattern of the digits in both sets of paddles are similar. Their overall structures embody different kinds of force transmission, so while it is fun to compare and explore – they have not evolved to be the same; or entirely different. We can stand on our hands, and we can improve ability in the feet and toes to advantage – however, their respective structures are naturally constrained and organized to excel at different things.

According to Jaap van der Wal, the mandible might be considered the uppermost limb, fused (only) in the human jaw structure (in all other species with a jawbone, it is formed of two bones joined via a symphysis). This is a fascinating consideration; that the feet rotate outward and cannot be joined wholly – while the mandible rotates inward and is fused. The arms then become the median limb-set, since they can be held together or held apart. They can functionally achieve some of what the other two sets of limbs are organized optimally for, but are not fully constrained to either.

Joanne Avison

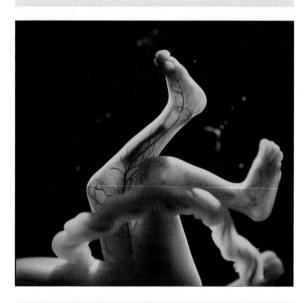

FIGURE 1.24

Human fetal legs at 16 weeks. The fetus can now grab and pull the long umbilical cord. The skeleton consists mainly of flexible cartilage, the soft precursor to bone.

(Lennart Nilsson, TT/Science Photo Library)

1.7 A more useful neutral

All this talk of foot fingers can leave you feeling a bit upside down and back-to-front! To reset the view, let's stop to consider the so-called

Across anatomy

anatomical position. The AP, such as it is defined in the study of anatomy, is the place at which we have arrived for determining anatomical terms of movement and position of human parts. It makes perfect sense for bipeds planning to walk exclusively on two feet, and for patients being discussed in the third person.

Having a consistent reference position means that two practitioners, for example, can refer accurately to specific points on the body, or particular actions/ranges of motion, relative to a common denominator. This is vital for doctors looking at scans to find pathology. For yoga practitioners considering the full spectrum of movement, however, the standard anatomical position becomes less useful.

Key concept 15

For a positional basis of yoga anatomy, we often need something that is less preferential regarding which end is up.

For the living yoga practitioner, perhaps a neutral position is more usefully considered a ready stillness that allows us to formulate a language of useful landmarks. It's like having the car in gear, the clutch with bite, prepared to release the handbrake. In a state of continuous preparedness, the pre-tensioned system is spiral bound and poised to balance itself from equilibrium, independently of its position relative to the ground and gravity.

Taking the body into a handstand position is a reminder that the upper limbs can manage

ground reaction force similar to the lower limbs (given appropriate circumstances). Handstand is another option for an anatomical position that illuminates positional polarity. The **vestibular** sense tells us when we're upside down,[60] and along with clear physiological cues (your face going red, for example), it is evident that the head has evolved to be on top. But hear this: the body self-organizes independent of gravity. In asana, we are playing with the **hierarchy** to find equilibrium in every position.

Biologic tissue lets living organisms, unlike skyscrapers and buses, adapt when overturned. When we consider the human body as a biped able to walk on either pair of its legs, its ultimate adaptability is easier to foster and explore. Yoga practitioners are, in particular, interested in pushing the boundaries to explore our relationship to gravity in all 360 degrees. The new paradigm offers the language we need to talk about it (head to Appendix A for more on biotensegrity).

As capacity increases, asanas can progress toward inversion. This inverse relationship continues as a defining experience, keeping the human body sprung regardless of position relative to the earth. In short, it doesn't matter which end happens to be up, on its side, front, or back. A neutral position is something of a shifting goalpost as we start seeing the body as a matrix of spirals rather than a collection of levers and pulleys in continuous compression following Newtonian laws of linear proportionality (see Table 1.2).

Table 1.2 Newtonian mechanics			
Newtonian law (approx. date)	Subject	Conventional assumption	Comparison in anatomy
Euler's formula (1757)	Buckling of slender columns	This law says that taller columns are weaker and less stable, so that very tall columns will bend under their own weight.	The spinal "column" should not be able to hold itself up if this formula applied.
Galileo's square-cube law (1638)	The bigger things get	This law describes proportionality in terms of surface area to volume: as the surface area of a structure squares, its volume cubes, crushing under its own weight.	Anything larger than an elephant would thus implode.
Hooke's law (1678)	as ut tensio, sic vis "as the extension, so the force"	This law talks about proportionality of how a material behaves when exposed to a force; it says that the stress-strain curve of a material is constant (linear).	Bone stiffness and brittleness is constant in animals of all sizes; why don't the long bones of humans fracture more easily than mouse bones?
Poisson's ratio (1807)	Relation to elastic moduli in isotropic solids	Describes the fundamental elasticity of a material. 1. A material stretched out gets thinner. 2. A squashed material bulges.	Biologic materials such as foams and crystals exhibit a negative Poisson's ratio (auxetic) making them resistant to shear and fracture.

 Role Play

On the spectrum of postural yoga, what are we doing with the feet? When we aren't standing on them, we can explore, within reason, the unfolding of the feet into hand-like gestures with gradually increasing supination. It seems there is value in integrating their dexterity with foot exercises that make them more subtle and aware ears to the ground when they are in the more usual gait mode.

For me, this is about finding neutral and exploring it – rather than finding opposition. In other words: balance is the result of being ABLE to supinate and pronate; invert and evert. We explore both, but not in an attempt to make them into each other; instead, to choose balance more eloquently for them, arising between their plausible extremes. A cartwheel is fun to do, but it isn't a requisite for functional health/morphology or self-expression. Balance *is*, however.

Joanne Avison

Across anatomy

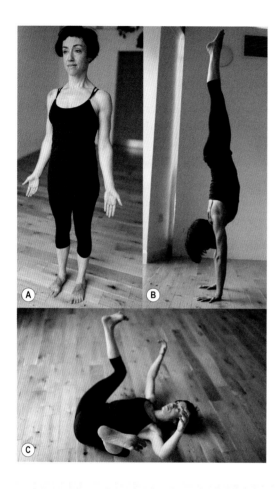

FIGURE 1.25

(A) Anatomical position; (B) bipedal on hands; (C) supine quadruped.

(Demonstrated by Amy Hughes)

So, what is the value of making the shift into working with the body as spiral-bound? Such a system is versatile on its hands and feet. Further, we can make feet out of anything in contact with the ground: forearms, bottom, belly, crown – all take on at least a sense of the foundational foot. A neutral position is where the polar body primes itself for movement, balanced in its spirality in a state of readiness. Understanding the winding, helical nature of joint systems gives you a way to discover positional virtuosity, the beauty of neutral, and how to teach from constraints safely and intuitively no matter what style you practice.

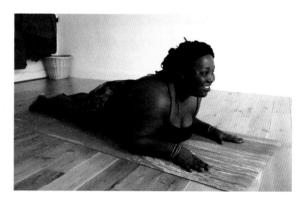

FIGURE 1.26

The activated prone position: in Danurasana, the anterior surface effectively becomes the foot.

(Demonstrated by Fadzai Mwakutuya)

This chapter opened with an anecdote about the subtle body versus Western anatomy in the study of yoga. We asked ourselves if there could be any middle ground. Toward finding that place of integration, I dropped our pin in the embryological origins of limb rotation in human development. Considering the limbs as continuities of their original rotation in utero gives an enriched picture of the system in the long arc of its development. Keep in mind that the human organism, once emerged from its neonatal beginnings, develops in constant gravity at a relatively stable pressure. Since it does so within constraints that are continuously balancing push and pull at every scale, it makes sense that things might likely continue as they started.

CHAPTER ONE

References

1   Kumar S. Swami Vivekananda: Complete Works. LBA; 2018.

2   Swatmarama Muktibodhananda, Yogi Saraswati. Hatha Yoga Pradipika. Bihar School of Yoga; 1450.

3   Gheranda Samhita. Adyar Library; 1933.

4   Mohan AG. Yoga Therapy: A Guide to the Therapeutic Use of Yoga and Ayurveda for Health and Fitness. Shambhala Publications, Inc; 2006. p. 240.

5   Charaka A. Charaka Samhita: Handbook on Ayurveda. Independently published; 2016.

6   Patwardhan K. The history of the discovery of blood circulation: unrecognized contributions of Ayurveda masters. Advances in Physiology Education. 2012;36(2):77–82.

7   Endo J, Nakamura T. Comparative studies of the tridosha theory in Ayurveda and the theory of the four deranged elements in Buddhist medicine. Kagakushi Kenkyu [Journal of the History of Science, Japan]. 1995;34(193):1–9.

8   Rastogi S. Building bridges between Ayurveda and Modern Science. International Journal of Ayurveda research. 2010;1(1):41–6.

9   van der Wal J. The architecture of the connective tissue in the musculoskeletal system – an often overlooked functional parameter as to proprioception in the locomotor apparatus. International Journal of Therapeutic Massage & Bodywork. 2009;2(4):9–23.

10 Newman SA. The Turing mechanism in vertebrate limb patterning. Nature Reviews Molecular Cell Biology. 2007;8:508.

11 Pohl C. Cytoskeletal symmetry breaking and chirality: from reconstituted systems to animal development. Symmetry. 2015;7(4):2062.

12 Prigogine I, Lefever R, Goldbeter A, Herschkowitz-Kaufman M. Symmetry breaking instabilities in biological systems. Nature. 1969;223(5209):913–6.

13 Zhao P, Teng X, Tantirimudalige SN, et al. Aurora-A breaks symmetry in contractile actomyosin networks independently of its role in centrosome maturation. Developmental Cell. 2019;48(5):631–45.e6.

14 Holló G. Demystification of animal symmetry: symmetry is a response to mechanical forces. Biology Direct. 2017;12:11.

15 Risbud MV, Schaer TP, Shapiro IM. Toward an understanding of the role of notochordal cells in the adult intervertebral disc: from discord to accord. Developmental Dynamics. 2010;239(8):2141–8.

16 Rustenburg CME, Emanuel KS, Peeters M, et al. Osteoarthritis and intervertebral disc degeneration: quite different, quite similar. JOR Spine. 2018;1(4):e1033-e.

17 van der Wal J. Not by bones, ligaments, and muscles alone. Biotensegrity Dissection, University of Dundee. 2017.

18 Bakkum BW, Bachop WE. Chapter 12, Development of the Spine and Spinal Cord. In: Cramer GD, Darby SA, editors. Clinical Anatomy of the Spine, Spinal Cord, and ANS (Third Edition). St Louis: Mosby; 2014. p. 541–65.

19 Jo Y, Kim HM, Lee J, et al. Fluid–matrix interface triggers a heterogeneous activation of macrophages. ACS Applied Bio Materials. 2020;3(7):4294–301.

20 Benias PC, Wells RG, Sackey-Aboagye B, et al. Structure and distribution of an unrecognized interstitium in human tissues. Scientific Reports. 2018;8(1):4947.

21 Bordoni B, Simonelli M. The Awareness of the Fascial System. Cureus. 2018;10(10):e3397-e.

22 Avison JS. Yoga: Fascia, Anatomy and Movement. Edinburgh: Handspring Publishing; 2015. p.376

23 Shea CA, Rolfe RA, Murphy P. The importance of foetal movement for co-ordinated cartilage and bone development in utero : clinical consequences and potential for therapy. Bone & Joint Research. 2015;4(7):105–16.

24 Pitsillides AA. Early effects of embryonic movement: 'a shot out of the dark'. Journal of Anatomy. 2006;208(4):417–31.

25 Mammoto T, Ingber DE. Mechanical control of tissue and organ development. Development. 2010;137(9):1407–20.

26 Nowlan NC, Sharpe J, Roddy KA, et al. Mechanobiology of embryonic skeletal development: insights from animal models. Birth Defects Research Part C, Embryo Today: Reviews. 2010;90(3):203–13.

27 Heegaard JH, Beaupré GS, Carter DR. Mechanically modulated cartilage growth may regulate joint surface morphogenesis. Journal of Orthopaedic Research. 1999;17(4):509–17.

28 Ingber DE. Integrins, tensegrity, and mechanotransduction. Gravitational and Space Biology Bulletin. 1997;10(2):49–55.

29 Baker R, Schnell S, Maini P. A clock and wavefront mechanism for somite formation. Developmental Biology. 2006;293:116–26.

30 Stecco C, Pirri C, Fede C, et al. Dermatome and fasciatome. Clinical Anatomy. 2019;32(7):896–902.

31 Kelly Kuan CY, Tannahill D, Cook GMW, Keynes RJ. Somite polarity and segmental patterning of the peripheral nervous system. Mechanisms of Development. 2004;121(9):1055–68.

32 Keynes RJ, Stern CD. Mechanisms of vertebrate segmentation. Development. 1988;103(3):413–29.

33 Gracovetsky S. Function of the spine. Journal of Biomedical Engineering. 1986;8(3):217–23.

34 Dupin E, Calloni GW, Coelho-Aguiar JM, Le Douarin NM. The issue of the multipotency of the neural crest cells. Developmental Biology. 2018;444 Suppl 1:S47-S59.

35 Shyamala K, Yanduri S, Girish HC, Murgod S. Neural crest: the fourth germ layer. Journal of Oral and Maxillofacial Pathology. 2015;19(2):221–9.

36 Muñoz WA, Trainor PA. Neural crest cell evolution: how and when did a neural crest cell become a neural crest cell. Current Topics in Developmental Biology. 2015;111:3–26.

37 Khataee H, Czirok A, Neufeld Z. Theoretical analysis of neural crest cell migration. bioRxiv. 2020:2020.03.04.976209.

38 Duband J-L, Nekooie-Marnany N, Dufour S. Establishing primary cultures of trunk neural crest cells. Current Protocols in Cell Biology. 2020;88(1):e109.

39 Dupin E, Calloni GW, Le Douarin NM. The cephalic neural crest of amniote vertebrates is composed of a large majority of precursors endowed with neural, melanocytic, chondrogenic and osteogenic potentialities. Cell Cycle (Georgetown, TX). 2010;9(2):238–49.

40 Calloni GW, Glavieux-Pardanaud C, Le Douarin NM, Dupin E. Sonic Hedgehog promotes the development of multipotent neural crest progenitors endowed with both mesenchymal and neural potentials. Proceedings of the National Academy of Sciences of the United States of America. 2007;104(50):19879–84.

41 Levin SM. The tensegrity-truss as a model for spine mechanics: biotensegrity. Journal of Mechanics in Medicine and Biology. 2002;2:375–378.

42 Sheth R, Marcon L, Bastida MF, et al. Hox genes regulate digit patterning by controlling the wavelength of a Turing-type mechanism. Science (New York, NY). 2012;338(6113):1476–80.

43 Catavitello G, Ivanenko Y, Lacquaniti F. A kinematic synergy for terrestrial locomotion shared by mammals and birds. eLife. 2018;7:e38190.

44 Barna M, Pandolfi PP, Niswander L. Gli3 and Plzf cooperate in proximal limb patterning at early stages of limb development. Nature. 2005;436(7048):277–81.

45 Onimaru K, Marcon L, Musy M, et al. The fin-to-limb transition as the re-

organization of a Turing pattern. Nature Communications. 2016;7:11582.

46 Giffin JL, Gaitor D, Franz-Odendaal TA. The forgotten skeletogenic condensations: a comparison of early skeletal development amongst vertebrates. Journal of Developmental Biology. 2019;7(1):4.

47 Zuniga A. Next generation limb development and evolution: old questions, new perspectives. Development. 2015;142(22):3810–20.

48 Yano T, Tamura K. The making of differences between fins and limbs. Journal of Anatomy. 2013;222(1):100–13.

49 Leite-Castro J, Beviano V, Rodrigues PN, Freitas R. HoxA genes and the fin-to-limb transition in vertebrates. Journal of Developmental Biology. 2016;4(1):10.

50 Blechschmidt E, Freeman B. The Ontogenetic Basis of Human Anatomy: A Biodynamic Approach to Development from Conception to Birth. Pacific Distributing; 2004.

51 Stooke-Vaughan GA, Campàs O. Physical control of tissue morphogenesis across scales. Current Opinion in Genetics & Development. 2018;51:111–19.

52 Mongera A, Rowghanian P, Gustafson HJ, et al. A fluid-to-solid jamming transition underlies vertebrate body axis elongation. Nature. 2018;561(7723):401–5.

53 Ingber DE. The Architecture of Life. 1998. Available from: http://time.arts.ucla.edu/Talks/Barcelona/Arch_Life.htm.

54 Martin DC. Living Biotensegrity: Interplay of Tension and Compression in the Body. Kiener Verlag; 2016.

55 Young NM, Wagner GP, Hallgrímsson B. Development and the evolvability of human limbs. Proceedings of the National Academy of Sciences. 2010;107(8):3400–5.

56 Keil D. Functional Anatomy of Yoga: A Guide for Practitioners and Teachers. Lotus Publishing; 2014. p. 383.

57 Chen S, Mahadevan L. Rigidity percolation and geometric information in floppy origami. Proceedings of the National Academy of Sciences. 2019;116(17):8119–24.

58 Wang P, Meyer TA, Pan V, et al. The beauty and utility of DNA origami. Chem. 2017;2(3):359–82.

59 Dudte LH, Vouga E, Tachi T, Mahadevan L. Programming curvature using origami tessellations. Nature Materials. 2016;15(5):583–8.

60 Jenkin MR, Dyde RT, Jenkin HL, et al. Perceptual upright: the relative effectiveness of dynamic and static images under different gravity states. Seeing and Perceiving. 2011;24(1):53–64.

2.1 Into the round: mapping movment — 38

2.2 Kinematics of coupling — 43

2.3 Rotational redux — 51

2.4 The meso story — 56

2.5 The Five Filaments rubric — 58

2.6 From coupled to throupled — 73

2.7 The spirals as patterns of movement — 78

2.8 Guiding the glide — 82

The Five Filaments

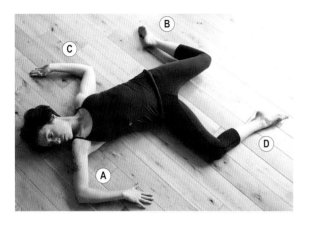

FIGURE 2.1

Mahaswastikasana: (A) the grounding upper limb; (B) the grounding lower limb; (C) the opening upper limb; (D) the opening lower limb.

So'ham
I am that.

Key concepts

1   Closed kinematic chains (CKCs) are whole interlinked systems that form the basis of biologic movement, connecting everything in the body to everything else as a closed (enclosed) volume.

2   Constraints like rotational patterns give us a means of understanding how best to work with our bodies in space and how to honor their limitations to preserve our resilience wisely.

3   Spirality is an approach to anatomy that is congruent with embryological origins and observable helical arrays of tissue in the CKC structure.

4   CKCs in helical constraints are the founding feature behind the Five Filaments (5F).

5   Rotations can describe the localized appearance of movement within the spiral flow of body tubes, such as your upper and lower limbs.

6   Humans, although currently bipedal (walking on two legs), are classified as Tetrapoda (having four feet); both hands and feet are platforms for standing, and we can also balance unipedally.

7   Imagining various positions, such as Downward Dog, it is easy to see why it is useful to consider (appropriately) the limb pairs as reciprocal to some extent in their rotation patterns.

8   The 5F aim to put all the pieces together into a simple, graspable, pragmatic set of movement cascades based on rotational spirals intrinsic to biomotional integrity.

9   The concept of myofascial slings is 2D-3D, whereas the human body is multidimensional.

10 CKCs can be considered as coupled. However, their coupling naturally gives

rise to a third entity, or plane, by the laws of so-called coupled motion. We have called this a "throuple" to distinguish the experience of coupled motion, always giving rise to motion in the third plane.

11 A spiral approach to anatomy emphasizes the importance of virtual space, or continuity, resilience and openness, within the harmonious whole.

12 The 5F rubric adopts and embraces many recognizable models of classical biomechanics, such as the scapulohumeral rhythm; while contextualizing them as part of a more profound expression of rotation – innate to our forming.

2.1 Into the round: mapping movement

Chapter 1 introduced the character of developed anatomy through the lens of its unfolding as an embryo. This story of development is truly epic. What we experience as anatomy in any moment is just a snapshot from that still-unfolding journey. This is a tale that didn't start at birth, or even in the womb, but much earlier than we can imagine. Let yourself become carried away with the mind-blowing scope of this legendary (yet completely ordinary) process.

Also, consider that these first moments are mainly the same for all complex organisms. I sense that we all *get* that, but what holds us back is that the embryology can be so intensely confusing. The cumbersome nomenclature involved is enough to stop anyone in their tracks. It can be incredibly daunting for those seeking to make sense of classical biomechanics from studying embryology.

Organicism and organismic constraints deal with, unsurprisingly, organisms. The first is the position that sees the universe as orderly and alive, much the same as life on earth as we know it is alive, with parts that are connected into the whole.

The latter, organismic constraints, include factors built into an individual's actual body. These include personality factors (e.g., risk-taking behavior), personal fitness, mental skills such as concentration and emotional control, individual anthropometrics (height, weight, and limb lengths), as well as perceptual and decision-making skills.[1] **Morphological constraints** are organismic constraints that arise from our body plans during embryonic development and show how the shape of a body guides its movement.

The Five Filaments

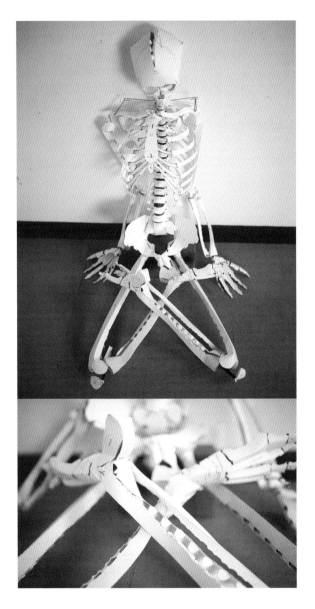

FIGURE 2.2

Origami skeleton: its shape and movement emerge as a consequence of its constraints – the dotted lines indicating where to fold the paper.

(With thanks to Fergus Murray, the intrepid constructor)

Let's leap straight to the point. Because rotation and spirality give rise to our body blueprint during formation, it follows that these patterns – **constraints** – can guide the way for intentional movement to flow. I touched on the constraints that arise from human morphology in Chapter 1. These are the most efficient paths for natural human motion, characterized by the feeling of "good space" or *sukha* that we will explore here as rotational patterns.[2]

The iconic source for the how-what-and-why of yoga is embedded in *The Yoga Sutras* of Patanjali,[3] where asana is said to be characterized by the experience of this spatial quality of sukha. Furthermore, these rotational patterns persist into archetypal kinematics evident in the embryo. They are underpinned by a helical arrangement of filamentous connective tissue fibers that have been observed and identified by anatomists for decades.[4–7]

So, does it follow that the subtle body system might resonate with the *obvious* body anatomy? How does moving my physical body influence an "imaginary" set of invisible structures whose only evidence seems based in folklore? To see how embryonic development gives rise to tissues with a subtle aspect, we'll explore the interlinking of structure in the physical body, and give this mechanism a name that suits our view (there are countless interpretations).

Continuing into Chapter 3, the story builds on these interconnected patterns from the gross to the subtle. In essence, the story is both pervasive and subtle. It is expressive of our chirality and evident in the pretensioned nature of the embryonic architecture. This is where we cross the great divide and begin to seek new terms for non-linear biologic forms.

CHAPTER TWO

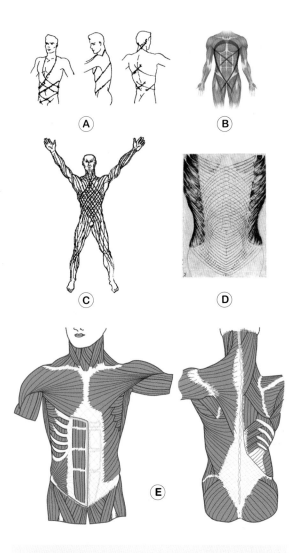

B Dr Kurt Tittel's Muscle Slings in Sport, 1956.
C Russian anatomist, Shaparenko, referred to the enantiomorphic (from enantios, or "opposite") arrangement of myofascial tubules circa 1980. **D** Askar's "aponeurotic expansions".[41]
E Scarr's schematic drawing of the cross-ply evident in the torso.

(C, courtesy of the Kozyavkin Method. E, courtesy of Handspring Publishing)

Here is where the fascination with geometry comes in. Geometry maps the invisible forces that hold our soft-matter architecture together *as a subtle body* – in a gross one! Biotensegrity maps that archetypally and kinematically; and it naturally gives rise to spiral forms – via the *invisible* forces that the fascia transmits. (None of us can see gravity – only its impact!) We ask ourselves: how did the ancient Vedic sages understand these subtleties to the extent that they *became* folklore?

Joanne Avison

FIGURE 2.3

Myofascial cross-ply in body culture. **A** Dart's "double spiral arrangement" with regard to human anatomy and embryology was originally published in the Journal of the Institutes for the Achievement of Human Potential in 1967.

These patterns come up in one way or another across disciplines.[8–11] They constitute a new way of talking about movement in terms of relationships as *biomotion* rather than as *biomechanics*. We pointed out in Chapter 1 that there are no open chains in the human body, however popular the misconception. (Recall that a lever is a rigid bar pivoting about a fulcrum forming an open two-bar chain). Instead, these helical patterns connect in continuous relationships referred to mechanically as **closed kinematic chains** (CKCs).

The Five Filaments

CKCs are coupled, modular elements in the body. They are closed, in that there are never any loose ends and movement is thus attenuated and integrated throughout the system.[12,13] Here, we'll look at CKCs as a structural form of coupling. Coupled elements are those of a closed loop, and coupling is a term used in a wide variety of contextual applications from engineering to biology and beyond.[14–17]

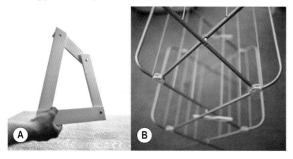

FIGURE 2.4

A four-bar linkage demonstrates the coupled, integrated motion of closed kinematic chains. **A** A model of the four-bar. **B** The four-bar in action as part of a drying rack in situ.

Biological couplings refer to integrated systems, such as CKCs, that are embedded throughout and amongst individual bodies.[18,19] These interconnections express **coupling functions**, and they are essential to the underlying modus of biologic movement, from oscillations that drive circadian rhythms to the hive mind of collective behavior (think starlings in murmuration or a peloton of cyclists).[20] In practical terms, couplings are what link the tiniest movements within a living structure (at a microscopic level) to far-reaching effects in the whole macrocosmic organism (and beyond).

These effects arise as emergent properties in the whole body (from organelle to organism) and extend beyond the individual into group dynamics and rhythms in nature. Such coupling functions take the form of resonant phenomena in organisms, such as bioluminescence and biological electron transfer (ET),[21,22] cardiac rhythms,[23,24] neuroendocrine loops[25] and dopaminergic systems with widespread effects on our neurobiology.[26] The coupled oscillatory systems within individuals can resonate within self and amongst others. Resonance is the connector of the interconnected universe, within which our fascial envelope vibrates rhythmically with nature.

Biomotion

Biomotion has been suggested by Avison, augmenting the meaning of the term biomechanics when applied to the living body, particularly suited to movement practitioners.[27] *Biomotion* takes into account the helical flow of tissues and the energy to move them (e-motionally) as living beings, animating them uniquely as expressions of our archetypal morphologies. Let's consider biomotion alongside the four classical categories of motion.

Motion is classically defined as the change of position of one body with respect to some reference body. The living body in motion (biomotion) changes within itself in a way that incorporates all the other types of motion at once across timescales.

Linear (translational) motion

Linear motion is also referred to as translational motion. When you move something from one place to another, it experiences linear motion.

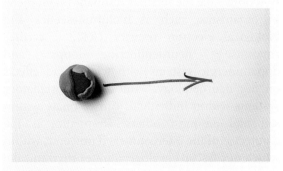

FIGURE 2.5

Linear motion.

Rotary (rotational) motion

When something rotates around a well-defined geometric axis, like a merry-go-round, it has rotational motion. The wheels of a bicycle, spinning around their hubs, are another example.

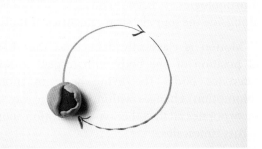

FIGURE 2.6

Rotatory (curvilinear) motion.

Reciprocating motion

Motion is reciprocating when an object is translated (moved linearly) back and forth along one path, as in when we saw wood, in a straight line.

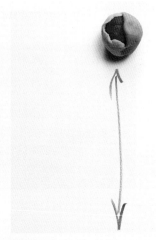

FIGURE 2.7

Reciprocating motion.

Oscillating motion

Essentially, oscillation is reciprocating motion with a rotary path that traces an arc.

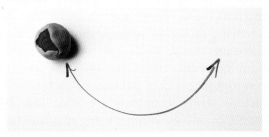

FIGURE 2.8

Oscillating motion.

The Five Filaments

Biomotion

Biomotion: When compared to the previous ball of clay, notice that this one is not moving relative to a fixed "other." Rather, the ball has folded in on itself as a continuity - a multidimensional, invaginating flow of an organism within itself.

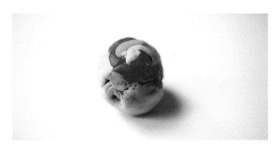

FIGURE 2.9

Biomotion.

Key concept 1

Closed kinematic chains (CKCs) are whole interlinked systems that form the basis of biologic movement, connecting everything in the body to everything else as a closed (enclosed) volume.

2.2 Kinematics of coupling

How do CKCs link up with spirals? As organisms, each species unfolds in a certain way. We unfold in a pattern that is actually like un*furl*ing as much as it is un*fold*ing (and *in*folding!). From the outset, in describing how we inhabit our form, furling and unfurling become a useful treatment for how we continue to move.

(i) Movement of oneness

Kinematics is a term for the geometry of coupled motion; the law of which gives rise to a third entity. We're referring such an entity as *throupled*, since it defines how movement in any two planes of motion inevitably gives rise to motion in the third plane (see Section 2.6) and consequently animates the volume in its wholeness.

In complex adaptive systems, such as biologic forms, coupling functions permeate the system with information at every level,[28] including our mental, emotional, and social selves.[29,30] This phenomenon is an exciting aspect of the literature reflecting developments in neuroscience, cardiac dynamics, and circadian rhythms,[31] as well as collective behavior. This meta-coupling invites resonance, a central theme and one we will revisit throughout this book.

The cross-ply of fibers in our fascial matrix spiral one way and counter-spiral the other. That is evidence of chirality as introduced in Chapter 1. These cross-ply fibers further define nested tubules formed out of tissue-helices woven together into coupled relationships throughout the body elements – and on every scale. This means it happens from the smallest nanofilaments of protein right up to the macro level of the torso structure with the limbs woven through it.

As we examine the fabric, the weave is the same across tissue strata throughout the locomotor system. Myofascia is tubular tissue with innervation following the same filamentous, fascicular organization (see Fig. 2.12). In such tissue, collagenous tubes ensheathe contractile fibrils that perform work as a result of myosin crawling around the spiral staircase of actin. Potential energy is stored in elastic fascial fibers with an array of **biopolymers** similarly bent on a spiral loom.

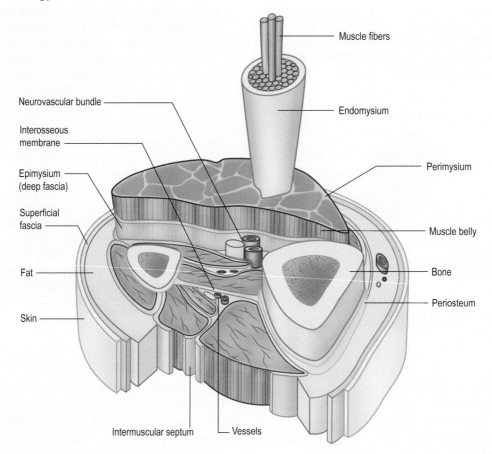

FIGURE 2.10

Compartmental arrangement of tubes typical of the limbs.

(Courtesy of Handspring Publishing)

 Collagen

Collagen, the most abundant protein in the human body, is a helical fiber woven out of triple-helical spiral filaments, right down to the sub-molecular level.[32] The hallmark of collagen is its elegant structural motif in which a right-handed triple helix arises from the coiling of three parallel left-handed polypeptide strands twisted into a helical conformation.[33,34]

The Five Filaments

These collagenous couplings are *closed* in the sense that there are no loose ends; we are whole and complete volumes. They're kinematic because they're self-animated (moving one bit moves all the other elements), and the term chain refers to the linking together. As a simplified postural example, think of Trikonasana as a three-bar CKC. The body forms two closed triangular shapes in this example. Any other postures add extra bars to the so-called CKC linkages we create throughout the body. Changing one aspect of the form will change it everywhere else in the system, intrinsically rebalancing with every move.

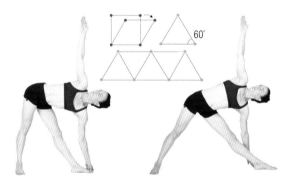

FIGURE 2.11

Trikonasana: a three-bar closed kinematic chain (CKC) is a stable triangle. Four-bar arrangements around flexible joints, by comparison, are mobile and unstable.

> CKCs have a fixed bar for stability and reference – gravity makes ours the ground. The gross postures include CKC attributes when their ground print is incorporated in the visual of the kinematic; which of course is an essential part of the functionality of the pose structure. The ground is the fixed bar that we take with us wherever we move.
>
> **Joanne Avison**

Resource

A useful and readable source for discussing CKCs is the paper by Levin, Lowell de Solorzano, and Scarr, "The Significance of Closed Kinematic Chains to Biological Movement and Stability".[12] To keep our current survey as conversational as possible, I'll let their paper be a starting source for the technical intricacies of CKCs. Here we can explore how they express our spiraling motion.

You don't have to be an engineer to get a feel for coupled kinematics. Your body awareness as a yoga practitioner comes with an inherent understanding of these interlinked chain motion-mechanisms. Our takeaway is that chains do more than simply bind things together. In the body, they link movement into countless, chiral reciprocities – they are tied into bio-couplings in a system-wide concert of continuous give and take.

It isn't just the locomotor system that forms the linkages. The fluid matrix of the fascia is a filamentous gooey-to-hard soft web that is spun through and around all tissue. Its molecular and cellular architecture co-create different aspects of our architecture, responding to forces through movement at different timescales, on and over the ground. Any biologic action is a result of various forces interacting within and through this interconnected, time-bending structure. It is our intrinsic, oscillating, networked structural organization that orchestrates elastic bounce both internally and in response to one's environment.

The resilience of the tissue matrix originates in this inherently prestressed architecture. It is what gives you the ability to jump back and stand on one leg without collapsing into a heap. Thus, our bodies store and release energy like a coiled spring. This repository of readiness springs back through your body, restoring itself in readiness for further actions. We oscillate around equilibrium in every held posture.

In this yoga context, we will venture beyond the notion that one muscle has to flex or pump to move, or ever does so in isolation. The kinematics of reciprocal patterns (along with our raw neurological reflexes) are the actuators of this animation; permitting motion that can happen without the need for our brains to lift a finger.

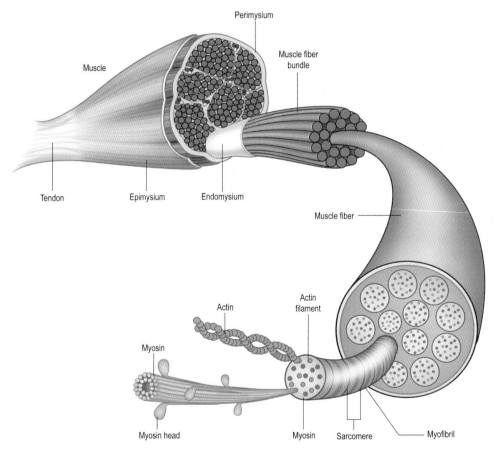

FIGURE 2.12

Fibrillar, helical structure of muscle. The action of myosin "crawling" around the spiral staircase of actin inside muscle fibrils is an essentially spiral movement inside spiraling collagenous myofascial chains. Braids of tightly wrapped collagen filaments scale up in their bundles and form a seamless continuity with the contractile lengths that we call "muscle." Collagen itself is structurally helical.

(Courtesy of Handspring Publishing)

The Five Filaments

As the body progresses in asana, the kinematics of our limbs are predisposed to spiral into ease as the bones and compartments make space in the tensional network for shapes of ever-deepening complexity. We'll soon see how the organ systems are tubes spiraling to coil around themselves and other tubes. Fig. 2.13 offers a simple suggestion for one such anatomical unit commonly suggested for the cruciate spiral matrix of the knee.

The classical cruciates are an example of the same motif: one coiling tubular fascial tissue. Ah, but the anatomy of yoga doesn't stop with the physical elements paused in three dimensions. Indeed, the physical level is but the tip of an invaginating iceberg. I'd like us to imagine those bar-based kinematics as a force model not just for the facility of fascia, but for how our movement in yoga might link into all systems of the body from gross to subtle. And we'll begin to see the bars as metaphorically wrapped in a filamentous, helical vitality in motion.

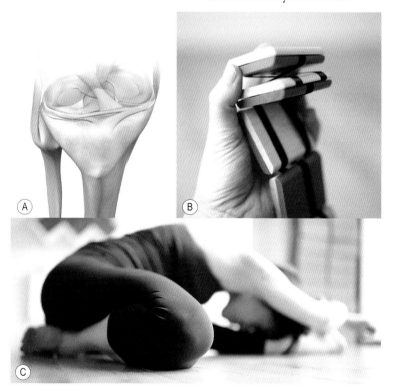

FIGURE 2.13

Helical couplings in anatomy. (A) Knee. (B) As a "uni-cruciate", the cruciate ligaments of the knee form a continuous helicoid structure that Levin likens to a "Jacob's ladder" four-bar CKC in their relationship with the articular surfaces of the femur and tibial plateaus. (C) Amy demonstrates the property of multistability as her knees manage a flow of continuous rotation in Viranchyasana B that defies the classical mechanistic description of knees.

CHAPTER TWO

 Morphologic constraints

The word constraint might sound a bit negative, synonymous with obstacles and restrictions. However, in the body, constraints are not only extremely valuable in our exploration, they are the stuff of the investigation itself. Constraints are simply the natural structural, organizational patterns, or lanes that guide movement. Without these structural directives, the body would flail and succumb to its own weight.[35]

Key concept 2

Constraints like rotational patterns give us a means of understanding how best to work with our bodies in space and how to honor their limitations to preserve our resilience wisely.

This becomes the basis of biomotional integrity – we have to learn to listen to the natural constraint. For example, the knee is normally optimized to a minimum of rotation (i.e. twist between tibia and femur particularly). We might consider that as a built-in architecturally protective and essential constraint, to preserve energy. It provides/endorses our containment, at the level of the cell membrane (to its organelles and between its neighbors) and the skin and subcutaneous tissues to the inner tube of the body and so on.

Joanne Avison

As an example, try medially rotating your hip while attempting to sit cross-legged. It just isn't going to happen, and that is down to the constraints specific to our shape (**morphology**). Movement practitioners across modalities interpret and play within the constraints we inherit as bipedal quadrupeds (more on this later).

A common thread

So far, we have seen how our tissues originated from a sphere, as the body plan first curled around axes in the embryo and found itself in the diaspora of somites. Perhaps we instinctually recapitulate our embryological journey on the yoga mat. Exploring the nature of spirality is a playful way of integrating the modern postural curriculum. As a continuum of this original spiraling pattern, our kinematic body fabric manages forces in a kind of chirality that makes the system **synergic** (responsive), resilient, and **minimal-energy** efficient. This behavior is the modus of all biologic form regardless of its embryonic origin.

The tissues default to responding in spiral patterns (as they were self-developed) to the forces of being alive. They are woven and interwoven as biological couplings at every level. Levin and Martin suggested the term mesokinetic organ to describe this pre-tensioned architecture and the geometry of motion/response patterns as a whole.[36]

The mesokinetic organ defies Newtonian constraints in its truss system of CKCs: semi-rigid segments connected by tensioned, flexible elements that keep the body segments floating snugly in place.[37] This truss architecture creates frictionless joints that factor out shear from the equation, as in the human body, a non- Newtonian vector space where structure takes shape as chiral trusses that spiral in response to the forces of tension and compression.

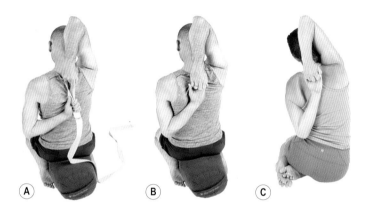

FIGURE 2.14

Gomukhasana is the binding of the two spiralities of shoulder flow: lateral rotation in the top arm (Opening), medial rotation in the bottom one (Grounding). Here shown in (A) with a belt; (B) clasping fingers; (C) increasing lateral flexion in the Axial Matrix.

Levin and Martin also describe a phenomenon they refer to as "poles of movement", illustrating regions of the axis within the tensional mesh where movement initiates.[36] They discuss in a biotensegrity context what we can feel in action as an intrinsic "polar quality" in motion. Illustrations of their poles of movement appear as spirals in the sagittal plane as applied to flexion and extension of the spine (see Fig. 2.15).

These poles of movement are kinesthetically subtle, but practical, nonetheless. As an anatomical structure is generally curved, we may experience momentum in opposite filaments as the structural constitution of our body fabric reorganizes itself responsively. The Anusara literature refers to a similar phenomenon in the "loops" proposed in their classic training manual.[38]

Rotation is intrinsic to the structure and movement of most animals. Emerging spirality leaves structural evidence within the cross-ply of tissue. The patterns of this cross-ply have been observed by many anatomists, therapists, and body enthusiasts over centuries (see Fig. 2.3).[6,39] This is despite the generalized reduction of the overall structural explanations into levers and pendulums as the more linear basis of human motion.[40]

The influence of coiling and spirals is also a central theme in subtle body anatomy that we will explore in Chapter 3. In this chapter, we continue

CHAPTER TWO

looking at how rotational patterns and embedded spirals influence structure and movement as an essential, if often ignored, theme. This theme is critical to non-linear, living forms, however difficult it might be to describe what happens on the mat. We struggle using classical anatomical terms and biomechanical theories for bodies that move in anything but 90-degree angles and lever-based mechanical postures.

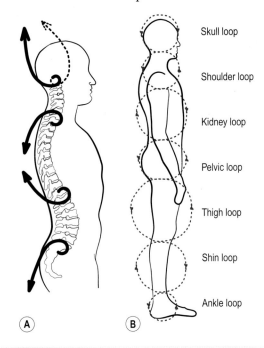

Skull loop

Shoulder loop

Kidney loop

Pelvic loop

Thigh loop

Shin loop

Ankle loop

Ⓐ   Ⓑ

FIGURE 2.15

Sagittal plane rotation: (A) Levin and Martin's poles of rotation[38]; (B) loops from the Anusara manual.[40]

Key concept 3

Spirality is an approach to anatomy that is congruent with embryological origins and observable helical arrays of tissue in the CKC structure.

Advancing in yoga practice can gradually reveal the body-wide kinematic patterns of rotation that we naturally understand more vividly through actual felt experience. By intentionally exploring these inbuilt spiral tracks with reasonable effort in harmony with the breath, the practitioner can maximize adequate flow while tuning in to minimize the risk of injury (acknowledging the natural constraints).

The system of Five Filaments (5F) for yoga described in this chapter does not single out or propose unrecognized anatomical structures. Instead, it is a constraints-led approach to anatomy based on filamentous kinematics, relevant to anyone interested in exploring the roots of our natural form. I'm drawing on a rich tradition of seeing spirality in tissue. It is a rubric that resonates with not only Martin's poles and Friend's loops and the Fourteen Body Segments of the Steccos (see Fig 2.46), but with what I can best describe as common sense (given our romp through the garden of embryology in Chapter 1). The 5F represent biomotional chirality as the natural expression of rotation, or spirals, via the paired nature of converging limbs.

Learning how to practice yoga deeply isn't something you can learn solely from a book! However, I hope that this guide provides useful basic directions for steering in the territory of both teaching and practice. Before we look at the 5F rubric, let's first revise some of the relevant anatomical terms.

Key concept 4

CKCs in helical constraints are the founding feature behind the Five Filaments (5F).

2.3 Rotational redux

What does rotation actually mean? In the classical sense, a rotation is one of a predefined set of moments available at a particular joint (such as flexion, extension, ad-/abduction, circumduction, etc.). Kinesiology offers classical terms for describing movement; for example, "rotation" describes how forces roll and glide through the fascial form, via joints, as part of a continuum.

> The law of coupled motion is already established and might be better named the Law of Tripled motion. Like it or not, when we move in any two planes, the third arises anyway.[41] It is a whole triumvirate of force transmission, by the most basic rules of biomechanics. What is rarely proposed (and is beautifully explored here) is the idea that the same law cannot (and does not) arc through the soft-matter of our tissues in linear transmissions: ever. It may do it in geodesic transmissions – which, given the closed kinematics of our motion-sequences – results inevitably in spiraling forms. It simply isn't possible for the body to produce a linear structure, due to the original primary biological emergence of the embryonic limbs. (Take a look at them!)
>
> We are, by nature, non-linear biologic forms. This point is crucial to safe practice. We are not trying to twist at a joint or rotate a distal limb on its proximal aspect (or vice versa). We are respecting its fundamental forming formula, in chirality (pre-bony formations). Thus, we need to become super-sensitive/self-aware to honor subtle flow through the tissues that naturally default to spiral constraints.

> While we animate the stream, we acknowledge the constraints to withhold the dangers of forcing forces through them. The body, as Karen demonstrates in her thoughtful and long-standing practice, gently responds to this exploration. It has been built over time into corresponding (as in co-responsive) tissues, and there is no "bash and dash" basis of these exquisitely developed asana explorations. Temporality is built into our tissues and honoring their relationships from ground to crown, through the limbs in any way up, is an art form. See Section 2.5 for more perspective on how this conversation takes us from coupled to throupled.
>
> **Joanne Avison**

My aim in this chapter is to join the thread of classical anatomy together with the embryology established in Chapter 1. First, we have to reckon with some of the classical nomenclature that comes with the territory – or rather, the *map* of the territory.

The term "rotation" normally gets stuck in the reductionist sense. I hope that by looking at rotation up close and then from a broader perspective, we'll see how coupled kinematics animate rotation globally throughout the system. Even actions like flex and extend are part of spirality, it's just that they've been taken out of context and examined to the exclusion of the larger movement patterns of the gross body and its naturally spiraling forms.

Take the hip, for example. In the anatomy for yoga conversation, there is a hard focus on topics like hip-opening, often accompanied by visuals that zoom into the ball-and-socket joint of the hip, which is supposedly the ground zero of the apparent rotation. Much dialogue has emerged on angles of trochanters and depth of socket as if these calculations define the whole. How could they? They do not begin as isolated formations, and they don't even appear as a fully developed pelvis until post-toddler childhood.

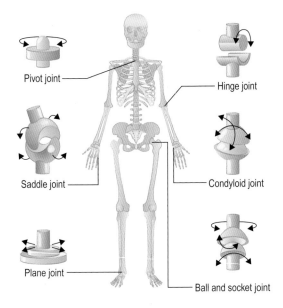

Pivot joint

Hinge joint

Saddle joint

Condyloid joint

Plane joint

Ball and socket joint

FIGURE 2.16

Classical synovial joint classifications.

(i) Anatomical motions

- **Angular motions** occur through synovial joints, changing the angles between bones such as when you flex your knee or elbow.
- **Gliding motions** happen between flat surfaces, such as the motion of the scapula along the thoracic cage, and the intervertebral discs.
- **Rotational motions** rotate a structure about its longitudinal axis, for example during twisting.

In the spiral-bound approach, we include angular and gliding motions into rotation, and see rotation as part of the broad trajectory of biomotion: spiral.

When you pan out and look at the whole organism, the "hip" is actually a stream of structures, through which movement spirals away and outward, inward and around, defying categorization in discretely functioning planes (however you classify the leverage or joint type). Although it is useful to reduce the hip to parts to get our language around it, we often forget to bring it all back together again.

Of course, it is useful and interesting to examine linear relationships of the hip joint and to correlate the data with potential implications for movement. My aim is for us to widen the context for that data. Hip tissue is formed in response to a flow of transmissions through adjacent tissue, rather than a list of separable parts joined together as if they were types of bolts (see Appendix B).

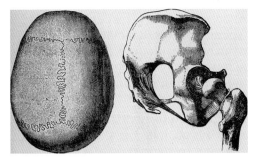

FIGURE 2.17

Poles apart: the cranial bones "fuse" along a fibrous joint that is not synovial, whereas the hip is a classic synovial joint with a host of densities to manage much different kinds of forces.

(Walker J. *Anatomy, Physiology and Hygiene*. Boston: Allyn and Bacon; 1900. p. 46)

The Five Filaments

Indeed, it is a common misconception that the hip is where the leg connects to the trunk, and that rotation is defined by the ball and socket of the iliofemoral joint. The legs, or lower limbs, actually include the hip-bones, and these attach to the axis at the sacroiliac joint. The SI joint in itself is just a word encompassing a massive complex of influence that invariably includes the soft tissue matrix as well, in a closed coupling (within another and another of varying densities) around it.

So, what we call hip-opening in yoga is exploring the angular-gliding-rotation of the lumbo-ilio-sacral matrix, which is profoundly and intimately related to the diaphragm and thoracolumbar fascia with its continuities as well. So, where do we start? Where do we stop? How do we talk about this stuff? It's no wonder that anatomy tries to break it all down into tiny parts to define them suitably. Tissues defy definitive definitions because of their roundness and spatiotemporal continuity.

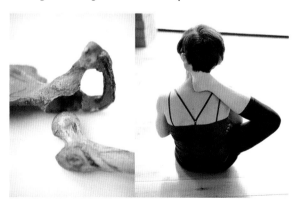

FIGURE 2.18

Virañchyāsana A is an expression of the Opening Hip Filament (the pelvifemoral rhythm).

(Demonstrated by Amy Hughes)

Key concept 5

Rotations can describe the localized appearance of movement within the spiral flow of body tubes, such as your upper and lower limbs.

Since we are stuck with the classical anatomical position as the control state, it is this model that we have to begin with for rotations within these spiral filaments for reference to yoga anatomy. Filaments are the natural result of linkages and continuities, large and small, gross and subtle, and we will use them in this personal research of spiral anatomy in asana.

ⓘ External/lateral and internal/medial rotation

Here is a quick reference for rotations, so that we are all located at the same starting point. Rotation is classically defined concerning the movement directionality of long bones around their long axis towards or away from the body as follows:

- **Medial (or internal) rotation** is the rotation of the limb towards the axis of the body.
- **Lateral (or external) rotation** refers to rotation of the limb away from the body axis.
- **Scapular and hip rotation** happen as these "flat" bones rotate about a central axis.
- **Axial rotation** has two modes, left and right (as we will see, flexion of the axis in any direction produces a concomitant rotation).

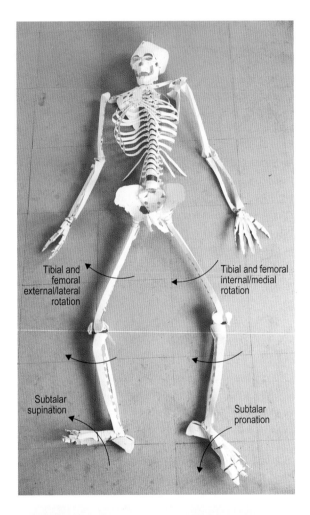

FIGURE 2.19

Rotation of long bones about their axis laterally and medially corresponds with supination and pronation in the ankles as shown.

(Demonstrated by Amy Hughes)

These terms are based on movement relative to the classical anatomical position. There is a certain symmetry between the upper and lower limbs when the arms rise overhead. This inherent symmetry is somewhat obfuscated because the terminology is based on the arms at one's side, the classical anatomical position for bipeds.

My suggestion is that it is useful to remember that although our species is bipedal, we also belong to the superclass Tetrapoda, having four "feet." Birds, snakes, and humans are all tetrapods because even though we don't *currently* have four legs, we have all evolved from a common four-footed ancestor. Recall the discussion on limb comparison from Chapter 1.

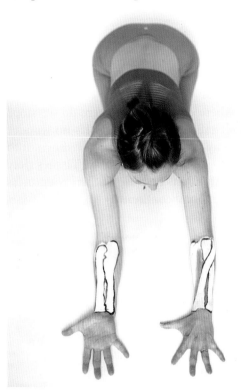

FIGURE 2.20

Forearm supination and pronation. Right palm facing up shows the anterior (flexor) compartment where the radius and ulna are in parallel (supination); where the palm is facing down, the radius rotates over the ulna (pronation) to make an X.

The Five Filaments

Levin suggests we are in fact unipedal![42] Given our explorations in yoga of one-legged postures and our ability to hop on one leg (our more obviously tetrapodal family hops on two), we might consider this proposal well worth exploring. Yoga so loves to explore rotational movements of the torso over the unipedal foundation of postures such as Garudasana (Eagle pose).

Joanne Avison

The point of this section is to see that rotation is not in and of itself a spiral; it is just the only word we have to describe a pattern in a much larger movement flow. Like any tube, our limbs are stabilized, or appropriately constrained by the pairing of opposite directionalities of filamentous flow. The inward-and-down spiral that presses down the balls of the big toes when you're standing up, for example, is paired with the upward-and-outward energy in the arches of the feet. (This relationship is explored later as supination/pronation in the Foot Filament.) This is just one example of the ways we can consider the organizations of rotational flow that are, in reality, continuities within a much larger arc of motion.

Key concept 6

Humans, although currently bipedal (walking on two legs), are classified as Tetrapoda (having 4 feet); both hands and feet are platforms for standing, and we can also balance unipedally.

We are currently stuck with the lexicon of "external/lateral" and "internal/medial" tagged to the less-than-natural "anatomical position" (AP). They aren't the ideal terms to describe the body in yoga, because the dynamic body is rarely standing still, or likely to stay in that position for long. To further complicate matters, the yoga body is quite often moving on *four* feet, or even turning upside down and backwards.

> Pronation = medial rotation = grounding.
> Supination = lateral rotation = opening.

As mentioned in Chapter 1, it would be informative to pin our movement references to a *quadruped* tetrapod, that is, a four-legged animal that currently uses all four legs for locomotion. Such a reference for the AP could be more relevant to multiple asanas than a *biped* tetrapod, or one that in theory is considered incapable of using (for weight-bearing) two of its four legs.

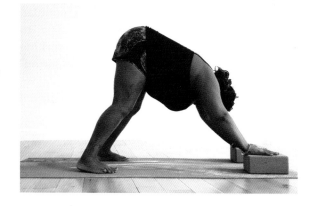

FIGURE 2.21

Downward Dog illustrates the principle of arms taking root in the thoracolumbar fascia as the body is effectively two pairs of limbs making a triangle with the line of the floor.

(Demonstrated by Fadzai Mwakutuya)

55

Key concept 7

Imagining various positions, such as Downward Dog, it is easy to see why it is useful to consider (appropriately) the limb pairs as reciprocal to some extent in their rotation patterns.

2.4 Spiral motion in yoga

By this point, we have seen clear evidence that we are structurally expressing the continuation of embryonic spiral inclinations. Everything joins up into one continuity. Coupling functions describe the whole body, kinematic within itself as one closed system, as well as the small networks within that one, closed system. By closed, I don't mean that the modules are not open to outside influence; on the contrary. In our narrative, closure is simply referring to the lack of loose ends. The pattern itself is scale-free and modular, casting connections amongst individuals to galvanize collective behavior. We have a working knowledge of the anatomical terms "rotation" and "anatomical position", but this agreement on words is something of a double-edged sword.

Given that the study of Western classical anatomy is fixed in terms of language and customs, it becomes problematic when we try to make it fit into the context of natural movement possibilities. The parts-list approach to anatomy makes cueing movement in a practical sense contradictory, complicated, and unnecessarily tedious. It doesn't reduce down. The loaf cannot be unbaked.

As teachers, we trip over these words. We get stuck in an old paradigm that was great for ushering in the much-needed scientific method. It might now be more of a limitation as we expand our sense of biology as based in the physics and chemistry of emotional, living, non-linear soft matter in all its variety of colors, cultures and morphologies – *to make it real*. What if we could harness all those old Latin words into a set of simple cues that incorporates everything we know to be real about movement – and make it *inclusive*?

Cue the Five Filaments.

Is this yet another style of yoga? No. The Five Filaments (5F) is first an approach to understanding spiral-bound anatomy. In this approach, the fascia and all the structures naturally arising from the embryo form the starting point and lens for looking at the anatomy of postural yoga.

This book is a manual intended to support students and teachers of yoga to focus on the commonalities amongst the many different styles. Such an approach gets us over the stumbling blocks of reductionist anatomy and deeper into the interconnected, sensory web that brings any posture to life. It seeks to experience that animation directly (particularly since *it is originally spiral bound*). It evolves the story, without excluding the more classical approach.

 Terms of movement and position

Kinesiology is hugely relevant to the Five Filaments approach. Each modality (style of movement) can approach the rubric utilizing its language for cueing the desired application. Developing any physical practice comes through an evolving understanding of agonist/antagonist relationships, contractility

The Five Filaments

modes, recruitment strategies, reciprocal inhibition, facilitation, and other reflex arcs.

My intention is not to downplay the importance of such terms; as yoga teachers, we should all know this stuff inside and out. My suggestion is that the felt-sense of these concepts can be explored with micromovement inspired by the nomenclature of kinesiology to deepen the experience of reinforcing our natural morphological constraints. This book aims to fold it all into the spiraling filaments. It's up to each of us as teachers to find the power of descriptive language to reinforce the constraints appropriately.

There is a spiral arrangement to the fibers of the living fascial system, the essential tissue of every single minuscule part of our entire architecture. It interweaves in non-linear patterns that are continuous at every scale, resulting from the cross-ply of the wrappings[40] formed in a triple helical structure. These united triumvirates invite us to consider tissues as tubular, cylindrical structures. We can study their development, from the tiniest particles up into joint systems that work in rotation-based movement orientations, including the muscles that spiral into place (they may be drawn in the anatomy books as if they are flat – they are not.).

These tubular chiralities we are referring to as body-wide patterns, work in actual motion, somewhat like finger traps. In essence, they form cross-ply patterns facilitating spiral movement – as volumes (i.e., tubular continuities). Any and every chirality unites to create a tube, the third force, the volume they enclose on every scale.

Spiral movement is not something we have a lot of names for. Anatomically, all we have is the linear term rotation from the lever system

as applied to single joints in one plane. Despite best efforts to simplify, you'll see how the parts-list rotations of classical biomechanics, while necessary for early learning, can be very confusing when we attempt to apply it to real live yoga bodies (or any other movement modality). The spiral-bound perspective offers a foundation to all these rotations, described individually, as part of an integrated approach to anatomy for yoga.

Key concept 8

The 5F aim to put all the pieces together into a simple, graspable, pragmatic set of movement cascades based on rotational spirals intrinsic to biomotional integrity.

From this approach, we propose that the tissue directionality of these spirals guides harmonious motion: that is, movement in tune with the pattern underlying our morphology (shape development). The pattern is in the tissue itself, and the forms it forms, dominantly based in chirality. Which, in turn, invites us toward naturally constrained spiraling movement patterns. It makes sense that moving in harmony with underlying patterns is more likely to lead us to ease and integrity.

The 5F approach suggests a method based on this principle of **vinyasa** in the broad sense. Vinyasa finds its home in the convergent-divergent movement of a structure in the round. It is the center-outward, and back-into-center (flow of breath) made manifest in practice (see more about breathing and vinyasa in Chapter 5). Inhale, exhale; expand, draw inward; opening, grounding – in spiral-bound motion patterns. These opposing pairs find countless iterations in tissue, and in yoga, we balance and unite oppositions by recognizing their spiral volumetric wholeness.

So, where are the actual spirals? Well, in a word, *everywhere*. (We explore the ubiquity of spirals further in the online Reflection and Growth chapter.)

They're in the particles at the micro level, the cross-ply of the fibers, and scaling up we can see spirals in the way our limbs are organized on the macro level. That the body is so arranged will, of course, show up in how it moves: rotationally. And every rotation requires a pair of spirals for counterbalance and support (functionally) and tubular nature (structurally).

In my practice, on the gross level, I've found that the rhythms of movement can be broadly interpreted into rotational families that correspond with certain posture groups. If you stand back and look at these rotational families as spirals, all the Latin terms and biomechanical descriptions flow into them seamlessly. Simplicity emerges. It isn't always easy – however, it is worth the exploration to reveal the simple!

2.5 The Five Filaments rubric

A caveat: reductionist, Western, classical anatomical language is still the intellectual solvent we have for the analysis of structure and function. There is currently no other way to write about physical postures critically than to use the Latin-infused biomechanical descriptors. Furthermore, a rubric of any kind is always going to challenge something of the wholeness that is our authentic natural reality.

Accepting that reduction of any kind is a compromise, I am rounding up the anatomy and using it (and the images) to get us all onto the same page. Once we have common ground, we can go where we don't stumble so much over endless jargon. Until then, please take the following as my earnest embrace of the classical anatomy, if only for as long as it takes to weave this thread into the new tapestry.

All Five Filaments are paired rotations giving a total of ten spirals, demonstrated in the pairs of images below.

1. Shoulder Filament: The Scapulohumeral Rhythm

Pairs:

1. **Opening spiral**: upward and outward rotation of the arm/upper back.

2. **Grounding spiral**: downward and inward rotation of the arm/upper back.

Anatomical basis

The scapulohumeral rhythm classically refers to the lateral humeral rotation with upward scapular rotation as the arm flexes at the shoulder. It involves clavicular rotation as well as coupled rotation of the associated softer tissues (see Fig. 2.45).

Opening

The **Opening Shoulder Spiral** is activated in movement elevating the humerus out and up as one does when the arms are reaching overhead. The further upward the arm goes, the deeper the coupled flexion and the more crucial and all-encompassing the lateral humeral rotation becomes. Along with the spiraling upward trajectory of the scapula and clavicular rotation, the lateral humeral rotation is definitive of flexed-shoulder backbends.

The Five Filaments

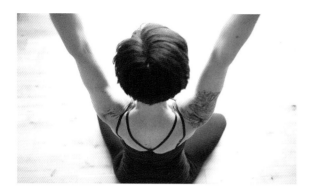

FIGURE 2.22

Opening Shoulder Spiral. As the upward/ outward spiral of the arms deepen their flexion at the shoulder (such as in Downward Dog and Urdhvadanurasana), the glenohumeral joint laterally/ externally rotates in conjunction with upward rotation of the scapula and rotation of the clavicle.

(Demonstrated by Amy Hughes)

This spiral accommodates various combinations of scapular protraction and retraction, and axial extension and flexion. The Opening Shoulder Spiral is commonly associated with ushering in what little extension is available in the thoracic spine. Opening Shoulder Spiral is also involved in all the formal flexed shoulder arm balances.

Examples: Downward Dog, Urdvha Danurasana (Wheel), Handstand, Virabhadrasana (Warrior) A.

Grounding

The **Grounding Shoulder Spiral** involves medial humeral rotation, and downward scapular rotation as the arm extends at the shoulder. The Grounding Spiral is activated in arm movement down and around the back, elevating the humerus posteriorly as one does in taking the arms downward and back behind the body. The further behind and up the arm goes, the deeper the extension and consequently, the rotation intensifies.

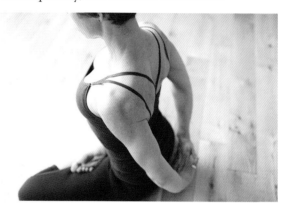

FIGURE 2.23

Grounding Shoulder Spiral. As the downward/ inward spiral of the arms deepen their extension at the shoulder (such as in bridge and Prasarita Padottanasana C), the glenohumeral joint internally rotates.

(Demonstrated by Amy Hughes)

This spiral accommodates various combinations of scapular protraction and retraction, and axial extension and flexion. Keep in mind that the shoulder is often medially rotated and retracted simultaneously, a situation that can at first look like external rotation, i.e., Suptavajrasana (see Fig. 2.26).

Examples: Ustrasana (Camel), Purvattonasana (Upward Plank), Prasarita Padottanasana, Marichyasana A.

2. Hand Filament: Supination/pronation

Pairs:

1. **Opening spiral**: supination.

2. **Grounding spiral**: pronation.

Anatomical basis

The Hand Filament describes arm spirality continuing through the elbow, radius and ulna, and into the hand through the flower spray flow of the wrist bones into the stems of the fingers. It has two spirals that can be paired with the Shoulder Filament for a continuing or countering spiral.

Opening

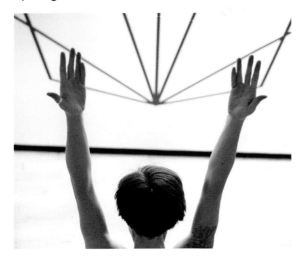

FIGURE 2.24

Opening Handstand. Supination of the forearm continuing into the turning hand with radius and ulna in parallel.

(Demonstrated by Amy Hughes)

Supinating the forearm (radius stays parallel to the ulna) is found most often in postures involving an upward-reaching arm. An **Opening Hand Spiral** is simply the continuation of the Opening Shoulder Spiral distally into supination. OH can offer a counterspiral to the Grounding Shoulder Spiral in a few postures, but this scenario is limited in formalized postural yoga.

Opening spiral of the forearm/wrist/hand works with any kind of hand position and a range of wrist movement when **the radius stays parallel to the ulna.** Opening can be paired with meeting or grasping any substrate and is optimized for rotating unopposed into the sky. This filament rolls out to continue the opening spiral of the shoulder.

Examples: Upward and open-reaching postures when intentionally supinating, Parsvakonasana (the reaching hand), Trikonasana (both hands when grasping the big toe). Supported Shoulderstand is one of the only inversions using supinated forearms. Mayurasana, Peacock Feather, is the only formal arm balance (that I know of) using supination.

Grounding

Pronating the forearm (radius rotates over the ulna) is most often organized with appropriate wrist extension to explore making the hands, functionally, behave more like feet. A **Grounding Hand Spiral** is the continuation of the Grounding Shoulder Spiral distally drawn into pronation, and in yogasana, it often appears as a counterspiral to the Opening Shoulder Spiral. Indeed, this is the case for almost all the traditional handstanding postures (Mayurasana is the notable exception) (see Fig. 2.26).

The Five Filaments

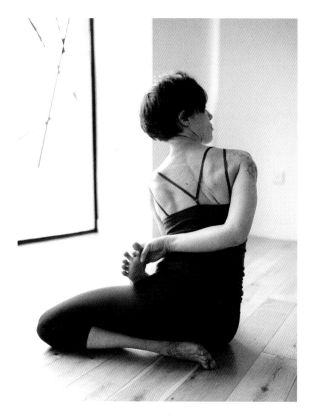

FIGURE 2.25

Grounding Handstand. Pronation of the forearm continuing into the turning hand with radius crossed over the ulna, as Amy is doing with her right forearm here as she binds her toe (Vamadevasana B).

(Demonstrated by Amy Hughes)

the stop sign (palm facing forward) that counters lateral humeral rotation with an opposing spin.

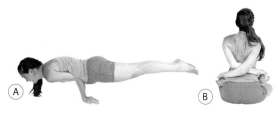

FIGURE 2.26

(A) Mayurasana, the Peacock: unique amongst the arm balances in that it uses an Opening Handstand (the body is balancing on supinated forearms!). (B) Suptavajrasana, example of grounding shoulders in retraction.

(Demonstrated by the author)

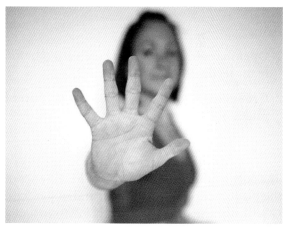

FIGURE 2.27

Pronation with wrist extension, the universally recognized "STOP".

Grounding Hand Spiral is optimized for weight-bearing but works with any kind of hand position and a range of wrist movement, so long as **the radius stays crossed over the ulna**. It pairs with meeting/grasping any substrate. The opposition increases integrity by stiffening the forearm, reinforcing it to become more like the feet. Think of the cross of the forearm bones as

The grounding hand reaches to the ground and almost through it. Hands are alternating as feet to deal with ground reaction force (GRF), so they must spiral into the floor and be poised to spring back – it is their nature as a pre-tensioned architecture. In other words, while the forearm strongly pronates in a tighter spiral, the hands un-spiral to flatten to the floor, and while weight-bearing the hands are micro-spiraling to manage GRF. They release back into their natural curled cup when they stop weight-bearing.

Examples: All forms of Handstand (except Mayurasana (see Fig. 2.26)), Urdvhadanurasana (Wheel), Kapotasana, Downward Dog, Purvattonasana (Upward Plank), Prasarita Padottanasana C, Pincha Mayurasana (Forearm Stand; an interesting variation of the HS that makes the forearm and hand a functional unit, when pronated).

3. Hip Filament: The Pelvifemoral Rhythm

Pairs:

1. **Opening spiral**: upward and outward rotation of the leg/lower back.

2. **Grounding spiral**: downward and inward rotation of the leg/lower back.

Anatomical basis

The pelvifemoral rhythm refers to kinematics of the pelvis, sacrum, lower back, and upper legs. Classically, the pelvis is thought of as virtually fused to the sacrum in the anatomy of mature humans via the relatively immobile sacroiliac joints (SIJs). During early development and in the maternal years, the SIJs are known to have more give than in their "normal" state. Here, we look at the spectrum of tissue surrounding joints when considering their range, which includes from hard to soft. In the embryo, there is a ring of cartilaginous potential, and in

childhood, this becomes denser through force-transmission (in other words – use!).

With loading, the pelvis gradually becomes the familiar adult bony arrangement. However, it remains responsive to force and neuroendocrine influence. Thus, it has the advantages of strength and suitable stiffness to hold us together – and just enough yield to allow pregnancy and birth in the female. It does all this to allow the giant human cranium to emerge from the relatively narrow human female pelvis while still managing the contralateral motion of our walking blueprint (the so-called "obstetric dilemma").[43] Its filamentous arrangement is not as delicate as that of the draped shoulder girdle that reaches upwardly, as its density is fit for purpose. However, we emphasize the spectrum of condensation here to reiterate earlier discussion that the anatomy of the hip and shoulder girdles are comparable (but not interchangeable).

Recall that the Shoulder Filament (scapulohumeral rhythm) talks about flatter bones rotating about a central axis in association with the arm rotating around its long axis during flexion and extension. Similarly, the Hip Filament describes how the ilia rotate in association with the movement of the femur and how this action flows through couplings of adjacent tissues (and beyond), referred to as the pelvifemoral rhythm.

Opening

The **Opening Hip Spiral** activates in movement involving flexion of the hip tending toward abduction (widening of the legs). This lateral spiral includes the action of opening the legs out to the sides from approximately hip-width and becomes fully expressed as flexion pairs with abduction. The Opening Hip Spiral can be paired with lumbar flexion

The Five Filaments

or (given enough range of motion) lumbar extension and can work with either spiral of the Footstand. Continued opening broadens the pelvic inlet, and results in sacral counternutation, bringing spaciousness to the pelvis.

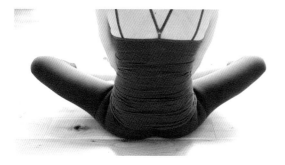

FIGURE 2.28

Opening Hip Spiral. As the upward/outward spiral of the legs deepen their flexion at the hip (such as in wide-legged forward bends), the iliofemoral joint laterally/externally rotates in conjunction with a corresponding rotation of the iliolumbar region and counternutation of the sacrum.

(Demonstrated by Amy Hughes)

Examples: Forward bends, Downward Dog, seated and standing hip-openers, Baddhakonasana, legs behind the head, Janusirsasanas.

Grounding

The **Grounding Hip Spiral** involves medial femoral rotation with the associated rotation of iliolumbosacral tissues. The Grounding Hip Spiral includes medial rotation of the femur that increases as the femurs adduct (or draw toward one another). This medial spiral of the adducting femurs rounds from hip flexion through extension and into hyperextension with lumbar extension for increasingly acute backbending postures.

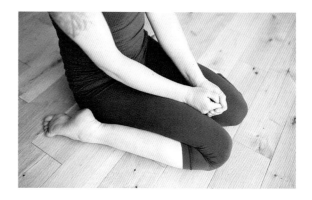

FIGURE 2.29

Grounding Hip Spiral. Medial hip rotation is easy to see in Virasana. As the downward/inward spiral of the legs deepen their extension at the hip (such as in backbends), the iliofemoral joint medially/internally rotates in conjunction with a corresponding rotation of the iliolumbar region.

(Demonstrated by Amy Hughes)

These movements are classically coordinated with a narrowing of the iliac crests, sacral nutation and widening of the pelvic outlet.

Examples: Virasana and its one-legged variations, the flexed knee side of Parighasana, lunges, kneeling backbends, Urdvhadanurasana (Wheel), all prone backbends such as Shalabhasana (Locust).

4. Foot Filament: Supination/pronation

Pairs:

1. **Opening spiral**: supination.

2. **Grounding spiral**: pronation.

Anatomical basis

The Foot Filament describes leg spirality continuing through the knee, tibia and fibula, and into the foot. It has two modes that can be paired with the spirals of the Hip Filament for options in a continuing or countering spiral from the hip. Compare with the Hand Filament to see the reflection of the evolutionary and embryological journeys. In pronation, the tibia-fibula never cross as the ulna-radius do, an arrangement that shows our quadrupedal adaptation for bipedalism. Reflecting the common embryonic unfolding of all four limbs, Foot Filament spirals follow the same pattern as those of the Hand Filaments: supination and pronation.

Opening

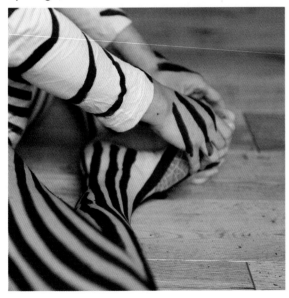

FIGURE 2.30

Opening Spiral. Supination continuing the Opening Spiral of the Hip Filament as pictured here in Baddhakonasana.

(Demonstrated by Amy Hughes)

The **Opening** Spiral of the Foot Filament involves supination of the foot and pairs with either spiral of the Hip Filament. In Opening mode, the foot is effectively a continuation through the talar mortise and can coordinate with whatever rotation is happening in the lower leg. In seated postures, for example, the flexed knee in medial rotation can continue medially rotating through the ankle and foot (Virasana), twirling back on itself in pronation towards eversion. The flexed knee in lateral rotation can rotate laterally through the ankle and foot, supinating with inversion in the Opening spiral, such as in Baddhakonasana as pictured in Fig. 2.30.

In the extended (straight) leg, the Opening Spiral of the Foot continues the directionality of the Hip Filament. Like the Opening mode of the Hand, the Opening mode of Foot is optimized for spiraling unopposed and is not so good for weight-bearing. In effect, the Opening Foot Spiral removes the stand and makes the foot more like a hand. You can challenge this arrangement with educational effects, as when attempting Downward Dog on pointed toe.

Examples: Inversions, Virasana, Padmasana, Dwipada Sirsasana.

Grounding

Grounding Spiral of the Foot Filament is the act of "normal" standing on the feet when pronation is continuously counterbalanced with supination via the coupled talar mortise of the ankle. Continuing in pronation deepens the Grounding Spiral. Classical descriptions give us the story of how the Grounding Spiral of standing involves dorsiflexion of the ankle

The Five Filaments

and activation of pada bandha in something called the windlass mechanism (see the next sections for a more detailed discussion). Activating the Grounding Spiral out of weight-bearing has a powerful effect, as the dorsiflexed ankle can both magnify force and stabilize with a stirrup-like impact through the knee and into the rest of the body.

When compared to the Grounding Hand Spiral, which is simply pronation of the forearm with the radius crossed over the ulna, the difference is that in the legs the tibia and fibula are always parallel and never crossed. In normal pronation of the lower limbs, the Grounding Footstand, there is simply "normal standing."

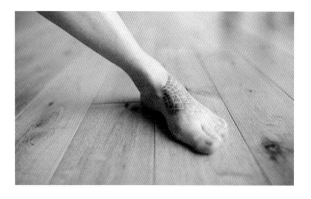

FIGURE 2.31

Grounding Footstand. The ankle stabilized in the Grounding Spiral of the foot, stabilized in standing with the Windlass Mechanism.

(Demonstrated by Amy Hughes)

Examples: Samasthitih and all standing postures, Urdvhadanurasana (Wheel), Downward Dog.

5. Axial Matrix Filament

Pairs:

1. **Twists (contralateral).**

2. **Flexion (multidirectional).**

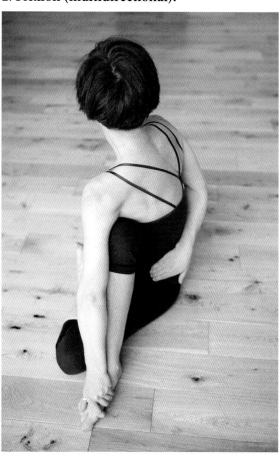

FIGURE 2.32

Axial Rotation, or Twist. Closed: rotating the axis to "close the loop" with flexion by bringing together contralateral limbs. For an example of an Open Twist, see Fig. 2.25.

(Demonstrated by Amy Hughes)

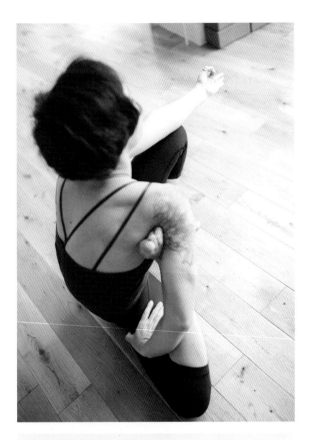

FIGURE 2.33

Axial Flexion. In this demonstration of
Yogadandasana, Amy demonstrates how the
Grounding shoulder and Opening hip can cocreate
axial flexion.

(Demonstrated by Amy Hughes)

Anatomical basis

The trunk is a hub of helical convergence
at various timescales, densities, depths and
directionality. The axial vectors are the first to
form in the embryo, with the limb buds emerging
later in gestation. In postural yoga, flexion/
extension (backbends and forward bends) are
powered through limb kinematics converging in

and *around* the axis. The 5F rubric regards this
crux as a multilevel integration of limb pairs.

 Epi- and Hypo-

In a sense, the somites launched a back-
to-back campaign. Part of each somite
wrapped around your front body to become
the **hypaxial** structures. In contrast, a smaller
contingent of somitic material wound
around the opposite way to contain what
would come to be known as the **epaxial**
structures (Fig. 2.34). The 5F look at how
the limbs, hypaxial structures, coordinate
rotationally to influence both hypaxial *and*
epaxial posturality: backbending and forward
bending. In this sense, holding a posture
consists of balancing the opposition of
flexions *in the round*.

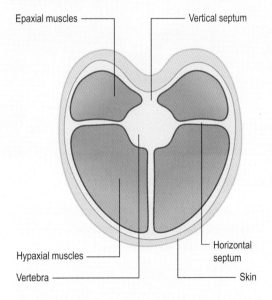

FIGURE 2.34

Epaxial and hypaxial: a diagram of wrapping. Epi
(above) -axial refers to the somite material that
wrapped up the dorsal myofascial structures,

The Five Filaments

those that arose "above" the notochord; hypo (under) -axial refers to the somite material that wrapped up the ventral myofascial structures, those that arose "below" the notochord. Back and belly; dorsal and ventral; back and front; posterior and anterior.

Downward Dog (see Fig. 2.21) comes up again as a clear illustration: a triangle with three functional bars. In this posture, the hands-arms-trunk is one bar, the legs another, and the ground forms the third in what is essentially a (temporarily) stable triangle – a three-bar CKC mechanism. The arm pair unit is a V that integrates with the V of the leg pair unit, effectively making the tissue wrappings of the torso into a spiral, contralateral pattern – in other words, they don't end there, they continue as an X arrangement. This integration coordinates differently depending on the posture. Wheel pose (see Fig. 4.6) illustrates the same concept, except that lumbar spine extension has to be negotiated quite differently (since, after all, we are not reversible).

The scapulothoracic and iliolumbar rotations are authoritative in that they have a corresponding interaction of ground reaction force that directly informs the axis. Posturally, the trunk is essentially doing what the limbs tell it to, and vice versa. At no time in asana are they (the limbs and axis) decoupled, separate or without a role in negotiating force transmission through and around the whole body. Trunk movement is a question of coupling and how we manage the helical constraints, and this is analyzed differently depending on whether you're looking at gait or posture.

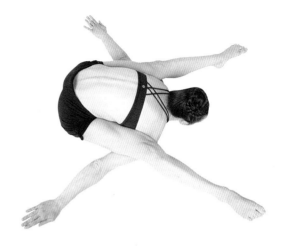

FIGURE 2.35

Kūrmāsana: pose of the tortoise, morphological foil for Kapotasana. Medial shoulder rotation with retraction flows spirally through both upper limbs, especially once the forearms pronate fully to turn the hands skyward during binding (see Suptakūrmāsana compared with Kapo in Chapter 4); hips are in their full opening spirals as they flex and abduct, eventually far enough to circumnavigate the trunk.

(Demonstrated by Sarah Hatcher)

Flexion (multidirectional)

Because of its basic segmentation pattern, the trunk can flex and extend laterally as well as rotate. In this context, all bending of the trunk that is not rotation is simply *flexion*. As this story continues, bear in mind that the original curvature of our axis is in the sagittal plane. And any two planes of motion give rise to the third, as we experience our trunk in all its volumetric wholeness – hold that thought.

You can hang backwards over props like the yoga wheel and focus on flexion passively,

CHAPTER TWO

bending as if limbless like a worm. I highly recommend it when you are ready for it and if the appropriate constraints are in place. But you can only drive the shape kinematically and topologically, and by that, I mean deepen the asana without props, using work from the arms and legs through the shoulder and hip girdles.

The "X" of the thoracolumbar fascia (TLF) is one basis for the 5F rubric as applied to what some consider as more extreme asanas. In this model, arms and legs are contralateral continuations of one another. Deepening our own felt-sense of constraints gives us access through the continuous recognition of the body's original logic. The Shoulder and Hip spirals conspire to drive the extension and flexion of the spine, and their spirality encompasses the back bend/forward bend.

Recall Fig. 1.20. The TLFX diagrammatically explodes further into an axial matrix. Thus, the X includes not only TLF but its deep neighbors, the structures lining the posterior abdominal wall and its continuities. Further, the X also encompasses the fibers interiorly, anteriorly, and laterally. This is the integrated X or the deeper X (a pattern at every level of the tissues). This model takes into account the effect of all the cross-ply epaxial and hypaxial tissues plus their visceral continuities throughout the tube at every level.

This mega cross-ply isn't limited to the macro, and it incorporates a scale-free self-assembled body plan. In the big picture, it isn't just the TLFX (the all-encompassing cross-ply of thoracolumbar fascia composite) that provides insertion and a fibrous cross-ply hub for the contralateral limbs; it is indeed happening right through the whole tubular network. Functionally, the torso is a hyperboloid in the round (so are the limbs).

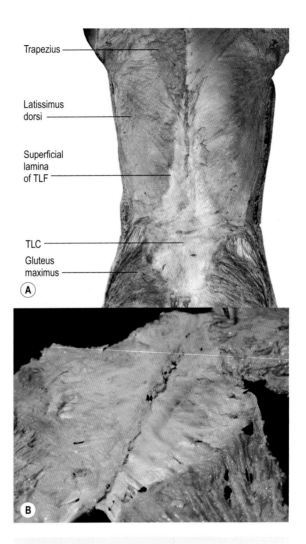

FIGURE 2.36

Thoracolumbar continuities. (A) Posterior view of the back showing connections with the lattisimus dorsi, trapezius and gluteus maximus to the TLF and thoracolumbar composite (TLC). (B) Thoracolumbar fascia with gluteus maximus in situ.

(A) with permission from the Willard/Carreiro Collection, University of New England. B) courtesy of Stecco C, Sharkey J, Schleip R. Fascia Net Plastination Project/von Hagens Plastinarium, 2018.)

The Five Filaments

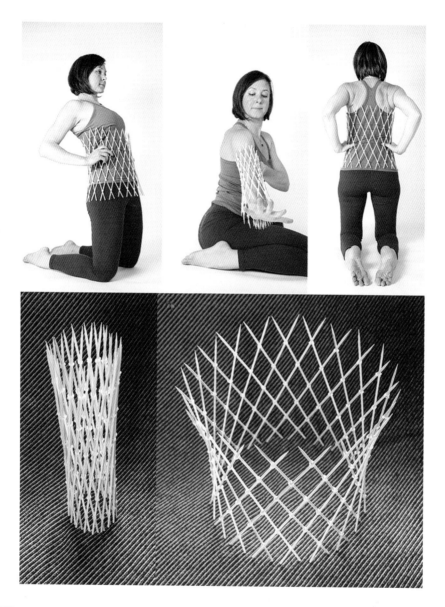

FIGURE 2.37

Hyperboloid structures are based on volumes defined by doubly ruled surfaces, creating curvaceousness out of cross-ply straight lines that can spring to life with twisting and flexion. This model was woven from skewers and hair bands by the author.

CHAPTER TWO

In yoga, we learn to feel the body in its caterpillar sense, i.e., free to bend segmentally, yet with a balance of inward pull and outward push to maintain structural integrity. The appendages are helical tubes whose power lies in their ability to coil as matrices of interconnected, volumetric spirals responding to forces. In this organization, each of these spiral geometries corresponds to the familiar joint systems and expresses behavior according to their situation of connectedness no matter which end is up.

The limbs converge into a kinematically coupled, meta cross-ply within the metameric array of motion segments. Since that cross-ply of limbs *is* the trunk, it follows that driving axial movement in all forms of flexion involves gearing up the limbs. The same perspective guides an integrated approach to axial rotation (Twists).

(i) *Topology*

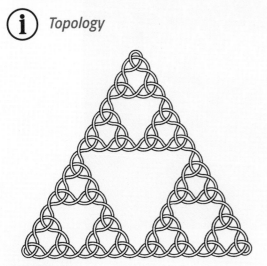

FIGURE 2.38

The Sierpiński Triangle: knots, triangles and fractals.

Topologists study knots. They are looking for which properties of a shape can be retained

during bending, twisting, and squeezing so that the form stays continuous and doesn't break (considerations especially suitable for the yogi).

Twists (contralateral)

The Twist is rotational movement through the axis (see Fig. 2.32). The Twist Filament shifts our view of the tetrapod from seeing the arms and legs as comparable pairs to seeing the left and right sides in the contralateral counterbalance. This relationship can be explored from various perspectives, such as:

- the X across the lumbosacroiliac region via the thoracolumbar fascia

- the X across the anterior thoracopelvic canister

- the X across the diaphragmatic crura into contralateral hip flexors

- the X throughout the oblique layers

- the visceral ligaments, i.e., endopelvic fasciae

- the neurovascular bundles coursing continuously.

What we are referring to as a closed twist is one that flexes onto itself, joining the oblique ends of the lines in the X into a continuous loop. This is one thread of the X band (the latissimus dorsi, the thoracolumbar fascia (TLF), the fascia of the sacral and gluteal region through the contralateral iliotibial band (ITB)).

The closed Twist Spiral aims to bring the humeral attachment of one latissimus dorsi anteriorly and across the body towards the tibial attachment of the contralateral iliotibial

The Five Filaments

thickening. Although classically contralateral, when you see the X, functionally, it is a loop as it brings together the ends of the same continuity.

The complete closed twist Möbius empowers the material involved to optimize recalibration of the torso tube via the breath.

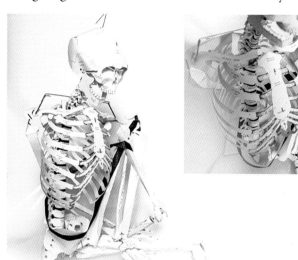

FIGURE 2.39

Paper skeleton demonstrating Marichyasana C, a closed twist. Here, the hyperboloid torso rotates around and down to bring the lateral knee (distal aspect of Iliotibial band) across to unite with the attachment of the contralateral latissimus dorsi (an experientially multidimensional loop).

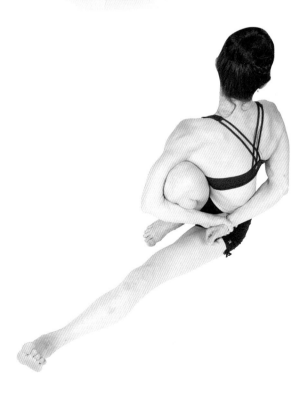

FIGURE 2.40

Marichyasana C.

(Demonstrated by Sarah Hatcher)

Inside and outside

Let's take another look at that closed twist we made by creating a loop by joining the ends of a line together onto itself. This is a window into oneness, when we move from models of tissue as discrete continuities with orientability[44] and into the nonorientability of the Möbius strip and the Klein bottle[45] (see Fig. 2.41). These latter two geometries are nonorientable in that they invaginate themselves, integrating the "outside and the inside"[46] as a whole and complete experience. Lines, so useful in two- and three-dimensional diagrams of anatomy, cannot express the multidimensional experience of having a body.[47,48]

CHAPTER TWO

Orientable surfaces are those for which a consistent orientation can be attributed to its surfaces. Any two-sided surface in space can be considered orientable, as we can easily see the sides are separate – top and bottom, inside and outside are distinctly and consistently separate features. Nonorientable forms are just that – you can't establish "vector normal" on its surface.

We can draw a line from the insertion of latissimus dorsi inferomedially across the myofascial sling to the insertion of the iliotibial band to make a simple loop. While this "sling" informs our understanding of how the parts relate to each other as bands, its surface separates outside from inside. If we consider this as a myofascial Möbius (rather than a sling), it allows us access to the continuous nature of the inside/outside.

All models of biologic forms are abstractions, but linear models by definition cannot incorporate the intrinsic multidimensionality of a self-organizing biologic form experiencing itself. The boundaried-thinking separateness threatens to distract us from the oneness of self-referential biologic coupling. The spiral-bound approach looks for models, such as the Klein bottle, that keep open that window into the fourth dimension.

Key concept 9

The concept of myofascial slings is 2D-3D, whereas the human body is multidimensional.

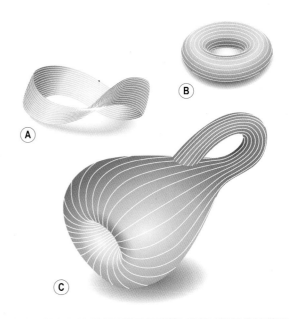

FIGURE 2.41

Non-orientability is hard to get our heads around! Here are three topological shapes relevant to multidimensional models of anatomy: (A) the Möbius band; (B) torus; and (C) the Klein bottle which shows a 2D surface making a space that looks 3D while interpenetrating itself. It is thus considered non-orientable, which means a system for determining a consistent vector cannot be defined. If you let ants loose on the surface, they would get around over its entirety as a surface without ever crossing a boundary, collapsing the distinction between Inside and Outside. Looking at animations of the Klein construct, you can see it contains the mobius as well as the torus, rotating into and out of itself in 4D. This curious arrangement may perhaps be experienced by feeling the continuities of our fascial system in movement.

What we are referring to as open twists, such as the supine/passive version, are those

The Five Filaments

that rotate away from the loop between the latissimus insertion on the humerus and the contralateral ITB attachment (the other end of the line in the X). Whether open or closed, all twists form a pair in that they have chirality (expressing right- and left-handedness, uniting as a pair). The Axial Matrix is an umbrella term encompassing contralateral cross-ply, an arrangement that has garnered quite a literature base investigating its implications for movement.[11,49–52]

2.6 From coupled to throupled

In the early 20th century, a medical doctor by the name of Robert Lovett introduced coupling to the scoliosis literature when he wrote about the induction of axial torque during lateral flexion, a phenomenon that became known as **coupled motion**.[53] He pointed out that side-bending and rotation of the spine are always associated, and you can't have one without the other.[54,55] The flexible spine bent in one plane cannot bend in another plane without rotating.

Think about it this way: since the spine is already curved in one plane (lordotic and kyphotic curvature in the sagittal plane), anytime we flex it in any other plane we automatically give rise to an unexpected complexity of segmental axial rotation. Harrison Fryette further developed this concept, a doctor of osteopathy whose three principles of spinal coupling have been influential in biomechanics over the last century.[56]

Coupled motion

Spinal coupling occurs as a consequence of the morphological shape (constraints), classically attributed to the facet joint surfaces and the interconnected tissue and spinal curvatures.

Panjabi et al. went further to show that pre-stress in the elastic spine under load produced three-dimensional motion consisting of three translations and three rotations.[57] Gracovetsky's visual Spinal Engine theory provides an analogy

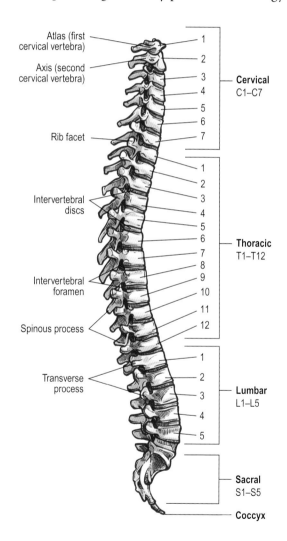

FIGURE 2.42

Standard bony arrangement of the spine, lateral view.

73

that brings the coupled motion concept to life as a "drivetrain" – something like the cogwheel gears of a bicycle.[58]

Gracovetsky shows that the three functional units of the spine – lumbar, thoracic, and cervical, cooperate in rotation as we walk. Since the pelvis and lumbar spine are coupled together, as the hips flex and extend, the pelvis rotates to allow the length of the stride. As the lumbar vertebrae don't much rotate due to their morphology, they send the rotation forces up the chain where they can be translated into motion by the thoracic motion segments. In gait, the rotatory action is harnessed and further "pumped" by the rhythmic swinging of arms[59,60] and "controlled falling" of legs coupled in rotational motion. Especially in running, stride is propelled by angular momentum,[61] essentially gravity-driven horizontal locomotion – controlled falling![61]

This coupled oscillation of counter-rotating filaments converges to drive locomotion. Gracovetsky's theory says that the legs aren't the drivers of gait, and in fact, we don't even need legs for walking. (Note: this is different from how we consider the limbs as drivers of shape in postural yoga.) The recoil of rotation from the shoulders via spinal facet arrangement and cross-ply in the TFLX propel us forward. Earls has explored the application of the Anatomy Trains to this model with insights well worth exploring.[62]

The idea follows that with side-bending to the right, the lumbar bodies rotate to the left and vice versa. Since these contra-directional couplings are synergistic, they form the drivetrain of gait as embedded in the form. The idea that motion can generate itself through the elastic recoil of coupled counter-momentum can be very relevant to yoga practitioners (see the Talking point below).

Throupled motion

Locomotion, an orchestra of rotation, is driven within the axis in response to flexion and vice versa. This swing-pump drivetrain is the mechanism of the orthograde strategy, unique to humans and our ape relatives, mentioned previously. The flexion-rotation drivetrain underlies the rotational contra-propulsion of gait, but the coupling (or throupling, more to the point) also describes the torsional balance we experience in postural yoga.

To extend the reach of coupling, I like the definitions offered by Stokes et al., that coupling happens when: "a primary (or intentional) movement results in a joint also moving in other directions".[63] In gait, we "pump" the action with limb-swinging as part of "interlimb neural coupling".[64] In postural yoga, we pump up the system for a different rhythmic effect with breath and movement.

During right leg weight-bearing, for example in Tree pose, the lumbar spine is drawn into side-bending and rotation by the TFLX structures. The pelvis synergistically counter-rotates to find equilibrium in flux. The flex/spin within an elastic matrix thus amounts to a third phenomenon: that of volumetric, self-regulating motion guided by the helical constraints evident from the onset of embryonic development. In our view, it isn't just the spine that works this way; indeed, it is the entire body that is an expression of continuous throupled motion and self-organization.

Talking point

The powerful engine of locomotion is easy to see in sprinters, especially, as they pump their arms and drive their stride to accelerate. The strategy is evident in cyclists as well as in runners, as they search their reserves to harness every scrap of gain to get up the mountain or over the finish line first. It is in those "do or die" moments that the side to side "pumping" action appears most obviously.

In yoga, we remain "still", and there is no mountain, no gait, and no finish line. Yet, is there something of this power at work in our bodies on the mat, when the breathing and movement are synchronized? Can expansion and retraction form a more subtle kind of drivetrain based in throupled motion? (Grab your Hoberman sphere ("breathing ball") and head to Chapter 5.)

Key concept 10

CKCs can be considered as coupled. However, their coupling naturally gives rise to a third entity, or plane, by the laws of so-called coupled motion. We have called this a "throuple" to distinguish the experience of coupled motion, always giving rise to motion in the third plane.

Handstand and footstand notes

When considering an asana biomotionally, we are always looking at a balance of spirals that have some relationship with a substrate. As earth-dwellers, this substrate is usually the ground via gravity, but can also be the wall, or another body part, or another human. As Tetrapoda, this relationship is quite often through the hands and feet, although in yoga it can also be the head, hips, front body, knees, knuckles, forearms, elbows, etc.

In the wild, it is grounding upon which we primarily depend. To support this, the limb

spirals that start in the trunk and continue distally (out through the endpoints of the hands and feet) need a counterspiral to match and constrain them. For example, when you twist a towel, it densifies and stiffens up with an evident "middle" limit. This is how the limbs know when to stop; this is how the structure of the deeper tissue matrix constrains them appropriately.

The simplicity of this arrangement is complicated somewhat by the differences evolved between our land-loving feet and our sky-loving arms (which are still called feet, technically, since we are Tetrapods). We have an evolved limb patterning that involves two long bones (zeugopod) joining the foot (autopod) (see Fig. 1.23), but their adaptations give them unique attributes. It is relatively easy to see rotation patterns in the hips and shoulders but codifying how they play out in the hands and feet took me long hours of puzzling.

Like the Hip and Shoulder Filaments, the Hand and Foot Filaments have two main modes that can each either continue the spiral of the proximal limb filaments or provide the opposition, like the wringing of that dishtowel. These spirals describe how the limb spirals communicate with a substrate, including space, and their relationships to proximal counterparts.

Handstanding

In the upper limb, Grounding mode is essentially pronation. Pronation is what happens when you flip your forearm over, so your palms face the ground. It means the radius is rotating over the ulna, creating a counterspiral when paired with the Opening Shoulder Spiral, or a continuous spiral with the Grounding Shoulder Spiral. The upper limb is in Opening mode when it is supinating continuously into external rotation, usually when the palms face upwards as if receiving a bowl of soup. Here, the radius is *not* rotating over the ulna.

Take Downward Dog as an example of the Handstand. You *can* supinate in Downward Dog, and it is an educational experience to feel Handstand on the backs of the hands. But it just takes one attempt to experience clearly why we preferably use pronation to bring the palmar surfaces into contact with the substrate in this pose. Tissues of the palm have developed the way they are to predispose palmar integration of GRF; it is part of the same argument in a way, i.e., a response to force transmission shapes the tissues.

The tissue presupposes the forces they transmit. The forearm twists into firmness as the radius crosses over ulna in forearm pronation, a reinforcement strategy required by the less-suited to weight-bearing limbs. In any arm balance, the forearm and hand are generally in Grounding mode (for the hand-standing side if it is an asymmetrical pose, such as side angle pose).

Interestingly, if you try Downward Dog with supination, the hyperextending elbow problem goes away. I put this phenomenon over to you for careful and conscious consideration!

It is easy to see Opening mode, when the rotation continues the Opening Shoulder and keeps the radius and ulna parallel and not crossed over one another, in postures that involve the arms reaching up into space. Taking the side angle pose as an example, the reaching arm is an Opening Shoulder Spiral and continues rotation in that direction from root to fingertips. The radius is moving away from its ulna-crossing, opening laterally. This supination can be thought of as a reprisal of the embryological journey of the arms.

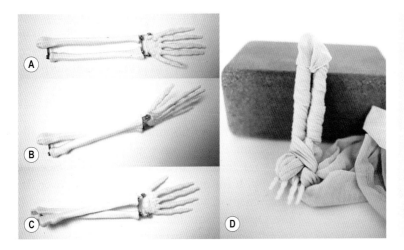

FIGURE 2.43

The radioulnar joints unite the proximal and distal ends of the two bones, forming a closed kinematic chain with rotation animating the system as shown in these images of forearm pronation (A–C). Image (D) shows the forearm as wrapped in fabric to illustrate the CKC in continuity (no bolts in the body!).

The Five Filaments

Both Opening (supination) and Grounding (pronation) of the Hand Spiral can give us a kind of standing hand, or one that is appropriately, intentionally stiffened or softened into various shapes (rather than just hanging there). In the case of a forearm stand, experience will contradict what theory may predict. It is possible to find a degree of unexpected stability on a supinated forearm provided the supination is adequately firm. In yogasana, the activated hand can also be used in mudra, as a seal, providing an endpoint for energy that reflects into the system. Experience for yourself the effects of a completely soft hand as a basis of comparison.

Footstanding

In the lower limb, Grounding mode is not as easy to differentiate because the lower leg is necessarily much more fixed in its arrangement. It pronated embryologically to carry out its destiny in weight-bearing. The fibula does not rotate over the tibia as the radius does over the ulna to make the X. Although tetrapodal, we have indeed evolved as bipeds. Whereas the arm can readily flip from Grounding to Opening, the loaded lower leg has developed effectively the grounded bearing of continuous pronation with its two bones anchored in parallel. The evolved density has stabilized the ankle in pronation without the need for the X. However, over-pronation with valgus (fallen arches) is a common example of constraints in need of reinforcement.

All biomotional spirals are paired in balance; as such, the evolved pronation is matched in its effect with supination potential. In equal human standing, you could say that, in a sense, we are supinating and pronating *at the same time*, even without the crossing of tibia and fibula. How might this be possible?

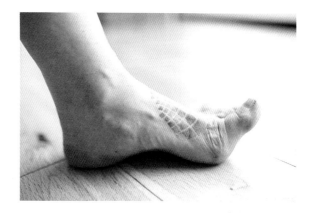

FIGURE 2.44

The term "windlass" to describe the foot is borrowed from the mechanics of sailing. Pressing down through the ball of the big toe whilst flexing and abducting the toes is correlated to stiffening the plantar aponeurosis, akin to the sail "stiffening" in sailing. The fascia of the sole supports the arches of the foot.

Together, the distal aspects of these two leg bones form a kind of spiral grip around the midfoot. This arrangement is known as the talar mortise, classically described as a mortise and tenon articulation. The upshot is that when the lower leg laterally rotates, the supination effect is like a gear turning the arches of the feet upward. Here again, we feel the coupling that generates the third. In yoga, we explore how this supination/arch lift effect coordinates with grounding the big toe, tensioning the plantar fascia, an effect known in biomechanics as the **windlass mechanism**. *Grounding* is the functional term I'm using for the cumulative impact of these actions in Footstand.

Grounding in the lower leg involves both supination and pronation in balance. In a weight-bearing Footstand, such as in Downward Dog, we are always in Grounding mode (but again, as with the hands, it is useful to explore the opposite.) In the lower limb, Opening mode is supination and pairs with external rotation in postures when the knee is flexing, such as in Padmasana (lotus pose).

That same talar mortise coordination is at work in pronation, making the foot effectively a continuity of the lower leg. Thus, if the lower leg is laterally rotating and the ankle is plantarflexing, then the foot follows that lateral rotation. If the lower leg is medially rotating in plantarflexion, the foot follows suit. Of course, all these directionalities can be reversed and challenged. Indeed, that seems to be the yogi's project (in particular the lineage of Krishnamacharya).

2.7 The spirals as patterns of movement

Breath-coordinated movement is the central theme driving the transformative process of

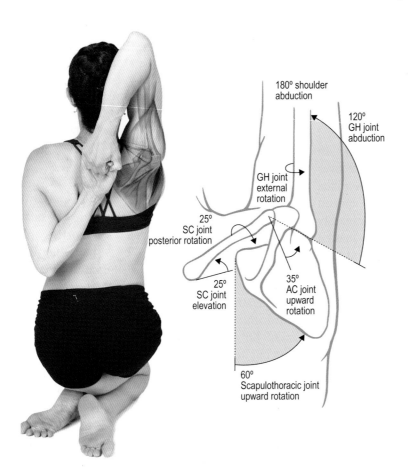

180° shoulder abduction

120° GH joint abduction

GH joint external rotation

25° SC joint posterior rotation

25° SC joint elevation

35° AC joint upward rotation

60° Scapulothoracic joint upward rotation

FIGURE 2.45

Space-making with the scapulohumeral rhythm: bringing awareness to drawing the humerus into the joint as it rotates will increase the sense of felt space as the movement progresses into greater complexity.

(Image by Joanna Darlington with BSIP SA/Alamy Stock Photo. Demonstrated by Sarah Hatcher)

The Five Filaments

yoga. Taken a step further, the in-and-out rhythmic movement attunes to the anatomical concept of CKCs and throupled motion. How can we apply this anatomical approach to the natural biomotion of yoga?

Ekam, inhale (arms up). A typical instruction we give in a yoga class is to raise the arms overhead. This presents Opening activation of the arms (upper limb spirals), as the humerus (upper arm bone) laterally rotates during flexion to bring the arms overhead (the scapulohumeral rhythm of classical biomechanics).

Intentionally pronouncing this rhythm will help keep the shoulder's joint capsule spacious around its core (as an invitation to sukha). Pushing the arms straight up, without deliberately pronouncing the subtle rotation, can lead to inflammation of the soft tissues resulting in rotator cuff damage (not uncommon in the injury list of powerful yoga-flow practices).

In the same cue, the legs (lower limb spirals) are in Grounding mode while the forearms and hands can be Opening, or Grounding into one another. These modes are consistent features that guide the 5F in all movement. Further research reveals that biomechanical principles based on coupling, such as the scapulohumeral rhythm, are embraced in each of the filaments. In the effort to unite the classical with what our bodies know to be true from experience, we are fostering the context of a multidimensional tubular tissue matrix rotating in coordination with the breath.

Recall that the *meso* is the tissue substrate that gives rise to the structural myofascial system. It

Teaching point

 Bear in mind that the standard cue most of us have used or heard at some point in the arms-overhead movement is for students to keep their shoulders down. When we look at how the scapula has to move to elevate the arms, it becomes apparent that if we try to keep them down, we'll be in for an impossible and quite painful task! The scapula upwardly rotates during the elevation of the humerus after 30 degrees as part of the scapulohumeral rhythm.

What other cues can we use to keep the shoulder filament spacious around the neck during practice? If we aim to remain accurate without resorting to jargon, in my experience, the most straightforward cue is the best one. "Keep the shoulders soft" is one of my favorites. "Draw the upper arm bones into the shoulder sockets" is another. "Rotate the arms up and the spine down" is an idea.

is wrapped in *ectodermal* skin and envelopes the *endodermal* depths in the torso walls. The 5F are seated in tissue arising from this substrate, with the **deep fasciae** intrinsic to it.

The Stecco family write about the convergence of spirality in their work on the Fascial Manipulation Technique.[65] Fig. 2.46 shows the Stecco "Fourteen Body Segments" model, that demonstrates the convergence of myofascial elements involved in fourteen functional segments of the body.[66] Their work reveals more about how all fascial segments participate in body-wide spirality both structurally and functionally.

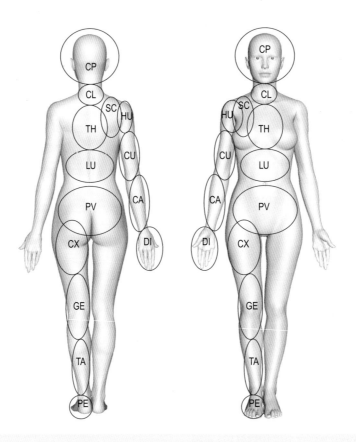

FIGURE 2.46

Fourteen body segments of the fascial system. CP: Caput, CL: Collum, TH: Thorax, LU: Lumbar, PV: Pelvis, SC: Scapula, HU: Humerus, CU: Cubitus, CA: Carpus, DI: Digits, CX: Coxa, GE: Genu, TA: Tarsus, PE: Pes. Each segment comprises joint(s), portions of muscles that move the joint(s), and the fascia surrounding these muscle fibers. Latin terms are used to distinguish these segments from simple joints.

(Redrawn with permission from Stecco C, Stecco AN. Fascial manipulation. 2012. https://www.researchgate.net/publication/288215443_Fascial_manipulation)

 Filamentous matter

A filament is a fine thread. Filamentous matter ranges from carbon nanotubes to filamentous proteins of biologic structure such as collagen. These are responsible for the exceptional strength of our tissues,[67] especially those of the fascial matrix where collagen is the star player. When we think of working with the deep fascia on a practical level, adjusting ourselves and our students

The Five Filaments

in asana, the material we're working with is composed of very fine threads both subtle and gross; fluidic to firm.

The term "filament" works as a reference to the bundles of filaments as we experience the polymorphism (many shapes) of deep fasciae around the joint complexes described in our rubric. The filaments are not only capable of shape-shifting, but also changing densities and states as liquid crystalline filamentous matter in motion. We need to factor in the interplay of innervation as the filaments of neural tissue are structurally spiral bound and contribute to the model as part of the fascial matrix.[68]

> This filamentous anatomy makes more sense of our earliest roundness. The embryo doesn't have a separate clavicle or a shoulder blade and glenohumeral joint as such. It has a suite of cartilaginous tissues (placeholders for the future formation of bone) with potential to become thicker, harder and denser at their core. We thus originate with a girdle that rotates when it moves.
>
> **Joanne Avison**

During yoga practice, we invite tissue to almost manipulate itself with smooth and rhythmic continuity from the inside out. We can employ any language to describe the invitation; I like Long's "Engage the prime movers to sculpt the pose and polish it with the synergists" (from p. 21 of the Bandha Yoga Codex[69]). Sometimes I describe it as micromovement, other times simply as wiggling. However you choose to describe it, intentional movement links profoundly into the web of rotatory kinematics of the helical tubular matrix. On the mat, we live in a place where the biology of motion integrates the energy as inseparable, rhythmical dialects.

The 5F rubric is a codification of constraints that originated during embryological development as the limbs spiraled into place. These ideas are an approach to anatomy for yoga. This is not a new style of yoga; merely a way to approach anatomy that is based on nature and guides us gently across the divide between 2D part-thinking and 3D-and-beyond systems of natural, non-linear, biologic forms. In other words, you and me on our mats! Flip to Chapter 4 to see these ideas come to life in formal asana, as demonstrated by Sarah Hatcher.

General ideas about the Five Filaments:

The 5F is an integrated approach to postural anatomy.

- The potential ways of playing with this rubric of particular spiral sets are limitless.

- The pairs of spirals in flow express from-center-outward and from-outward-into-center motion (integrating breath).

- Regions of the body-wide network have more self-limiting action when they are appropriately loaded and can naturally become stiffer/stronger.

- Yoga postures can progress in spirals toward increasingly sustainable states; this might look like extreme gymnastics but can be genuinely therapeutic with appropriate self-referencing skills.

- As the postures advance, the available rotation depth can increase accordingly, given appropriate constraints.

- Limb spirals are continuous into the trunk (axial matrix).

- Spirality is not representative of a discrete anatomical system; instead, it is observed in the body-wide transanatomical patterns at every size scale.

- The spirals are guides for directionally oriented shape-change.

- The 5F involve countless, continuous rotations through the limbs and torso in continuity (CKCs).

- In every style of yoga (in all their stylistic differences) the body and limb rotation patterns are based on spiral CKC biomotion.

- These rotation/spiral patterns follow the same grain in everybody no matter what level of yoga, age, gender, ethnicity, or level of fitness.

- Rotating in these patterns increases the space (sukha) around and flows with the fibrocartilages instead of against them, thus minimizing injury.

- Spiral action is a compelling basis for instruction because spirality and rotation tend to have the most significant positive effect with minimal intervention.

2.8 Guiding the glide

Understanding the embryonic roots of spiral movement in asana is essential because it is universally applicable to all styles of yoga. Tubular structure at the macro level allows joint systems to glide harmoniously, preserving the congruence and thus maximizing the resilience of their delicate inner surfaces. As we come to embrace the closed couplings and their kinematic dynamism, we can reconcile these with ancient yogic subtle body principles. In that moment of integration, a fresh perspective on functional anatomy emerges.

What we are doing here is pointing to a rubric of rotation, one that integrates aspects of anatomy especially relevant to yoga practitioners. This

space (kha) is never empty; it is a virtual space. It is a de facto element of anatomy in its own right. Spirality in anatomy draws emphasis around spaciousness, that is to say, regions of potential motion *appropriately constrained.*

heyaṁ duḥkham-anāgatam
The suffering which has not yet come should be avoided.

Patanjali, *Yoga Sutras*, 2.16

Learning to stiffen the spirals can help us reinforce our sleeves of stability, intelligently calibrating the matrix to allow shapes that appear only to involve flexibility. Crucially, this sleeving can provide a kind of brace (we might call it an appropriate tubular constraint) that is protective, even as part of increasingly extreme postures, as deformations from which we reform instinctively.

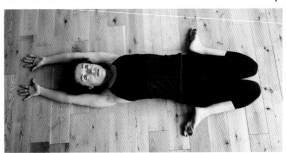

FIGURE 2.47

Postural yoga can be a playground of rotation where "rules" get bent. Paryangāsana (sometimes Paryankāsana, from *paryanka*, Sanskrit for "couch") from the Advanced (B) Series of Ashtanga Vinyasa Yoga. This is essentially reclined W-sitting with dorsiflexion, a therapeutic position given the right circumstance yet it goes "against" the Five Filaments rubric and is potentially devastating without adequate experience!

(Demonstrated by Amy Hughes)

The Five Filaments

Key concept 11

A spiral approach to anatomy emphasizes the importance of virtual space, or continuity, resilience and openness, within the harmonious whole.

ⓘ *Trans-leverage*

Considering the bones as space-makers rather than levers opens up new ways of experiencing movement through understanding the structure that permits and promotes it. Mindful, rotational movement can protect the more vulnerable fibrocartilages found within the joints, such as the meniscus of the knee and the labrum in the hip and shoulder. Without spiral biomotion, we would never even make it out of the womb.*

In this sense, the 5F rubric reconciles with classical principles of functional anatomy and biomechanics. Here, they evolve into something more congruent with our self-assembly as soft-matter, self-developing creatures.

Our bodies manage movement globally, whereas classical models attribute kinematics to kinetic leverage and other forces measured locally. And that rounds us back to the point: using all the technical, reductionist language to get our heads around the pieces of the puzzle does mean that we might temporarily lose the big picture. My intention in this book is to see the trees *and* the forest *at the same time* as we boldly embrace the integration of parts-list with the idea of whole-body attenuation.

*Head to my blog at karenkirkness.com/ blog/pelvifemoralrhythm for more about the pelvifemoral rhythm, the cardinal movements of birth, and other rotatory mechanisms inherent to the kinematics of humans.

Key concept 12

The 5F rubric adopts and embraces many recognizable models of classical biomechanics such as the scapulohumeral rhythm, while contextualizing them as part of a more profound expression of rotation – innate to our forming.

The 5F are like stockings for all these so-called biomechanical rhythms and couplings. We need these stockings because the terminology and technical jargon gets stuck and keeps us in a deadlock over details that will never resonate with real life. They can't – such terms are based on linear (therefore non-biological) forms. Notice that there isn't just one spiral for each limb; instead, the arms and legs operate as paired, double helices. This pairing of opposites (within which spiral oppositions reside) accommodates the push–pull required for our human homeostatic system to maintain itself as such. It's how we hug.

ⓘ *Firmness, the friend of yogis*

It has to be said: stiffness has a lousy reputation in yoga. But we need to get our heads around appropriate stiffness as an essential facet of shape-making. Without sufficient rigidity, or firmness, there is no support for the give, no bounce back from the deformation. Stiffness makes our bodies *al dente* rather than limp like a soggy noodle.

CHAPTER TWO

Stockings stuffed with spirals is an oversimplification, but to me, it is a welcome relief from all the technical talk about the anatomy of levers. I lost myself in terminology for several years as I grappled with anatomical principles, until I gave myself permission to drop the jargon and stay close to the pure experience. The principle itself is so simple: everything in anatomy wraps around in spirals, creating tubular structures. And what is the defining characteristic of a tube? Let's shift gears as we head into the next chapter and take a walk with yoga theory, over terrain in which that question gains traction and pretty much answers itself.

The human soul has sojourned in lower and higher forms, migrating from one to another according to the samskaras or impressions, but it is only in the highest form as a human being that it attains to freedom.

Swami Vivekananda[70]

References

1   Renshaw I, Davids KW. Task constraints. In: Eklund R, Tenenbaum G, editors. Encyclopedia of Sport and Exercise Psychology. Los Angeles: Sage Publications Inc; 2014. p. 734–7.

2   Mennell JMM. Joint pain: diagnosis and treatment using manipulative techniques. Little, Brown; 1964.

3   Iyengar BKS. Light on the Yoga Sutras of Patanjali. HarperCollins Publishers; 2012.

4   Tittel K. Muscle Slings in Sport: Analysing Movements in Various Disciplines from a Functional-Anatomical Point of View. Kiener Verlag; 2015.

5   DeRosa C, Porterfield JA. Anatomical linkages and muscle slings of the lumbopelvic region. In: Vleeming A, Mooney V, Stoeckart R, Wilson P, editors. Movement, Stability & Lumbopelvic Pain (Second Edition). Edinburgh: Churchill Livingstone; 2007. p. 47–62.

6   Shaparenko PF, Pshenichnyi NF. [Principle of spiral arrangement of the skeletal muscles of humans and animals]. Arkhiv Anatomii, Gistologii i Embriologii. 1988;94(6):55–9.

7   Myers TW. Anatomy Trains: Myofascial Meridians for Manual and Movement Therapists (Third Edition). Edinburgh: Churchill Livingstone; 2014. p. 332.

8   Maraziotis IA, Perantonis S, Dragomir A, Thanos D. K-Nets: clustering through nearest neighbors networks. Pattern Recognition. 2019;88:470–81.

9   Wang D, Lee K, Guo J, Yang C. Adaptive knee joint exoskeleton based on biological geometries. IEEE/ASME Transactions on Mechatronics. 2014;19(4):1268–78.

10 Cortés J, Siméon T. Sampling-based motion planning under kinematic loop-closure constraints. In: Erdmann M, Overmars M, Hsu D, van der Stappen F, editors. Algorithmic Foundations of Robotics VI. Berlin, Heidelberg: Springer Berlin Heidelberg; 2005. p. 75–90.

11 Ivaldi FAM, Morasso P, Zaccaria R. Kinematic networks. Biological Cybernetics. 1988;60(1):1–16.

12 Levin S, de Solórzano SL, Scarr G. The significance of closed kinematic chains to biological movement and dynamic stability. Journal of Bodywork and Movement Therapies. 2017;21(3):664–72.

13 Olsen AM. A mobility-based classification of closed kinematic chains in biomechanics

and implications for motor control. The Journal of Experimental Biology. 2019;222(21):jeb195735.

14   Lewis S. A new kind of coupling. Nature Reviews Neuroscience. 2020;21(4):182.

15   Ermentrout B, Park Y, Wilson D. Recent advances in coupled oscillator theory. Philosophical Transactions of the Royal Society A: Mathematical, Physical and Engineering Sciences. 2019;377(2160):20190092.

16   Cohen AH, Holmes PJ, Rand RH. The nature of the coupling between segmental oscillators of the lamprey spinal generator for locomotion: a mathematical model. Journal of Mathematical Biology. 1982;13(3):345–69.

17   Neu JC. Coupled Chemical oscillators. SIAM Journal on Applied Mathematics. 1979;37(2):307–15.

18   Ren L, Liang Y. Biological couplings: classification and characteristic rules. Science in China Series E: Technological Sciences. 2009;52:2791–800.

19   Winfree AT. Biological rhythms and the behavior of populations of coupled oscillators. Journal of Theoretical Biology. 1967;16(1):15–42.

20   Stankovski T, Pereira T, McClintock P, Stefanovska A. Coupling functions: dynamical interaction mechanisms in the physical, biological and social sciences. Philosophical Transactions of the Royal Society A: Mathematical, Physical and Engineering Sciences. 2019;377:20190039.

21   El Khamlichi C, Reverchon-Assadi F, Hervouet-Coste N, et al. Bioluminescence resonance energy transfer as a method to study protein-protein interactions: application to g protein coupled receptor biology. Molecules. 2019;24(3):537.

22   Zhang Y, Liu C, Balaeff A, et al. Biological charge transfer via flickering resonance. Proceedings of the National Academy of Sciences. 2014;111(28):10049–54.

23   Vaschillo EG, Vaschillo B, Pandina RJ, Bates ME. Resonances in the cardiovascular system caused by rhythmical muscle tension. Psychophysiology. 2011;48(7):927–36.

24   Taylor JA, Carr DL, Myers CW, Eckberg DL. Mechanisms underlying very-low-frequency RR-interval oscillations in humans. Circulation. 1998;98(6):547–55.

25   Maturana A, Van Haasteren G, Piuz I, et al. Spontaneous calcium oscillations control c-fos transcription via the serum response element in neuroendocrine cells. The Journal of Biological Chemistry. 2002;277(42):39713–21.

26   Grattan David R, Akopian Armen N. Oscillating from Neurosecretion to multitasking dopamine neurons. Cell Reports. 2016;15(4):681–2.

27   Avison JS. Yoga: Fascia, Anatomy and Movement. Handspring Publishing; 2015. p. 376.

28   Theise ND, d'Inverno M. Understanding cell lineages as complex adaptive systems. Blood Cells, Molecules, and Diseases. 2004;32(1):17–20.

29   Preise R, Biggs R, De Vos A, Folke C. Social-ecological systems as complex adaptive systems: organizing principles for advancing

research methods and approaches. Ecology and Society. 2018;23(4):46.

30 Shafir T, Tsachor RP, Welch KB. Emotion regulation through movement: unique sets of movement characteristics are associated with and enhance basic emotions. Frontiers in Psychology. 2016;6:2030.

31 Hannay KM, Forger DB, Booth V. Macroscopic models for networks of coupled biological oscillators. Science Advances. 2018;4(8):e1701047.

32 Juhan D, Quasha G, Dychtwald K. Job's Body: A Handbook for Bodywork. Station Hill Press; 1987.

33 Shoulders MD, Raines RT. Collagen structure and stability. Annual Review of Biochemistry. 2009;78:929–58.

34 Ramachandran GN, Kartha G. Structure of collagen. Nature. 1954;174(4423):269–70.

35 Kozyavkin VI. Kozyavkin Method for Cerebral Palsy Treatment. Available from: http://www.reha.lviv.ua/.

36 Levin DSM, Martin DD-C. Biotensegrity: The mechanics of fascia. In: Schleip R, Huijing P, Findley T, editors. Fascia: The Tensional Network of the Human Body. Elsevier; 2012. p. 138–55.

37 Gordon JE. Structures: Or Why Things Don't Fall Down. New York: De Capa Press; 1978.

38 Friend J. Anusara Yoga Teacher Training Manual. Anusara Press; 2009.

39 Askar O. Surgical anatomy of the aponeurotic expansions of the anterior abdominal wall. Annals of the Royal College of Surgeons of England. 1977;59:313–31.

40 Scarr G. Fascial hierarchies and the relevance of crossed-helical arrangements of collagen to changes in the shape of muscles. Journal of Bodywork and Movement Therapies. 2016;20(2):377–87.

41 Gracovetsky S. Stability or controlled instability? Movement, Stability & Lumbopelvic Pain. 2007;279–94.

42 Levin SM. Personal communication. 2018.

43 Washburn SL. Tools and human evolution. Scientific American. 1960;203:63–75.

44 Jockusch H, Dress A. Re: Jockusch and Dress 'From sphere to torus: a topological view of the metazoan body plan' (Bull. Math.Biol. (2003) 65, 57–65). Bulletin of Mathematical Biology. 2004;66:1455.

45 Rapoport D. Klein bottle logophysics, self-reference, heterarchies, genomic topologies, harmonics and evolution. Part II: Non-orientability, cognition, Chemical topology and eversions in nature. Quantum Biosystems. 2016;7:74–106.

46 Rapoport DL. Klein bottle logophysics: a unified principle for non-linear systems, cosmology, geophysics, biology, biomechanics and perception. Journal of Physics: Conference Series. 2013;437:012024.

47 Bissell MJ. Goodbye flat biology – time for the 3rd and the 4th dimensions. Journal of Cell Science. 2017;130(1):3–5.

48 West G, Brown J, Enquist B. The fourth dimension of life: fractal geometry and allometric scaling of organisms. Science (New York, NY). 1999;284:1677–9.

49 Gracovetsky S. Linking the spinal engine with the legs: a theory of human gait.

Movement, Stability and Low Back Pain – The Essential Role of the Pelvis. January 1997.

50 Lovett R. A contribution to the study of the mechanics of the spine. American Journal of Anatomy. 2005;2:457–62.

51 Edwards BC. Combined movements of the lumbar spine: examination and clinical significance. Australian Journal of Physiotherapy. 1979;25(4):147–52.

52 Cholewicki J, Crisco JJ 3rd, Oxland TR, et al. Effects of posture and structure on three-dimensional coupled rotations in the lumbar spine. A biomechanical analysis. Spine. 1996;21(21):2421–8.

53 Lovett RW. A contribution to the study of the mechanics of the spine. American Journal of Anatomy. 1903;2(4):457–62.

54 Gibbons J. Functional Anatomy of the Pelvis and the Sacroiliac Joint: A Practical Guide. North Atlantic Books; 2017.

55 Panjabi MM, Brand RA, White AA. Three-dimensional flexibility and stiffness properties of the human thoracic spine. Journal of Biomechanics. 1976;9(4):185–92.

56 Fryette HH. Principles of Osteopathic Technic. Academy of Applied Osteopathy; 1980.

57 Panjabi MM, Krag MH, White AA 3rd, Southwick WO. Effects of preload on load displacement curves of the lumbar spine. The Orthopedic Clinics of North America. 1977;8(1):181–92.

58 Gracovetsky S. The Spinal Engine. Aardvark Global Publishing; 1988.

59 Ogawa T, Sato T, Ogata T, et al. Rhythmic arm swing enhances patterned locomotor-like muscle activity in passively moved lower extremities. Physiological Reports. 2015;3(3):e12317.

60 Bruijn SM, Meijer OG, Beek PJ, van Dieën JH. The effects of arm swing on human gait stability. The Journal of Experimental Biology. 2010;213(Pt 23):3945–52.

61 Kanstad SO, Kononoff A. Gravity-driven horizontal locomotion: theory and experiment. Proceedings of the Royal Society A: Mathematical, Physical and Engineering Sciences. 2015;471(2181):20150287.

62 Earls J, Myers T. Born to Walk: Myofascial Efficiency and the Body in Movement. North Atlantic Books; 2014.

63 Stokes IAF, Wilder DG, Frymoyer JW, Pope MH. Assessment of patients with low-back pain by biplanar radiographic measurement of intervertebral motion. Spine. 1981;6(3):233–40.

64 Mu Z, Zhang Q, Yang GY, et al. Development of an Improved rotational orthosis for walking with arm swing and active ankle control. Frontiers in Neurorobotics. 2020;14:17.

65 Stecco C, Day JA. The fascial manipulation technique and its biomechanical model: a guide to the human fascial system. International Journal of Therapeutic Massage & Bodywork. 2010;3(1):38–40.

66 Stecco C, Stecco AN. Fascial manipulation. 2012. Available at: https://www.researchgate.net/publication/288215443_Fascial_manipulation.

67 Martinez-Torres C, Burla F, Alkemade C, Koenderink GH. Revealing the assembly

of filamentous proteins with scanning transmission electron microscopy. PloS One. 2019;14(12):e0226277.

68 Jones JB, Safinya CR. Interplay between liquid crystalline and isotropic gels in self-assembled neurofilament networks. Biophysical Journal. 2008;95(2):823–35.

69 Long R. Anatomy for Hip Openers and Forward Bends. Bandha Yoga; 2011.

70 Ashrama A. What Religion Is: In the Words of Swami Vivekananda. Advhaita Ashrama; 1985.

3.1 Steady and comfortable — 92

3.2   A hole in the middle — 93

3.2 Gross and subtle — 96

3.4 Gastronomical — 101

3.5 The mystery — 103

3.6 Prana — 105

3.7 Srotamsi: many rivers — 107

3.8 Akasha by Kate O'Donnell — 110

3.9 Srotas: subtle kinematics — 111

3.10 Weaving threads — 115

3.11 Subtle body, spiral bound — 118

3.12 Vayu — 120

3.13 Integration — 125

Srotas-kinematics (tubular movement)

3

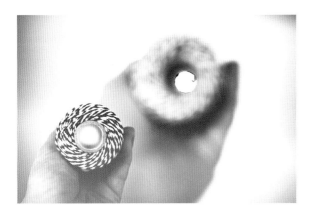

FIGURE 3.1

Two depths of field: one with a focus on the positive space of the tube, the other with a focus on the hole

Then Gargi (daughter of Vachaknu) posed her questions. "Yajnavalkya," she said, "tell me; since this whole world is woven back and forth on water, on what, then, is water woven back and forth?"

Brihadaranyaka Upanishad, 3.8[1]

Key concepts

1   Asana by Patanjali's definition is that which is easy (*sukha*) and steady/comfortable (sthiram).

2   The concept of *sukha* (spaciousness) is fundamental to asana.

3   The 5F rubrics show how the body's spiral movement patterns maximize spaciousness; working within these constraints can help yogis progress in the safest and most energy-efficient way.

4   Comparing the symmetry and shape of animals helps us understand the bigger picture of animal development as a valuable resource in understanding our natural structural template.

5   All animals develop embryologically from a single hole; in complex animals, the hole eventually continues right through the cell mass to the other side, forming the gut tube.

6   A srotas is a tube in Ayurvedic anatomy.

7   Each *srotas* has a root (*sroto mula*), a passage (*sroto marga*), and a mouth (*mukha*).

8   Every living body is a physiology of tubules (*srotamsi shareera*) made up of systems of tubes (*vaha srotas*) that each carry different substances/information.

9   Srotas-kinematics (tube movement) is a new term that describes the body's natural spiral movement and formation patterns, influencing all tissue and especially relevant in the tissue of the *mamsa vaha srotas* (myofascial system).

CHAPTER THREE

10 The *mamsa vaha srotas* is the tissue level from Ayurveda that encompasses the structural myofascial system.

11 While the body is alive, it is subtle; so-called subtle body anatomy is vital for teachers and students of yoga.

12 The Ida and Pingala course between the nostrils (Ida, left, and Pingala, right) and the base of the spine, spiraling around the filament of Sushumna like a double spiral staircase.

13 Vayu are the "pranic airs" or "winds" that are directionally oriented flows of Prana through the subtle srotamsi: the *nadis*.

14 Vayu-breath-bandha is a basic unit of practice within the subtle body; understanding this triumvirate is a foundation of integrated anatomy for yoga.

15 Srotas-kinematics explains routes of sensation and force that interplay throughout the *srotamsi shareera* (body matrix).

16 The *vayu prana* and *apana* refer to inward pull and outward push, respectively. They have a special relationship (dynamic reciprocity) that relates to the synergic, expansion-retraction rhythm of the breath.

3.1 Steady and comfortable

Asana practice is a playground for experiencing theory. As we look beyond all the theory and practice of shape-making, why would anyone bother with the effort in the first place? What might motivate people to experiment with different ways of moving? I'm certainly not the first to point this out: seeking spaciousness and ease in our bodies is a common thread not just amongst yogis. Movement and **therapeutic modalities** are all tuned into the fundamental idea of finding spaciousness.

As we mature, yogis often look more intensely for meaning and guidance from source texts on the journey towards spaciousness, and Patanjali's advice for asana practice is straightforward:

sthira-sukham-āsanam
Asana is steady and comfortable.

Patanjali, Yoga Sutras, 2.46

By this definition, referenced simply as *sthira-sukham*, asana is simply a state of steadiness and comfort. The etymology of *sukha* comes out of the chariot. Ancient Indo-European peoples influenced customs across the globe from India to Ireland. The Aryans brought their horse and cattle customs to India, and thus the chariot made its way into Indian culture as an essential vehicle, both practically and allegorically. The *Bhagavad Gita* is one such example, using the chariot as a rich metaphor for personal transformation (see p. 303 of the Eknath translation).[2]

Key concepts 1

Asana by Patanjali's definition is that which is easy (*sukha*) and steady/comfortable (*sthiram*).

Srotas-kinematics (tubular movement)

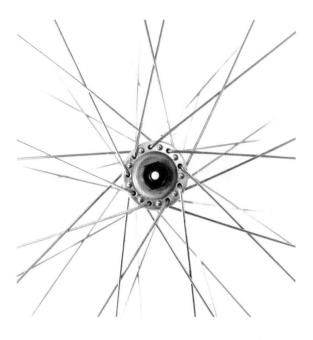

FIGURE 3.2

Sukha-dukha: the dvandva of physical pleasure and pain is represented allegorically in the quality of the axle hole.

The word breaks down to *su* (good) and *kha* (hole). It refers to the quality of a good chariot wheel, one with a "good axle-hole". Sukha is the foil of *duḥkha*, similarly translated to "bad hole", which means "bad space" or "pain". Where a chariot wheel articulates with the axle is a metaphor for the joint space (and other potential spaces both gross and subtle).

Sukha: A movement that is biomotional results in sukha, or pleasure, bliss, good space, a sense of ease.

Duḥkha (dukha): A movement that is not biomotional results in duḥkha, or pain, lacking space and locked in *conflict*.

Biomotionally appropriate = sukha.

Biomotionally inappropriate = duhkha.

Khecara: moving in the ether

Kha is the void, philosophically inviting the nothingness that precedes distinction. Here it is referring (in the physical sense) to the dorsal cavity in which flows **Suṣumṇā-nāḍī**. Finding kha, the hole, or space, is the critical pursuit for yogis, intrinsic to all forms of practice; be they physical or philosophical. Many hatha yoga texts refer to the unlocking or removing of obstacles, so the consciousness floods toward itself, into the nothingness from which it came. *Khecara* is the state of "moving in the ether".

One may question the validity of invisible structures such as nadis and vayus; however, in **Āyurveda**, yoga's allied science, all components of existence are considered in understanding the body, which includes the subtle energy of space. Because of its origin from the space element, bodily channels are also known as kha, which is a synonym for spaciousness.[3]

We saw it in the first chapter as the embryo folded in itself to become a tube, and around its axis to continue the process. The tubular concept is fundamental to existence from an Ayurvedic point of view, and what a tube needs to be a tube is a hole in the middle – a spaciousness around which it forms.

3.2 A hole in the middle

This pursuit of sukha happens in yoga as we learn to sense and feel the rotational, wrapping motion of the tissue. Take, for example, the

CHAPTER THREE

scapulohumeral rhythm discussed previously. Where the movement of elevating the humerus is accompanied by the gliding upward rotation of the scapula, bones maintain adequate spaciousness (sukha) between the roof of the acromion process and the humeral head for the soft tissues of the rotator cuff; thus, there is sukha. Further, we learn

FIGURE 3.3

The subacromial space. (A) Recall that two chiral coils (meaning of opposite handedness) come together to make a third entity: a spacious tube. (B) In the shoulder, the subacromial space is normally occupied by the rotator cuff soft tissues, here represented by the green 3D-printed supraspinatus muscle in situ. (C) We use the Shoulder Filament to reinforce this spaciousness especially through the subacromial space. (D) The hole in the middle is metaphorically referring to the spaciousness created when the two directionalities are balanced (grounding and opening/internal and external rotation).

to draw in the spiraled tissues, a subtle motion I cue with "suck the upper arm bones into the shoulder sockets" when I'm teaching backbends. Like unlocking the finger trap, we "untension" the cross-ply to increase spaciousness, allowing for more carefully constrained rotation without strain.

Where the bones are unable to glide and rotate due to an imbalance of forces, the result is usually pain. In simplified terms, the biomotion of moving in spiral patterns creates a kind of wrapping-around action that allows for *gliding* rather than *stretching*. In asana, we are always looking for sukha, assuming that the body network can self-regulate if given sufficient allowance. Sukha is related to the middle path, *sattva guna*, or balance.[4]

Key concepts 2

The concept of *sukha* (spaciousness) is fundamental to asana.

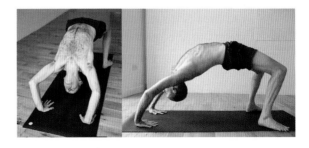

FIGURE 3.4

Urdhvadanurasana with duhkha with elbows out is often a sign of duhkha.

(Demonstration by Simon Kirkness)

Srotas-kinematics (tubular movement)

The bodily systems seem to flow more freely and give rise to increasing movement inside supportive tunnels of tissue. In other words, feeling into their original patterning seems to nourish those same patterns. Postures that appear very advanced *can* simply be an extension of what may be possible for a khecara, a yogi moving deeper into their self-supported spaciousness. Patanjali provides remarkably little advice on the stylistic aspects of asana, but what guidance exists speaks volumes: asana is sthira-sukham (steady and comfortable).

In this sense, *spaciousness* is simply that which can move or can be moved through/around. As round things, it serves us to consider this literally and metaphorically. And here we get to the crux: *how can moving my physical body give me access to something called a subtle body?*

Moving within the rotational tension-compression matrix of tubes and progressing

further in body intelligence means learning to facilitate spaciousness, or what we might call *structurally supported give*. Through coupled functions, we receive the means to avoid future suffering and increase the circulation of *prana* that we will explore in this chapter.

Key concepts 3

The 5F rubrics show how the body's spiral movement patterns maximize spaciousness; working within these constraints can help yogis progress in the safest and most energy-efficient way.

The roundness or spaciousness through the middle of tubular structure allows it to resonate with the experience of oscillation, what we might call Prana, energy, and Chi. Given how all the tubes are filamentous, embedded in webs and threads (on a spectrum of gooey to hard), it may be useful to think of this vibration as music. Whether we are referring to the drumskin over the tubular drum or movement through a tubular wind instrument, motion flows through the structure, as well as within and around it.

Yoga techniques improve the resonance of the bodily tubes and strings in the same way we would tune a musical instrument – based upon the pre-tensioned nature of all aspects of the soft tissue architecture. This tubularity was established in the very first days of life, giving rise to a meta-structure that is tubular from the micro to the macro and from subtle to gross and back to subtle. In the next sections, we'll continue talk of tubes and see the tubularity arise embryologically, and then consider how it is embodied in an Ayurvedic anatomical perspective.

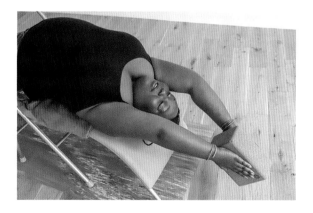

FIGURE 3.5

Supporting the Opening Shoulder Spiral, finding sukha.

(Demonstration by Fadzai Mwakutuya)

CHAPTER THREE

3.3 Gross and subtle

If you're starting to suspect that this anatomy book is more concerned with the potential space of body materials than with the actual muscles and bones themselves, then we're on the same page. But don't the basics of anatomy teach us that muscles pull on the bones to make movement happen? What about all those attachments and insertions we spent years trying to memorize?

It turns out that things in the body aren't so easily segregated. As you might have noticed already, the story of anatomy involves much more than the discrete (meaning separate) actions of muscles pulling on bones. The story transcends the (more recently) venerated fascial system. Our story involves becoming tuned in – to the tube.

This tubification isn't something I'm just making up, nor is it anything particularly "woo-woo" or novel. All we have to do is keep going back to embryonic development. It reveals just how similar we are to every other species (and the conservation of fundamental geometric strategies which are beyond the scope of this book, but valuable to the shift we are invited to make).[5,6]

It is useful to pan out and contextualize our species. The big-picture journey we inherit from our ancestors is even more astonishing for its ancient and continuing tubular theme. It is a story that we share in common with the body plans of other multicellular organisms.

Key concepts 4

Comparing the symmetry and shape of animals helps us understand the bigger picture of animal development as a valuable resource in understanding our natural structural template.

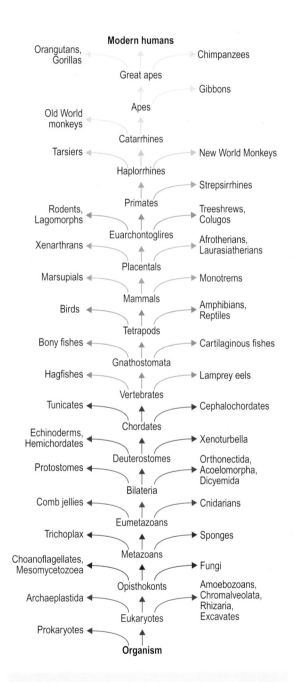

FIGURE 3.6

Phylogenic Tree: a diagram of selected evolutionary relationships.

Srotas-kinematics (tubular movement)

Anus first

Body plans are a basis of categorizing, exploring, and comparing the evolutionary development (evo-devo) of life forms. How life organizes itself is evident in what happens during embryogenesis. Step one is a very levelling action: every animal has to reorganize the spherical nature of its first moments to grow (known as symmetry breaking): thus, chirality appears.[7–11] All in, it is the (w)hole that matters. This is the **blastopore** – the keyhole through which *flow* can spiral through the sphere.

A hole by any other name: the blastopore

Just after implantation, a dimple appears in amphibian embryos as a dorsal lip. The dorsal lip is widely considered to be the equivalent of the primitive node in humans. The primitive node is contiguous with the primitive pit, like a raised rim or backstop. The pit is the "hole" (blastopore) through which migrating cells from the epiblast invaginate.

These early movers pour into/along the streak, effectively burrowing their way into becoming the notochord (the rod-like mass of mesenchymal cells introduced in Chapter 1). In chick embryos, the same inductive hole is referred to as the "Spemann Mangold organizer" (named after the early 20th century embryologists who described its significance). There are many names for this vortex, the first portal that draws into it the cells that swirl to become a tube that induces the formation of more tubes.

This tubularity is related to the formation of Animalia's more complex organisms, ones with true tissues: the **eumetazoans** (everything that isn't a sponge, basically). Of these tissue-sporting eumetazoans, there are two broad divisions: the Radiata and Bilateria. Radiata are classified by radial symmetry and two germ layers in the embryo, and Bilateria by bilateral symmetry and three germ layers. Bilateria are further divided into the clades **protostomes** (P) and **deuterostomes** (D), all of whom have a common ancestor and a blastopore that can't wait to make itself useful.

Game of pores

The fate of the blastopore is one way of classifying the body plans of animals. Recall from Chapter 1 the first infolding of the sphere, as the embryonic disc starts to cave in on itself during gastrulation

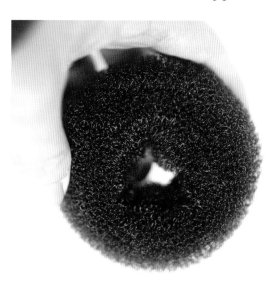

FIGURE 3.7

The "bun doughnut" is used for styling hair into voluminous buns... and in my world elegantly represents the triumphant blastopore.

CHAPTER THREE

to form a longish dimple. In development, negative space is every bit as relevant (if not more so) than the so-called positive space induced by the dimple. This dimple, the primitive pit (blastopore), becomes a funnel for the migration of cells down the spiral staircase described there. Picture the water vortex as you drain your bathtub: so swirls the invaginating primitive ectoderm through the pit (blastopore) from along the primitive streak. This, the nodal flow, describes the spiraling movement of migrating cells that continues breaking the symmetry and ushers further embryonic rotations into play.

The flow of cells from the epiblast (primitive ectoderm) will differentiate and prime the endoderm for its next act. The adventures of the blastopore will play out as the uniting characteristic of the Ps and Ds: a true body cavity (coelom). This is momentous for the Bilateria, as what the hole does next will determine if the organism is to be a P or a D.

Protostomes means "first mouth" in Greek. The Ps are the organisms in which the blastopore develops into the mouth of the organism, such as molluscs and arthropods. As you might surmise, *deuterostomes* means "second mouth", meaning the mouth comes subsequently. After what, exactly?

The Ds, phylogenetically including us humans, are organisms in which the blastopore develops and subsequently burrows through the folding creature to form the mouth. Evolution has changed somewhat the order of events in our human gut development. The body cavity linings fold around the yolk sac to zip up and enclose the gut tube (remember the burrito ballet from Chapter 1). The primitive human mouth is created as the buccopharyngeal membrane (formed out of the foregut) is perforated during the 4th week of development.

The first hint of the human anus arises before all that, at the caudal (tail) end of the primitive streak. It becomes a membrane, then a cloaca (common chamber for urogenital and anal opening). The anus proper finally opens to the world at about eight weeks, at which point the embryo is considered *toroidal* (**torus**: doughnut-shaped) in structure.

Although the mouth technically perforates before the anus in humans, the primitive streak/node is regarded as the first hole, as part of it does eventually turn into the perforated anus we know and love. Our very own phylum Chordata shares a common Deuterostome ancestor with the starfish (an Echinoderm). All of us: toroidal, tubular, and anus first.

Key concepts 5

All animals develop embryologically from a single hole; in complex animals, the hole eventually continues right through the cell mass to the other side, forming the gut tube.

Srotas-kinematics (tubular movement)

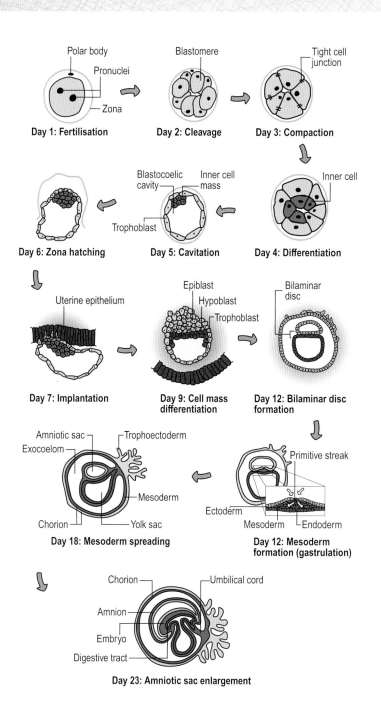

FIGURE 3.8

Embryogenesis.

(Image by Zephyris, labels modified by author. https://creativecommons.org/licenses/by-sa/3.0/deed.en)

Day 1: Fertilisation
- Polar body
- Pronuclei
- Zona

Day 2: Cleavage
- Blastomere

Day 3: Compaction
- Tight cell junction

Day 4: Differentiation
- Inner cell

Day 5: Cavitation
- Blastocoelic cavity
- Inner cell mass
- Trophoblast

Day 6: Zona hatching

Day 7: Implantation
- Uterine epithelium

Day 9: Cell mass differentiation
- Epiblast
- Hypoblast
- Trophoblast

Day 12: Bilaminar disc formation
- Bilaminar disc

Day 12: Mesoderm formation (gastrulation)
- Primitive streak
- Ectoderm
- Mesoderm
- Endoderm

Day 18: Mesoderm spreading
- Amniotic sac
- Exocoelom
- Trophoectoderm
- Mesoderm
- Chorion
- Yolk sac

Day 23: Amniotic sac enlargement
- Chorion
- Umbilical cord
- Amnion
- Embryo
- Digestive tract

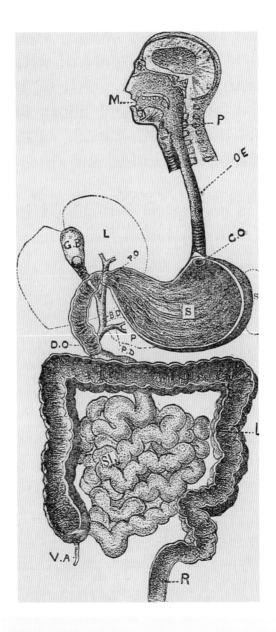

FIGURE 3.9

The gut tube: perforation happens as the anus and mouth become apertures, and in humans, the mouth actually perforates first, at four weeks.

(Walker J. *Anatomy, Physiology and Hygiene*. Boston: Allyn and Bacon; 1900. p. 46)

Torus

The torus is a core shape in sacred geometry. It depicts the form of electromagnetism. It is ubiquitous and has many representations, including an energy vortex that can be described

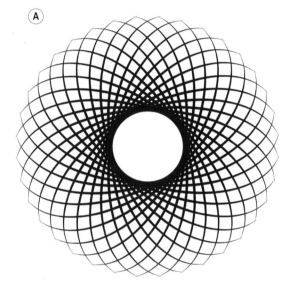

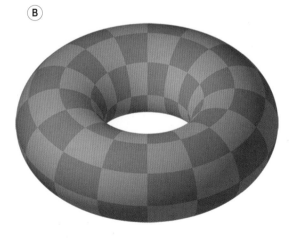

FIGURE 3.10

The torus: topological map of all complex organisms.

by cross-ply logarithmic spirals constantly writhing into and out of themselves. Thinking of it as a doughnut is useful at first. As you get your head around the solidity of that doughnut, you might then have the headspace to consider just its glazy-flaky outer layer. This surface layer, a two-dimensional spread of sweetness, carries with it our interest in the experience of manipulating our surfaces in a dance uniting the inside and outside.

Talking point

The torus is topologically orientable as it has two distinct surfaces that are continuously discrete. There is the doughy inside surface, and there is the surface that meets the air outside the donut (the glazed surface). Look further at the body as a living torus to see that its writhing donut shape describes another kind of inner/outerness. The toroid of our gut tub (a virtual space) is functionally distinct from the area outside the body.

Biologically, we draw the outside inwards and integrate with its material (and vice versa), such as when we consume food and drink and when we breathe and interact with others in our environment. Does this interaction between our inside and outside blur the boundaries between our self-space and the space of others? Here is an important distinction: biologically we are open systems, but biomechanically we remain enclosed within countless, coupled continuities.

3.4 Gastronomical

So why have we dived back into the embryo? In a word: tubes. The formation of the spiraling gut tube is fundamental to anatomy for yoga. The presence of the gut, an ultimately asymmetrical tube within a tube of a bilaterally symmetrical tube, is perhaps the defining characteristic of complex multicellular animals such as ourselves. (The internal organs are another story of spirals and rotations as they come to settle in their developed asymmetrical configuration.) The notochord is much more specialized, appearing only in relatively complex organisms.

The gut, or alimentary canal, is first known as the *archenteron*. It develops various regions of specialization on its route from mouth to anus. With it, we take in food, sort out the nutrition from the waste, process the former and eliminate the latter.

 Spiraling mesogastrium

The stomach appears first as a fusiform dilation (an elongated pouch shape) of the foregut in the 4th gestational week. It distends out of the endoderm and performs a 90° rotation in which the right side moves dorsally, and the left side moves ventrally, taking with it the attendant courses of the vagus nerve. The spiraling of the foregut tube is evident as the dorsal and ventral mesogastrium give rise to the spleen and the liver, respectively.

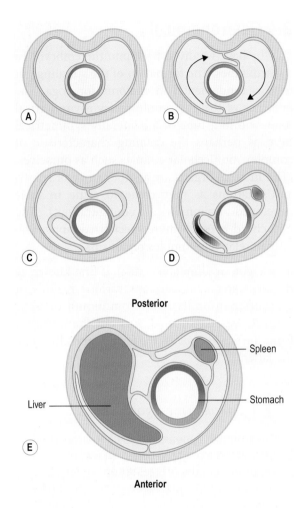

Posterior

Spleen

Liver

Stomach

Anterior

FIGURE 3.11

Spiral mesogastrium. Here you can see the spiraling of the foregut tube as the dorsal and ventral mesogastrium give rise to the spleen and the liver, respectively: (A) the gut tube held in its dorsal (back) and ventral (front) mesogastria; (B-C) rotation continues; (D) the spleen and liver emerge in the ventral and dorsal mesogastria; (E) the organs in their eventual positions.

So, it follows then that we all started as ambitious buttholes? Where can we possibly

go from here? Indeed, seeing tube-making as nature's earliest act is not where we end up, but where we start. And that is good news. Now that we are feeling perhaps a bit humbled, let's take a look at this tube through eyes tuned into subtlety. Here we spiral back to that chasm between subtle and gross, weaving a rope bridge across the divide.

A fiery tube

To the Ayurvedic physicians (acharyas), there is no anatomical structure more critical to human health than the gut, the *māha vaha srotas* (the *maha*, or "great" tube: the gastrointestinal tract). The fire of digestion is viewed as the engine of health and the origin of tissue, holding a balance of subtle constitutional determiners referred to as *doshas*. These three biologic energies, *vata, pitta*, and *kapha*, influence all health outcomes and longevity in every individual.

Anatomy is indeed as subtle as it is gross, and these ancient physicians duly recognized this paradox of seemingly opposite features. The acharyas of Ayurveda went about their consideration of human anatomy and embryology as a function of cosmogony (the origin of the universe and reality). In their world, the body materials are part of a phylogeny of all matter in the universe as it crystallizes from subtle to gross (known as the evolutes of **Prakrti**). Explore the spirality of this process with me in the Online Chapter.

From a modern perspective, the details of these Ayurvedic descriptions often sound esoteric,

Srotas-kinematics (tubular movement)

rooted as they are in cultural mores. However, the overall gist of ancient Eastern physicality links the human body intrinsically to the same principles as found in their ideas of the universe. As the torus is homologous to the body plan of our tube-within-a-tube anatomical structure, Ayurvedic physiology is gut-centric in its approach to health. From my current perspective, the great Ayurvedic classical works such as the *Charaka Samhita*[12] and *Sushruta Samhita*[13] become less like interesting mythology and more like compelling observations that dovetail elegantly with modern developmental biology.

3.5 The mystery

Before we venture further down the rabbit hole, I'll declare my limitations. Although a map ends definitively at its edges, the territory itself is boundless. My broad-brush approach gets us talking about the linking potential of helical couplings and their kinematics. We are looking at the mechanism by which things might be initially (and continuously) connected in the body, and this "everything is connected" message often shows us just how much we don't know.

We are taking in glimpses of embryology to appreciate a selection of subtle body concepts to illuminate our understanding of anatomy. Subtle body processes baulk Western account,[14] and the study of subtlety for its own sake is well worth the exploration.[15,16] Energy fields and quantum models of anatomy are relevant to kinematics, keeping us rooted in organicism (recall that organicism is the idea that what we experience as developed anatomy is emerging through a holistic process originating in the embryo and connected through universal patterns).

Where the subtle body is concerned, I often feel like I'm holding a fragile set of handwritten directions on a wet napkin, so humble is my grasp on what it means to have a body. I don't think that sense of adventuring into uncharted territory will ever be resolved by trying to navigate with the conventional maps.

Anatomy in its gross and subtle aspects hold core questions for us in the yoga world. It isn't just the anatomical information that compels, but the whole concept of knowing: how do we come to learn about ourselves? Where does the story start, and where is it going? On a practical level: what are the circumstantial variations that make some asanas, so easy for some, virtually impossible for others? Many of us go through a phase of memorizing body parts and bagging degrees out of a gnawing hunger to know more.

From my own experience in working with all kinds of body nerds both institutionalized and freelance, I've noticed there is a kind of continuum of knowing. One aspect of this knowledge is personal, and we can feel it in our bones. The other element is abstract, including everything we have memorized or learned from books. This book seeks integration of those forms of knowledge: i.e., to encourage feeling it practically while also appreciating some of the academics. No matter the differences in our respective practices, what unites us is that we want to know the *how* and *why* behind the increasingly detailed anatomical presentations appearing in the instruction of yoga.

The more we study, and the more things we think we know, the danger is we forget that the mystery of life is just that. Its totality is unknowable. So that's the branch from which we

CHAPTER THREE

are all dangling: we can become tricked into believing that the pieces and parts we have managed to memorize are all there is to the puzzle. As someone who has invested much into the academic shades of this anatomy continuum, I'm here to tell you that the scalpel (and theoretical frameworks, for that matter) can get you only so far. At some point, you have to listen to the ultimate instrument of learning beyond words: the Self.

 ## No scalpel required

The term anatomy comes from late Latin *anatomia*, a joining of *ana* with *tomia*, from the Greek root *temnein* "to cut": our understanding of anatomy is thus derived from cutting up dead tissue. This unfortunate order of operations in classical dissection means that in the pursuit of understanding the body, we have to destroy the very qualities that brought it to life. Movement gives us a means of feeling anatomy from the inside out. In this book, we find a route into an understanding of the body, without breaking the skin, by observing surface landmarks and movement patterns in real life.

The Self

Self-reflection is the excellent mystery which has occupied mythology, philosophy, religion, and science for millennia. Who are we? What are we made of, and where did we come from?

Ancient cultures never saw their anatomical origins as separate from the geometry of the cosmos. As many of us now look eastward for our

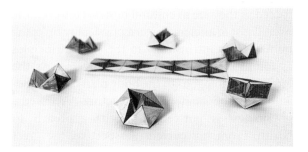

FIGURE 3.12

Flexagons, now in vivid color! We introduced the 3D flexagon in Chapter 1 to get an understanding of constraints (the creases in the paper are the morphological constraints). Here I've colored them to show how these folded paper polygons invaginate themselves topologically, just like the embryo. This in-color example shows how 32 triangles meet into a hexagon that can flex into and around itself continuously in both directions. You can make one yourself using just one sheet of paper, a ruler, a pen and markers. Head to www.karenkirkness.com for instructions on how to make this version.

health advice – physically and spiritually – yoga, Ayurveda, Tai Chi, and **Traditional Chinese Medicine (TCM)** have appeared prominently on the radar of popular lifestyle modalities. These modalities are based on the prevailing view that the human body is intrinsically woven into the fabric of life, part of a vast tapestry that includes all the elements. In this view, the health of any thread comes from inter- and intra-connectedness to the more extensive web.

The shift toward well-being for individuals, families, communities, and the planet at large still tacks against the prevailing winds of the mainstream, and yet the research community offers evidence-based connections between lifestyle and something called "natural health." The literature abounds with research looking at how actions and reactions of behavior are implicated in epigenetic processes that come to bear on health outcomes.[17–21] In making these connections, we can once again see our bodies as reflections of the cosmic whole, rather than separate from the natural world around us.

As we continue this survey of anatomical concepts, let's acknowledge that the body "baulks account."[22] All we can do in the face of this vast unknowableness is accept the mystery for what it is. A playground, a prison, a temple, a vessel: the body is many things to many people. For the yogis ancient and modern, it remains a tubular web of spiraling Prana.

3.6 Prana

Srotomayam hi shariram: the living body is a channel system

The yogic way of understanding anatomy is as a system of tubes animated by **Prāṇa**, *energy,* or *life force.* That's right: the humble tube is what connects Eastern and Western anatomy. Tubes! Their roundness, spirality, chirality, constraints, subtlety, grossness, fractality, invagination, connectivity, stiffness, springiness, glide, biotensegrity, nature of their walls, space inside, weave, wetness, flow-through/over/within: a tube can do it all. As Wainright says about soft-bodied crawlers like the caterpillar, so too are the bodies of vertebrates: "a set of pliant collagenous membranes."[23] In that sense, it is useful to keep the caterpillar in mind.

In the next sections, we'll look at the internal transport system of Hatha and its Ayurvedic anatomy: the **srotas** (singular form, meaning channel or tube). *Srotas, srotamsi* (plural), *srotomaya* (clinical/pathological application) all refer to the tubular nature of the body (*shariram,* or *shareera*). We'll also see how this tubular transport system is understood to be the organ of hearing (*sravanam*) in the Ayurvedic science of life.

Prana (with a capital "P") is the general life force energy that is divided fivefold into five vayu, the specialized directionalities of Prana of which prana (with a lowercase "p") is one.

Key concepts 6

A *srotas* is a tube in Ayurvedic anatomy.

 Vayu

In yoga, the potential directionalities for the flow of this *maha* or great Prana are called *vayu* (root *va,* "that which flows") as outlined in the *Hatha Yoga Pradipika.*[24] In short, vayu is a way to talk about how we experience movement (or how movement experiences us?). In the subtle body, vayu participates in this cross-ply matrix at all levels as "movement winds" that animate and govern all aspects of the system. Before we head deeper into the subtle body, we'll take a closer look at the anatomy of tubular structure.

CHAPTER THREE

 Cross-ply

Think of the cardboard tube inside a toilet roll. You can dissect it to find the best, cheapest way to make a basic tube with some inherent stability is a spiral. And the easiest way to reinforce the strength of the spiral is to lay across it another spiral going in the opposite direction. This is the anatomy of cross-ply.

As in Fig. 3.13, the cross-ply of helical fibers is much more suited to shape change than orthogonal arrays of inextensible fibers. Inextensible, in this case, means that because its fibers are at right angles to each other, the fabric can't elongate and bounce back to its original shape. Not all tubes are created equal! Without oblique cross-ply, a tube can't change shape because the longitudinal arrangement with its set lengths is not responsive and cannot bend without kinking.[25]

The body is a matrix of cross-ply helical tubes of unlimited interconnectivity. Cross-ply is a way of saying that two directionalities are offset and thus in balance. Recall the matrix of cross-ply interconnects via the coupling principle that we looked at in Chapter 2. This is a crucial concept for making and connecting tubes, the gift that keeps on giving. And the crux is that these coupled couples give rise to the third: a structural element that self-stabilizes in motion as a volume.

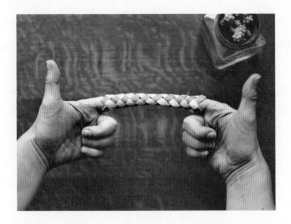

FIGURE 3.13

The Finger Trap provides a vivid experiential example of the concept of cross-ply. The different coloured spiral threads aligned orthogonally co-create a resilient weave that is extensible, expansive and convergent, doesn't buckle under loading and serves to constrain the space that it fosters. The same can be said for the weave of the Shoulder Filament, for example. The scapulohumeral rhythm fosters a spaciousness around the joint that both mobilizes and constrains the joint space. The same effects are not achieved with a ply of right-angled threads, as a tube made with threads at right angles will buckle under stress and is neither extensible or compressible.

Srotas-kinematics (tubular movement)

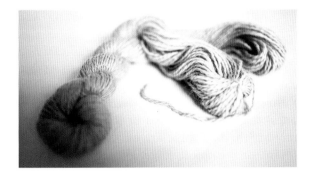

FIGURE 3.14

Ways of winding yarn around an axis. The hank method of winding yarn shows how a helical thread in one direction pairs with another in the opposite direction to make bundles of thread that can be further twisted in one direction and paired with another bundle of opposite-handedness to form a structurally stable twisted configuration.

3.7 Srotamsi: many rivers

In Ayurvedic anatomy, the living body comprises of a network of srotamsi (body channels) with unlimited connectivity. The etymology of the term is related to the Sanskrit root *stru-strabane*[26] and *srugatau*. Both sources point to various meanings related to flow, exudation, oozing, filtration, permeability and movement.

 A srotas refers to an individual channel, i.e. *anusrotas*. *Sthula srotas* refers to the various organ systems.

No structure in the body can grow and develop or waste and atrophy, independent of srotas...

Charaka Acharya

According to the *Charaka Samhita*,[12] the body is Sravanata Srotamsi, and that a srotas is a structure through which **Śravaṇam** (hearing, listening to wisdom) occurs.[27] Forces, nutrients, tissue elements (dhātus), waste (*mala*), and sensory information flow through the srotamsi: cellular apparatus on the gross level; nadis and vayu on the subtle level. Srotamsi are structurally modular and hierarchical, scaling to the microscopic level as well as forming macro systems like the māha vaha srotas (the maha, or great tube: the gastrointestinal tract).

Key concepts 7

Each *srotas* has a root (*sroto mula*), a passage (*sroto marga*), and a mouth (*mukha*).

Like any tube, each srotas has a root (*sroto mula*), a passage (*sroto marga*) and an opening, or mouth (*sroto mukha*). According to Ayurveda, blockages, as well as deranged and excessive flow at the local level, are the source of systemic pathology referred to as *srotomaya* (disease).

CHAPTER THREE

 Srotomaya

A classic example of srotomaya is the build-up of cholesterol, causing high blood pressure and associated symptoms.[3] Lack of movement in the *mamsa vaha srotas* local to the knee, as another example, interferes with joint function and can result in further duhkha elsewhere in the myofascial system.

Vaha translates as "bearing" or "carrying" and is used in conjunction with singular srotas, e.g., *prāna vaha srotas*, the breath/energy-carrying channels or *anna vaha srotas*, the food-carrying channels. The srotamsi are organized in a set of thirteen channels (plus a few gender-specific ones) that follow the idea of root, passage, and mouth. The first three are on the receiving end (prāna or breath/life-force, *anna* or food, *ambu* or liquids). The subsequent seven srotas

TABLE 3.1 Srotamsi shareera: the tubular body

Srotas	Functions	Mula (root)	Marga (passage)	Mukha (opening)
Prana	Respiration, emotion, thinking, communication	Left chamber of heart, GI tract	Respiratory tract, bronchial tree	Nose (nasa)
Ambu	Basal temperature, lubrication, energy, electrolyte balance, selection of waste	Pancreas (*kloma*), soft palate (*talu*), choroid plexus	GI mucous membrane	Kidneys, tongue, sweat glands
Anna	Digestion, assimilation, absorption	Esophagus, fundus of stomach	GI tract, lips to ileocecal valve	Ileocecal valve
Rasa	Blood circulation, nutrition, affection, faith	Right chamber of heart	Venous system, lymphatic system	Microcirculatory junction
Rakta	Oxygenation, enthusiasm	Liver, spleen	Arteriole system	Microcirculatory junction
Mamsa	Plastering (*lepana*), form, movement, support, protection, strength	Fascia and small tendons, mesoderm, layers of skin	Entire muscle system, heart and involuntary muscles	Pores of skin
Meda	Lubrication (*snehan*), personal love, beauty, insulation, bulk	Omentum, adrenal glands (*vrukka*)	Subcutaneous fat	Sweat glands

Srotas-kinematics (tubular movement)

	TABLE 3.1 continued			
Srotas	Functions	Mula (root)	Marga (passage)	Mukha (opening)
Asthi	Support (*dharana*), structure, protection of vital organs	Pelvic girdle, sacrum	Skeletal system	Nails, hair
Majjā	Fill bone space, sensation, communication, learning, memory	Brain, spinal cord, joints, junctions between *dhātus*	Central, sympathetic, and parasympathetic nervous systems	Synaptic space, neuromuscular cleft
Shukra	Reproduction, produces *ojas*, emotional release	Testicles, nipples	Vas deferens, epididymis, prostate, urogenital tract	Urethral opening
Artava	Reproduction, produces *ojas*, emotional release	Ovaries, areola of nipple	Fallopian tubes, uterus, cervical canal, vagina	Labia minora/majora (*yoni oshtha*)
Purisha	Absorption of minerals, strength, support, formation and elimination of feces	Cecum, rectum, sigmoid colon	Large intestine	Anus
Mūtra	Electrolyte balance, urination, maintenance of blood pressure	Kidneys	Ureter (kidney to bladder), bladder, urethra	Urethral opening
Sveda	Elimination of liquid wastes, sweat, electrolyte balance, body temperature, lubrication	Sweat glands	Sweat ducts	Sweat duct, pores
Mano	Thinking, feeling, inquiring, deciding, discrimination, desire, memory, communication	Heart, five bilateral nadi pairs (one for each of the five senses)	Entire body	Sense organs, *marmani* (marma points)
Stanya	Lactation	Lactiferous glands	Lactiferous glands	Duct openings in nipples

correspond to the seven *dhātus*, or tissue elements (*rasa, rakta, māmsa, meda, asthi, majjā, shukra*) that form a progressive passage of nourishment.

Key concepts 8

Every living body is a physiology of tubules (*srotamsi shareera*) made up of systems of tubes (*vaha srotas*) that each carries different substances/information.

Finally, the three root srotas are for expelling waste (mala) from the system (*sveda* or sweat, *purisha* or feces, *mūtra* or urine). *Ārtava* and *sthanya* regulate menstrual flow and breast milk, respectively, and are the two female-specific srotamsi. Within the srotamsi of mind, *mano*, every emotion and thought has a smaller srotas.

3.8 Akasha by Kate O'Donnell

The concept of srotas is fundamental to Ayurveda's understanding of the body. Across the board, Ayurveda considers not only physical structures such as tissue types and fluids but also those aspects that can't be seen: energy and consciousness. The philosophical system that underlies Ayurveda, the *Samkhya*, concerns a basic relationship between consciousness and matter and a particular ordering of the universe that results.

Of the physical attributes of the universe, *akasha*, space, is primary. It provides the field in which the other elements, air, fire, water, and earth, begin to move and form physical structures. Without space, movement is not possible. The Sanskrit word *kha* means space, or cavern, and is the root of the word akasha, "space element." Kha also appears as the second letter of the Sanskrit alphabet, which points to the fundamental nature of space as a starting point in the evolution of structure. Space is a foundation for both matter and consciousness.

In understanding the human body, the relationship between space and movement is also at the forefront. Srotas means channel, or river. The srotas are also sometimes referred to as kha, or space. These tubular structures, both energetic and physical, are spaces through which energy and matter travel. The word srotas implies, however, not only space but also movement. When is a river ever still? Those who have made an initial study of Ayurveda likely would have heard of *Vata dosha*, the compound of space and air elements that governs all movement processes in the body.

Vata means "that which moves," and is responsible for the currents in the body, as the air element moves along pathways of space. For example, the digestive tract is a space containing a current that leads from the mouth to the anus. The form is the srotas, the big tube between those two openings. The function is vata, or movement in a specific directionality, between the two openings. The speed, direction, and quantity of vata, as well as the state of the space it moves in, are vital aspects to maintaining digestive health.

In the topic of human bodies in motion, as in Ayurveda, an understanding of space is fundamental. Experiential knowledge of the relationship between space and movement is one of yoga's gifts. A dynamic system where form and function both hinge on interconnectivity could not be well understood without taking into account the nature of movement and the nature of the field within which it is occurring.

3.9 Srotas: subtle kinematics

Notice in Table 3.1 that the *māmsa* srotas level is highlighted. Mamsa corresponds to the meso, the proto-tissue of the embryo that gives rise to the myofascial system as described in Chapter 1. I suggest that yogis become familiar with the mamsa as the systemic equivalent (or co-conspirator) of the so-called myofascial system. Structurally, there are more architectural similarities than we can perhaps afford to ignore.

As we have previously established, movement within the body on a gross level happens as a result of closed kinematic chains (CKCs) operating within this matrix of tubular tissues. The mamsa is coupled with all the other srotas in the same CKCs, and in the srotamsi shareera, there is connectivity to all srotas gross and subtle via coupled functions.

Let's pause and take a deep breath. There are many more conceptual distinctions than there are actual differences in overall patterning in the living body. While these aspects are studied very distinctly in the anatomy laboratory, the matter of the living matrix uses very similar patterning to enclose potential space and create a facility for things like food and drink and energy forces to move through it.

Srotas-kinematics is a term I've been using to link gross-to-subtle tubular anatomy with spiral movement as we experience it on a practical level in the Five Filaments for yoga. The basic translation is "tube movement". The concept is related to the mamsa vaha srotas, the srotamsi system encompassing tissues of the embryological meso (bones, muscles, tendons, ligaments and variations on the theme of fascia) and kinematics (movement).

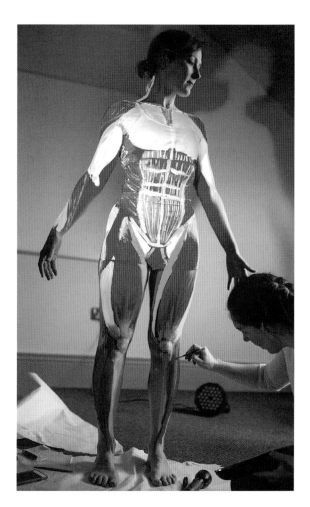

FIGURE 3.15

Mamsa vaha srotas: the myofascial system. Pictured here is physicist–Iyengar-yoga-teacher Louise Belshaw. She is showing off the classical musculoskeletal system applied in the UV anatomy body painting technique developed by Gabrielle Finn, Professor of Medical Education.

(Photo by the author, UV paint applied by Gabrielle Finn and the author at the Northern Ireland Science Festival, 2019)

CHAPTER THREE

Srotas-kinematics goes beyond the mamsa (and the meso) to include system-wide tubularity across the spectrum of subtle to gross. It refers to the whole body and transcends the separation of movement within and without. Srotas-kinematics as a term incorporates all levels of tubularity to describe *how* biomotion coordinates the inside with the outside, as we do.

Crucially, for yoga practitioners, this movement map ties together all levels of anatomy from gross to subtle that are known as *kośa*, or the *koshas* (see Fig. 3.20). Srotas-kinematics is a lens for modern yoga practitioners as we develop the therapeutic potential of movement, and it constitutes another aspect of our theoretical basis for the practical application of the 5F.

Key concepts 9

Srotas-kinematics (tube movement) is a new term that describes the body's natural spiral movement and formation patterns, influencing all tissue and especially relevant in the tissue of the *mamsa vaha srotas* (myofascial system).

Moreover, srotas-kinematics offers a simplified way to explain how yoga seems to reach across strata of bodily experience. The research shows what we experience anecdotally: yoga changes you, and it even happens on the level of gene expression.[28] Yoga has been shown to support better sleep, quiet the mind, support the nervous system,[29] improve mood and, of course, it can make the body beautiful and promote longevity.[30–32]

On the other end of the healthy spectrum, trauma experienced anywhere in the body is also felt everywhere, consciously or otherwise.[33] It is the tubes, or tubular networks, that connect *everything* in the body, subtle and gross, translating behavior into structure and function (and vice versa). Further, the interconnection happens not only within one body but also amongst multiple organizations and across timescales.

Talking point

Our generation is living through a time when the tools of science are quantifying the physiological effects of yoga and mindfulness on individuals and communities. Do you think the resulting literature base will generate enough momentum to make long-lasting changes in mainstream health care? Will we see more movement therapies regularly available alongside the modern menu of interventional, allopathic medicine?

Research into the neurobiology of compassion tells of the invisible linkages we experience via behavioral patterns.[34] Kim et al. show that while practicing compassion, "neural networks associated with threat are reduced".[35] The same threat-associated networks were heightened when being self-critical. Conversely, an increased parasympathetic response to compassion-cultivating activity was measured "by an increase in heart rate variability (HRV), versus the resting-state."[35] Perhaps there is more subtle patterning in the matter of us than can be readily separated into the function of the physical and biomotional nature of the being animating it.

Srotas-kinematics (tubular movement)

(i) Although this may be a new portmanteau, the mechanism of srotas-kinematics is primary, and the concept is ancient and universal. The term srotas-kinematics means tube movement. The srotas-kinematics are simply CKCs as applied to yoga anatomy based in the fascial matrix. They naturally resonate with the most ancient principles of ayurvedic wisdom.

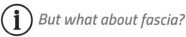

(i) *But what about fascia?*

Tissues arising from the mamsa vaha srotas are functionally equivalent to those of the embryological meso, drawing in the srotas (tubes) of all other systems. All tissue interconnects in a helical matrix[36] that shows up in the rotational, spiral movement patterns of the body in motion. Srotas-kinematics give us a way of talking about this functional arrangement in a way that acknowledges the subtle body integrated with principles of classical systems anatomy.

Mamsa refers to your muscles, bones, and connective tissues, but not in the conventional or classical anatomical sense of separate structures. The tubular nature of biologic systems is given full credence in the srotamsi shareera of Ayurvedic anatomy, where each srotas twirls into a larger srotamsi

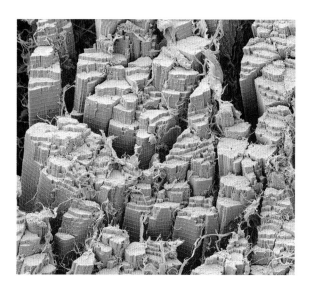

FIGURE 3.16

Muscle fiber. Colored scanning electron micrograph of a freeze-fractured skeletal (or striated) muscle fiber. The fracturing of the fiber has revealed that it consists of a bundle of smaller fibers called myofibrils. The myofibrils are crossed by transverse tubules (horizontal lines), that mark the division of the myofibrils into contractile units (sarcomeres). (Magnification: x8000 when printed at 10 cm wide.)

(Steve Gschmeissner/Science Photo Library)

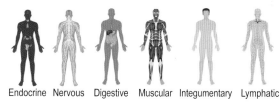

Endocrine Nervous Digestive Muscular Integumentary Lymphatic

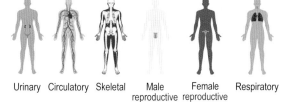

Urinary Circulatory Skeletal Male reproductive Female reproductive Respiratory

FIGURE 3.17

Classical systems anatomy.

(https://www.canstockphoto.com/eula/)

CHAPTER THREE

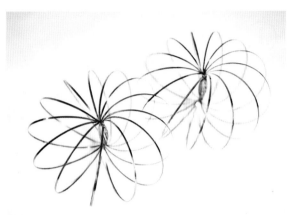

with a *mula, marga,* and *mukha* of unlimited interconnectivity. We are giving the mamsa a proper handshake here because it is a huge deal to anyone involved in functional movement, and a central theme to this work. We are inviting in an ancient established context, to re-contextualize the latest in contemporary understanding of fascia.

Key concepts 10

The *mamsa vaha srotas* is the tissue level from Ayurveda that encompasses the structural myofascial system.

The 5F concept is an algorithmic movement map consisting of directionalities that operate in states responsive to breath, bandha (more on these in Chapter 5), weight-bearing or non-weight bearing. Meridians describe lines in the body, whereas the 5F codify movement constraints as srotas-kinematics inherent in the volumetric living system. Dissection reveals the widespread helical pattern distributed throughout the fibers and compartments of the fascial web.[37,38] These spiral guidelines describe the helical constraints of natural movement and offer the therapist/teacher a means of enhancing self-directed practice.

Further, a movement that goes along natural spiral patterns in the tissues could be described as srotas-kinematic: it is the way the body *wants* to move. Unhealthy movement (a movement that goes harshly against the grain of spiral models) is *not* biomotionally optimal, does not operate in harmony with the constraints, and can lead to

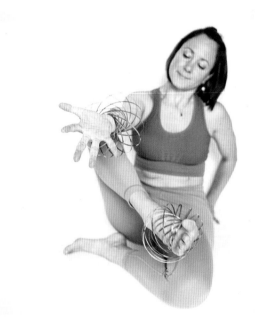

FIGURE 3.18

The Toroflux: a toy for feeling the power of spirality, chirality, invagination, and flow. It was originally developed by Jochen Valett in the mid–1990s, it is a kinetic toy made of one long, curly filament of metal that embodies all the resilient, auxetic, volumetric potential of spirals.

Srotas-kinematics (tubular movement)

duhkha (pain), especially under an increasing or inappropriate load. *Full Nelson*, anyone? Here is a crucial distinction, the paradox of our mysterious bodies: by learning to go with the flow, it may become possible to bend the rules and use the flow to make shapes that would be dangerous and pointless without such training.

(i) *More than a mouthful*

This a lot of terminology to be throwing around. It is a heady mix of Sanskrit, Greek, Latin, and some new terms I've taken some liberty in joining up in the spirit of integration. But by integrated, I don't mean complicated. As previously described, srotas-kinematics are simply the anatomical linkages flowing within the body's myofascial spiral patterns (and beyond), or simply, *tube movement*.

Understanding these rotating, spiral linkages is crucial for yoga practitioners to maximize the experience of spaciousness and stability (sthira-suhkham). A lynchpin in this model for yogis is that the CKC of the srotas-kinematics is a model for linking every level of tubular tissue on the spectrum of gross to subtle; macro to micro.

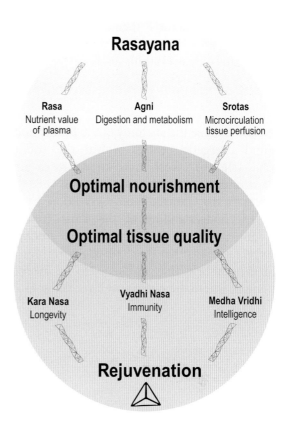

FIGURE 3.19

Rasayana.

Rasāyanā

The *rasayana* concept is the science of rejuvenation, part of the eight core clinical specialities of Ayurveda. Rasayana techniques look at the entirety of an individual's behavior to promote longevity through nutritional and behavioral interventions. Its approach is thought to act through a "psycho-endocrinological immune axis"[39] and illustrates the way kinematics link all our actions into a net effect via the coupled functions of srotamsi.

3.10 Weaving the threads

Hatha yoga offers a system of techniques for working with the body, to foster an awareness of all the tissues and tubes interacting through subtle connectivity. Essentially, this is happening on every level, within both the gross body and the more subtle systems throughout and amongst individuals. In our modern understanding, yoga can address and unravel toxic patterns that might not be serving the whole. It does so, once again, through the structural theme of the tubular network of which everything is made and by which patterning everything abides.

Koshas: subtle body anatomy layers in the round

We can visualize the anatomy of the Pranic body around energetic centers within the subtler koshas (sheath). Koshas are known as sheaths of anatomical structure according to Vedāntic sources.[40] The Tantrik/Tantric tradition has a different understanding of the same concept of coverings. What is common amongst interpretations is that these are the coverings of Atman or the Self. They are likened to the layers of an onion, where the outermost layer is the gross Self, and the interior is the subtlest aspect. The sheets are porous and interpenetrate one another. As Hareesh says about the pranamaya kosha, it "is a model for understanding the subtler aspects of our mental-emotional being and how it interpenetrates the tissues of the physical body."[41]

Let's not forget. While living, all aspects of anatomy are subtle. Bodies as we know them are a snapshot in time, evidence of these sheaths interacting. Across the timescale of one lifetime, the experiences of injury and disease may arise and influence all sheaths. Tuning in to the rotations of the srotas-kinematics can help protect the gross as well as connect us more intimately to patterns in nature that unite us all.

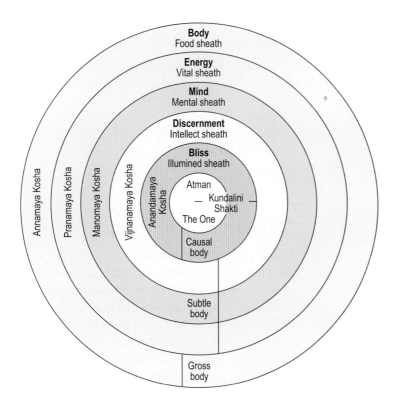

FIGURE 3.20

The Vedāntic version of the koshas from the *Taittirīya Upaniṣad*.

(Artwork by Joanna Darlington)

Srotas-kinematics (tubular movement)

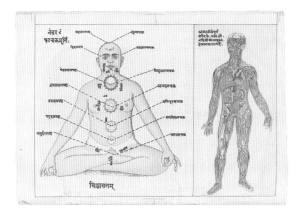

FIGURE 3.21

Illustration of the six chakras of Tantric yoga in Sanskrit and Hindi. One of eight colored plates, drawing explicit parallels between the yogic view of chakras etc., and the medical/anatomical view of the body. Svamihamsasvarupakrtam Satcakranirupanactiram: bhasyasamalamkrtam bhasatikopetan ca = Shatchakra niroopana chittra with bhashya and bhasha containing the pictures of the different nerves and plexuses of the human body with their full description showing the easiest method how to practice pranayam by the mental suspension of breath through meditation only.

(Svami Hamsasvarupa. Sanskrit MS 391. Drawings by Shri Swami Hansa Swaroop. Wellcome Collection. https://creativecommons.org/licenses/by/4.0/)

Now that we have established srotas as a framework for examining the structural foundation of subtle body tissue, what's next? It is time to develop a context for the energetic anatomy that follows, based on the yogic body of Tantra. Here again, we find the theme of channels and networks of tubes.

Tantra has recently garnered an erotic connotation, but the term comes from the Sanskrit for "loom"', or "weaving."[42] It was the dominant influence on religion in India from the 6th to 13th centuries.[43] As Hatha Yoga came into its own around the 12th century, naturally it would do so as infused with the Tantric first principles.

The Hatha yoga corpus brings together many threads of practice, including asana, pranayama, ritual, kriya, mudra, bandha, and yantra. All comprise ancient techniques to purify energetic channels within the srotamsi shareera known as *Nāḍī*, vessels of the subtle body (plural: *nadyaḥ*, simply *nadis*). As the practitioner cleanses the network of nadis, they are said to progress to Raja Yoga (the Royal path) toward the experience of *samadhi*. These practices were thought to conserve vital energy (seminal fluid) and ultimately draw said energy up the central channel of the yogic body.

Key concepts 11

While the body is alive, it is subtle; so-called subtle body anatomy is vital for teachers and students of yoga.

(i) Nadi

How is nadi different from the regular variety of srotas? Table 3.1 presented the gross anatomy of Ayurveda as outlined in the *Charaka Samhita*.[44] To find the nadi, we can

CHAPTER THREE

look to interpretations of classic yogic texts such as the *Hatha Yoga Pradipika*.[24] According to the HYP, the purpose of yoga is to awaken the subtle energy of *kundalini* through the purification of the nadi network (72,000 currents of subtle energy emanating from the navel and ending in the hands and feet; the appraisal varies as mentioned later). The nadis are the *pranic* srotamsi system.

Kundalini derives from the term *kunda*, the Sanskrit word for a vessel, "pit" or "cavity" within which shakti (latent energy) is allegorically "coiled like a snake" or, we could say "spiral bound". This imagery is compelling when you keep in mind the fate of the blastopore, the embryological pit that confirms the long, polar axis of the embryo.

3.11 Subtle body, spiral bound

The *Siva Samhitā* is a primary source of Tantric ideas regarding the subtle body.[45] According to the Tantric model, there are a total of 350,000 nadis in the human body (considerably more than the 72,000 of the HYP)[45]; of these, 14 are essential, giving branches that supply various systemic requirements throughout the body. Three of these 14 important nadis are considered to be the most significant: the *Ida*, *Pingala*, and *Sushumna*. Contemporary research looks at a neuroscientific rationale for its model of the nadis as "streams" through which the prana vayu circulate.[46]

Much of what we know of Hindu Tantra, now referred to as Kashmir Shaivism, comes to us through the writings of Abhinavagupta (c. 10th century CE).[47] In them, we find a focus on

Key concepts 12

The Ida and Pingala course between the nostrils (Ida, left, and Pingala, right) and the base of the spine, spiraling around the filament of Sushumna like a double spiral staircase.

the central importance of internal sensory signals in bodily experience. This focus has led Loizzo to conclude that the subtle body model serves "as an embodied, interoceptive neurofeedback aid"[48] in his comparative review of the literature.

We can thus understand interoception as our continuous experience of Self from an internal gauging of neural, immune and endocrine signals. Quadt et al. show that mind-body interactions influence both physical and mental well-being as a consequence of the "homeostatic reflexes and allostatic responses" of interoception.[49] In our view, these reflexes and responses are the stuff of coupling functions via the srotas-kinematics.

Sushumna originates in the bottom of the spine at the convergence of the principle nadis, Ida and Pingala, the region of latent energy known as kundalini, symbolised as a coiled serpent. This latent spiralling energy courses up through the center of the axis to the crown of the head. Ida represents the feminine principle, and Pingala represents the masculine principle, both winding around Sushumna carrying their pranic currents. These currents converge at Ajna (*command*) chakra. Chakras are energetic "wheels" in the subtle body.

When the nadis, most specifically Ida and Pingala, are balanced, for example through pranayama and other yogic techniques, kundalini

Srotas-kinematics (tubular movement)

TABLE 3.2 Nadis			
	Ida (comfort)	Pingala (tawny)	Sushumna
Gross equivalent	Parasympathetic nervous system	Sympathetic nervous system	Balance
Guna	Corresponds to Tamas	Corresponds to Rajas	Corresponds to Sattva
Course	Courses from left Muladhara to the left nostril	Courses from right Muladhara to the right nostril	Connects Muladhara to Sahasrara chakras via the spinal cord
Energy	Lunar energy	Solar energy	Channel for the flow of awakened consciousness
Gender	Feminine	Masculine	Neutral
Temperature	Cooling	Heating	Balance
Governs	Mental processes	Vital processes	Spiritual experience

is said to be awakened and rises spontaneously through Sushumna. As this ordinarily dormant, coiled kundalini energy circulates upward in its journey toward the crown (Sahasrara chakra), it pierces the *granthis* (energetic/pranic knots). It can subsequently further invigorate the nadis and chakras throughout the form.

Sushumna nadi is thought to operate autonomically at dawn and dusk, which is why these times of day are traditional times for spiritual practice. When the other nadis are flowing, Sushumna remains appropriately dormant. It becomes active only when the breath flows equally through both nostrils simultaneously, as an indication that *Ida and Pingala are in balance*. This distinction is crucial: the cross-ply (or chirality) of Ida and Pingala nadis, the subtle srotas, create a tube of potential space arising from their juxtaposition. This, essentially, recapitulates the notion of how two opposing forces unite to facilitate a trinity of wholeness flowing through – and toward – itself.

Since so many of the diagrams depicting this arrangement are relatively simplified, it does often look like the Ida and Pingala are just sort of "wavy gravy." It often appears that the central channel, Sushumna, is only a column in between the two wavy lines. Sadly, this misunderstanding loses the point entirely.

CHAPTER THREE

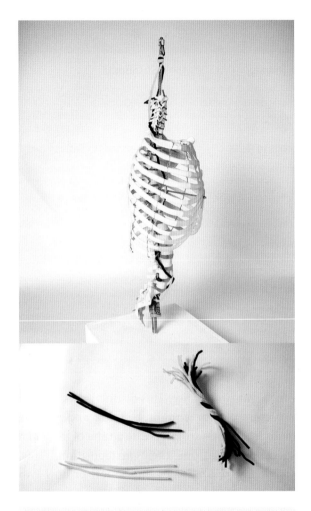

FIGURE 3.22

The principle nadis, Ida and Pingala, coursing around Sushumna. This activity allows students to wrap pipe cleaners around the skeleton, illuminating the structural relationships amongst the gross and subtle aspects. Using 3D materials helps us understand kinesthetically that Ida (blue) and Pingala (yellow) are chiral tubes coiling around the potential space of Sushumna.

The essence of the two chiral, 3D, helicoid nadis coming together to offset one another,

creating a tube, is something I like to explore kinesthetically with fellow students by making a pipe-cleaner model (see Fig. 3.22). In the spiral-bound model, the other nadis interconnect through their subtle srotas-kinematics to Ida and Pingala, who in turn align in balance. That alignment, in and of itself, *gives rise to the spatialization they form: Sushumna.*

As a diagram of srotamsi, this subtle body model shows us what happens when opposites complement one another in harmony and unity. Such opposites as masculine and feminine, sun and moon, **tension** and compression, prana and apana, attraction and repulsion, positive and negative, push and pull, can be considered symbolically in this idea. When these forces flow equally, in a kind of opposing balance, their inter-related coiling creates what we could think of as a dynamic tube.

Within this tubular arrangement, the central channel appears and invites the rising motion of subtle energy. This motion, metaphorically at least, also becomes the basis of animation in gross structure. In short, the subtle body model echoes what we saw on the gross level in Chapter 2 as the coordination of coupledness that gives rise to the throuple. Directionalities of flowing Prana balance the system; these are known in yoga as the **vayu.**

3.12 Vayu

As long as the vayu (air and Prana) remains in the body, that is called life. Death is when it leaves the body. Therefore, retain vayu.

Hatha Yoga Pradipika

In classical yoga, the Pancha (five) *pranadi* pranas flow in vayu as subtle directors with powerful effects in the entire subtle body system.[50]

Srotas-kinematics (tubular movement)

Think of vayu as specialized directionalities of Prana flowing through particular nadis. Vayu and nadi are the *sutra*, or threads (srotas), holding the pranas of all living things together to form an interconnected web of life,[14] as it is described in the Samvarga Vidya of the *Chandogya Upanishad*.[15]

Vayu are the winds that fuel the srotas-kinematics of the body, both gross and subtle. These winds (also called airs), flow in the nadis, the vaha srotamsi of the subtle body. The **Pancha (five) Prāṇa**, including prana vayu (not to be confused with Prāṇa with a capital "P") and its cohort of apana, samana, udana, and vyana govern different areas of the body, guiding physical and subtle activities.

Key concepts 13

Vayu are the "pranic airs" or "winds" that are directionally oriented flows of Prana through the subtle *srotamsi*: the *nadis*.

The vayu principle is a guide for voluntary movement within the srotamsi shareera where asana becomes a means of activating and refining the vayu. Exploring vayu as a kind of transanatomical route of force transmission within the body is to further appreciate where Eastern and Western insight dovetail.

 Maitrāyaṇīya Upaniṣad

The *Maitriyaniya Upanishad* is an ancient Vedic text from the "black" (or unorganized, motley) Yajurveda.[51] It contains an allegory about how life emerged as the vayu when Prajapati (lord of creatures) divided himself

fivefold and entered all living things.

The *Maitri* describes the vayu as follows:

- Prana is *the upward* breath.
- Apana is *downward* breath (exhale).
- Vyana *holds* the Prana and Apana in balance, giving strength to the whole body.
- Samana is that which *carries* gross food to Apana and then subtler food throughout the body.
- Udana is that which *delivers* food throughout the body.

Together with the substance (food), Prana and Apana provide the means which facilitate the production of heat for the body (as stated in paragraph 2.6 of *Maitri Upanishad*).[52] The Pranadi vayu are the five winds or Pancha (five) Vayu of the inner body. There are a further five vayu, the so-called Nagadi vayu. These are the winds of the outer body, sometimes referred to as the *upa pranas* outlined at the end of this section.[53]

What is so interesting about the vayu in a structural/anatomical context is that these energetic threads form a network of forces through the chakras animated in movement. Vayu are connected to the nadis of the srotamsi subtle body system. Recall the Klein bottle and our interest in reconciling the Inside with the Outside as a model for experiencing Self. The following is a description of the individual pancha vayu and ideas for working with them in practice.

Prana vāyu: inward, inspiring

The prana (not capital "P") vayu is the most fundamental of the five, governing inward motion, including everything we draw into our bodies. Physiologically, this vayu is associated with the

CHAPTER THREE

actions of inhaling, eating, drinking, smelling, etc. Prana vayu is the pathway related to tensional in-drawing, the intrinsic pulling in of body tissues we might think of as strengthening. Paradoxically, prana is associated with the in-drawing of the torso to let the out-breath happen.

The prana vayu also applies to the five senses and can be either weakened or strengthened by our choices in feeding them. Over-stimulation and overconsumption (food, drink, social media, loud music, etc.) interfere with the flow of prana vayu. A weakened prana vayu reduces the ability to concentrate. Potent prana vayu endows the practitioner with the inner fortitude required for meditation and self-regulation.

The prana vayu, positively charged energy, is carried in Pingala nadi. It has a heating and energizing influence on the body and mind when in balance.

Directing Prana through prana vayu

Activate prana vayu:

- Standing asanas with the arms directed upwards:
    * Virabhadrasana A
    * Utkatasana
    * Ardha chandrasana
- All back-bending stimulates the *flow* of prana vayu

- Meditation
- Savasana

Apana vāyu: down and outward

This vayu governs all elimination. Apana vayu governs everything that moves downward and outward at every level. As an element comes in, so it must eventually leave the body: breath, food and drink, metabolic waste, and bodily excretions. Apana is related to the functions of the female and male reproductive rhythms, including menses, female secretory functions, childbirth, and male ejaculation. A proper reproductive function depends on a healthy flow of apana vayu. A balanced excretory function is another sign of steady and robust apana vayu. Apana vayu can be experienced as the outward push (paradoxically the squeezing *in* of the exhale!) that resists or represents the opposite of the inward pull of prana.

Weak apana interferes with the ability to process and let go of experiences effectively and can lead to a sense of constant worrying and regret. Healthy apana regulates the proper flow of substances, emotions, experiences, illnesses and injuries *out of the system*. Where this flow is either too fast or too slow, apana vayu is out of balance. In the nadis, Ida represents the negatively charged, lunar, feminine energy of apana and has a calming, cooling and refreshing effect in the mind and body; ultimately to counter-balance Pingala.

TABLE 3.3 Pancha vayus					
	Prana	**Apana**	**Samana**	**Vyana**	**Udana**
Action	Inward	Outward	Assimilating	Pervasive	Upward
Location	Heart	Pelvis	Navel	Everywhere	Throat/head

Srotas-kinematics (tubular movement)

ⓘ The pelvic cavity (space below the arcuate line) is known as the Apanastan, home to the seed or essence of what David Garrigues refers to as "the out-breath pattern" related to apana vayu.[54]

Directing prana through apana vayu

Increase the flow of Prana through apana vayu by practicing twists in all forms, as well as seated forward bends. Abstaining from inversions during menstruation helps promote the flow of apana. Cleansing rituals such as juicing and Ayurvedic cleanses are considered part of maintaining the potential for the energetic flow of apana vayu.

Samāna vāyu: inward, assimilating

Samana vayu resides in the umbilical region as the pathway for the process of digestion, all-important in Ayurveda. Known as the "balancing air," assimilation is a crucial function of samana vayu. Balanced Prana flowing in samana brings strong powers of discernment as the subtle body works out what to keep and what to throw away.

Weakness and fatigue can be signs of a weakened samana vayu, as this pathway governs the way we process not only what we eat and drink, but also information and personal experience. It is not limited to the purely physical,

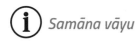 **ⓘ** *Samāna vāyu*

The HYP states that of all the vayu, samana is most important for yogis. Samana is the assimilating air that is charged by the convergence of prana and apana. We can support the cultivation of samana with continued practice of bandha.

or gross, experience – it includes the subtle body assimilation processes alluded to above.

Problems dealing with painful experiences can be characteristic of blocked samana. Difficulties with the processing of shock and trauma can overwhelm the system and prevent samana from flowing. When healthy and balanced, samana allows the individual to progress through stages of healing, to eventually be able to let go of residual excess via apana vayu.

Directing prana through samāna vāyu

To access samana vayu, direct the breath to the center of the abdomen, distributing it throughout the cylindrical trunk. Explore the inner surface and linings of the abdominopelvic cavity with each breath. Coordinate the lengths of inhalation and exhalation. As prana meets apana, samana is balanced and goes on to activate udana, the upward air.

Asanas that activate samana include:

- Arm balances.
- Standing, seated, and supine twists.
- Forward bends.
- Uddiyana bandha and Nauli kriya are incredibly powerful. These techniques stimulate apana vayu to unite it with samana and prana. (More about intensifying Uddiyana bandha for personal practice and teaching appears later in this chapter.)

Vyana vayu: pervasive, circulatory

Vyana vayu moves outward from the center. Known as the "omnipresent air," it permeates throughout the body and even extends into the surrounding area, also known as the *aura*. Vyana integrates and balances all the vayu and governs the movement of Prana through the nadis. These elements of subtle body anatomy give nomenclature to invisible forces that go by other names and interpretations elsewhere.

Vyana vayu relates to circulation on all levels, from the flow of food, water, and gaseous transfer throughout the body to the dissemination of postural information within the srotamsi shareera (and the circulation of balanced energy in and around the toroidal electromagnetic energy field). Optimal vyana promotes bioelectric flow through the nervous system, movement of fluid through the lymphatics, and the movement of the myofascial system, linking all systems together for homeostasis.

The flow of thoughts and emotions tie into vyana for processing and proper elimination. When vyana is out of balance, an individual may feel uncoordinated or out of control, as this vayu facilitates the flow of Prana in all the other vayu and results in a balanced and functioning whole. Consistent yoga practice leads to the flow of Prana in vyana vayu, resulting in a cascade of well-being factors. Balanced vyana leads to the ascension of Prana in udana vayu.

Directing Prana through vyana vayu

Inhale: Draw breath in from behind the eyes, ears, heart, and lumbar spine. Imagine that inhalation draws from every region of the body.

Exhale: Mentally follow the breath as it flows out through the arms, legs, trunk, and head. Feel how exhalation can exude from the pores, expanding the energetic body outwards omnidirectionally.

Practices that activate vyana vayu include:

- "Flow state" activities such as gardening, dancing, cooking, rock climbing, music.

- Surya namaskaras.
- Savasana.
- Yoga nidra.

Udāna vāyu: upward, creative

The udana pathway is known as the "ascending air." It is the expressive vayu governing the pharynx and associated tissues. The thyroid and parathyroid glands are particularly affected by udana. With udana in balance, our confidence is balanced and communication becomes more comfortable. Udana animates the urge to grow taller, express oneself, and rise to challenges.

Udana governs growth in all aspects. The flow of udana encourages Prana to flow from lower to higher chakras. Situated between the heart and the head, udana carries the energy of kundalini and is thought to channel it to higher levels of consciousness and self-expression. The pericardium of the heart is continuous with the tongue, tissue that invests the thyroid and regulates the communication of information as part of Jalandhara bandha (see Chapter 5).

Directing prana through udana vayu

To access udana, direct the breath from the feet (if seated, the pelvic floor) superiorly along the spine, exhaling through the throat. Follow the rise of the rib cage and sternum during inhalation and concentrate on the throat center. Inversions drive udana, primarily as the culmination of a balanced yogasana practice. Udana vayu is stimulated by vyana vayu. Vyana is promoted by samana vayu, which in turn is activated by the convergence of prana and apana vayu in balance.

For inverted postures:

- **Inhale:** Wherever the posture is grounded, breathe from this connection upwards. Whether it is handstand, shoulder stand,

Srotas-kinematics (tubular movement)

or headstand, start the breath from the base and use it to draw the shoulder and neck tissues toward the pelvis.

- **Exhale:** Direct the breath outwards along the legs and vigorously out through the feet.

Udana vayu brings lightness to the head, neck, and shoulders during inversions such as headstand.

Key concepts 14

Vayu-breath-bandha is a basic unit of practice within the subtle body; understanding this triumvirate is a foundation of integrated anatomy for yoga.

 Upa pranas

There are also five minor vayu, the *Upa* pranas:

1. Naga: burping, hiccup.
2. Kurma: blinking, eyelid movement.
3. Krukara: the induction of hunger and thirst; sneezing.
4. Dhananjaya: regulation of the heart valves; decomposition of the body postmortem.
5. Devadutta: yawning.

How the vayu stand for yogis

Nine the Vayus in body equal are Dananjaya, the tenth superior is, When the nine in their channels accord Life and body well accord, too.

Tirumandiram, Verse 653 [55]

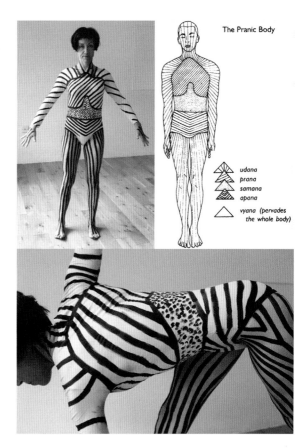

FIGURE 3.23

The Pancha Vayu (subtle srotamsi): udana, upward; apana, downward; samana, consolidating; prana, inward; vyana, expanding. Amy Hughes demonstrates the vayu in asana, with the body painted to draw awareness to vayu, "epistructural" routes (subtle srotamsi) of energy informing the felt sense of anatomy.

(Illustration of The Pranic Body from: S. Saraswati. *Asana Pranayama Mudra Bandha.* Bihar Yoga Bharati; 1997)

3.13 Integration

The vayu may have direct application in asana, giving yoga practitioners a feel for

CHAPTER THREE

the transanatomical structure introduced in Chapter 1. The force/energy of movement travels over gross structure in tubular arrangements at every level, whether voluntary or otherwise, in relationships I am referring to in a yoga context as *srotas-kinematics*, or tube movement.

Fascia researcher, Peter Huijing, has introduced the concept of "epimuscular pathways" into the literature, and I see these as intimately associated concepts.[56] Prana and apana are the coupled source from which all the other directionalities (airs, efforts, flows, forces?) emerge as a "thirdness" in volume and a "fourthness" of pure experience.

Infusion

Imagine a ginger spice teabag steeping in hot water. The plant essences are drawn into the hot water, and the water is drawn into the material of the teabag. A similar feeling arises as we breathe sensation into and around our bodies in movement. We experience forces as they flow along our filamentous body materials, but the flow doesn't take the predefined routes we see on the map. Sensation and motion are infused, as the ginger spice infuses our cup of tea; continuously and multidimensionally *trans-piste*.

Breathing in the direction of applied efforts is a crucial realization for anyone taking up a yoga practice and begins to reveal, experientially, the hidden interconnectedness within. Like the teabag and the water, prana needs apana and vice versa. Together, they are **prāṇāpāna**, the tension-compression architecture that makes life possible. In asana, pranapana is the prime energetic directive for all the standing postures,

particularly the more challenging balances. Pressing down and out against the tensioned matrix as if to push the earth away from you is a powerful means of stabilization. Breathing along udana vayu during inversions connects us to the internal upwardness for greater ease and an increasing sense of calm in the face of fear.

Key concepts 15

Srotas-kinematics explains routes of sensation and force that interplay throughout the *srotamsi shareera* (body matrix).

Through vayu, not only do we find a way of interpreting subtle kinematics, but we are also training and refining them as a practice during yoga. All the vayu flow simultaneously in dynamic yoga practice, leading to a balanced flow in vyana vayu (proper circulation). For example, in Downward Dog, prana vayu governs the in-drawing activity and physical effort (e.g., fronts of legs), apana vayu flows down and out of the legs to root the feet and samana charges through the natural inwardness (in-drawing) of the abdominopelvic membrane. Vyana describes the heightened circulation achieved in the balance of all these effects, leading ultimately to the ascending air of udana that raises latent potential. In this sense, postures such as Downward Dog (and indeed all asanas) are much more than the sum of their parts.

Prana + apana

In asana, the paradoxical actions of push and pull operate simultaneously. Without the push, there can be no pull and vice versa. Although prana and apana are said to be upward and

Srotas-kinematics (tubular movement)

downward moving energy, respectively, prana vayu is the energy drawing tissue inwards (resulting in compression). Apana vayu is the outward push (e.g., of the bones) which in turn, tension all that surrounds them (giving rise to prestress). In the round body, when tissue actively draws in, it *feels* like upward, as with the quadriceps during Downward Dog. Apana exists in the outward press of bones (the compression element) and that which resists the inward pull of tension (the tensional player) – their mutual opposition gives rise to the volume they co-create.

Verily by air, as by a thread, this world, the other world and all beings are held together.

Brhadaranyaka Upanishad[1]

Key concepts 16

The *vayu prana* and *apana* refer to inward pull and outward push, respectively. They have a special relationship (dynamic reciprocity) that relates to the synergic, expansion-retraction rhythm of the breath.

In the tubular system, prana and apana forces flow interchangeably to suit the moment in a state of perpetual tissue preparedness. Amidst the push–pull of individual asanas, the breath-centered movement of vinyasa churns the vayu with expansion–retraction. On a gross level, this churning agitates the tissues and changes their flow properties. This felt sense is that of **thixotropy**, from the Greek "touch-turn," which talks about how a material responds to the speed/scale of interactions.

Biological material is said to be non-Newtonian in its flow behavior,[57] which for our purposes means that our bodies respond differently depending on how fast/hard we meet a substrate (and vice versa; see Table 1.2). As body material warms up through vinyasa, it becomes increasingly conducive to flow. We can learn to *use* the ground (or any other substrate) to volley our energy to and fro intentionally. As Jo says, "how we greet the ground" has an enormous effect on the quality of feeling we might consequentially experience.

Thus, it follows that different speeds and intensities of practice will work with vayu in different ways. The convergence of prana with apana charges samana vaya. This promotes the all pervasive wind of vyana which represents healthy circulation, in turn stimulating udana to flow upwards, cleansing the throat, neck, and head. In the practice of yoga, balancing these pranic airs leads to Self-transformation.

Yoga as Self-transformation

The word transformation is a loaded term, as its implications are not limited to the physical experience. Transformation is a characteristic of the shape-shifting that we know to be intrinsic to soft matter. In yoga, this shape-shifting as a practice is something we *can* approach intentionally toward a spiritual purpose.

In an integrated view of anatomy, we look at how different appraisals of the body turn up with different ideas and terms for some of the same experiences. And, as it turns out, patterns are much the same, whether in the gross or subtle body. No form of terminology, in all its flawed humanity, is sufficient to pin down the experience of transformation. We are, after all, self-assembled and continue (via all these threads) to adapt ourselves and our resilience to the changes we meet daily. That may be

CHAPTER THREE

posture-by-posture or day-by-day. The pattern recognition is nevertheless key to both, whatever the scale – time- or space-based.

The deeper we go on this trail of transformation, the more we see the signposts pointing toward *the mystery*. Names and discreet structures with easy diagrams are so useful for reducing complex organic systems into linear relationships that we have a better shot at understanding. And the subtle body anatomy is undeniably beautiful. It is indeed a diagram befitting our interest as yogis in a physical practice that developed around ancient physiology.

However, just as the bones and muscles are much of a muchness, by this line of thinking, so too must be the numinous subtle body constructs of Ida and Pingala in their course around Sushumna, and the pranic airs called as such. These constructs as metaphors point to aspects of reality that can be explored in the context of biophysics and beyond. Suppose it is possible to adopt a seamless and fully integrated anatomy. In that case, as soon as we've digested a diagram, it is time to see it for what it is: a useful but ultimately incomplete human attempt at defining in 2D something that exists as multidimensional at least.

We have walked through the Tantric forest of kundalini and Prana, wandered along the vayu, only to arrive out on the other side and suggest that it, too, is a mirage. This we offer in the same whisper that asks us to consider that our reductionist anatomical terms are mythological ideas sanctioned into truths by declaration.

What I'm saying is that while subtlety is real, codifications of the subtle body are no different to codifications of the gross anatomy. Both are systems of nomenclature (worded codes) made up

over millennia. For now, we're going to love them and leave them. Our subtle and gross are both, more simply, considered as tubular kinematics, the formation of which is our embryological opening act.[58]

If we see the term *subtlety* without its cloak of implications, it is just a word for something so fine and delicate that it is hard to discuss. Something *nuanced*. I've come to think of it as a word for phenomena that are so very small, nobody in the Western conversation apart from physicists and spiritualists feel confident even considering them. But maybe we can at least reserve a space for the experience of subtlety as intrinsic to being alive (a fundamental right, so to speak). So, if you're still with me, let's set aside the formal subtle body for now, keep the concept of *subtlety* to hand, and get back to our yoga in all its nuanced experiential richness.

Yoga can happen by *not* doing, as powerfully as by doing. By choosing to stop the painful consequences of behavior going against the grain of nature, it might be possible to *experience* that grain of nature flowing through us. Once we find this middle path where there is good space (sukha), effort is *channeled with ease* so that we, as practitioners, can reap the myriad benefits of breath-centered movement.

This chapter opened by underlining the very simplest of actions as our embryonic selves first find their tubular shape in a seminal act of space-making. With a foundation in embryology, Five Filaments, and the tube movement of srotas-kinematics, our tubules are ready to meet us in an updated pedagogical space. Here we can talk anatomy in terms that are less linear and more interconnected. In such an integrated context, we'll look at patterns of spirality in practice.

Srotas-kinematics (tubular movement)

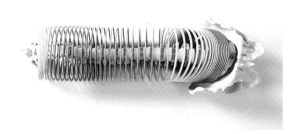

FIGURE 3.24

Rainbow pelvis.

This body is known as the Brahmanda (Microcosm)

In this body, the mount Meru – i.e., the vertebrae–

is surrounded by seven islands;

there are rivers, seas, mountains, fields;

and lords of the fields too.

Siva Samhitā 2.1 [45]

References

1   The Brihadaranyaka Upanishad: Sanskrit Text, English Translation, and Commentary. Divine Life Society; 1985.

2   Sargeant W, Smith H, Chapple CK. The Bhagavad Gita: 25th Anniversary Edition. State University of New York Press; 2010.

3   O'Donnell K. Everyday Ayurveda Guide to Self Care. Shambhala Publications; 2020.

4   Krishnamacharya T. Yoga Makaranda. Mysore: Madurai C.M.V. Press; 1934 (translation published 2006).

5   Blum M, Feistel K, Thumberger T, Schweickert A. The evolution and conservation of left-right patterning mechanisms. Development. 2014;141(8):1603–13.

6   Moukhtar J, Trubuil A, Belcram K, et al. Cell geometry determines symmetric and asymmetric division plane selection in Arabidopsis early embryos. PLoS Computational Biology. 2019;15(2):e1006771.

7   Lebreton G, Geminard C, Lapraz F, et al. Molecular to organismal chirality is induced by the conserved myosin 1D. Science (New York, NY). 2018;362(6417):949–52.

8   Sthijns M, LaPointe VLS, van Blitterswijk CA. Building complex life through self-organization. Tissue Engineering Part A. 2019;25(19–20):1341–6.

9   Zhang HT, Hiiragi T. Symmetry breaking in the mammalian embryo. Annual Review of Cell and Developmental Biology. 2018;34:405–26.

10   van der Gucht J, Sykes C. Physical model of cellular symmetry breaking. Cold Spring Harbor Perspectives in Biology. 2009;1(1):a001909-a.

11   Pohl C. Cytoskeletal symmetry breaking and chirality: From reconstituted Systems to animal development. Symmetry. 2015;7(4):2062.

12   Caraka, Kaviratna AC. Charaka-Samhita: Translated into English. Calcutta: G.C. Chakravarti; 1896.

13   Singhal GD, Singh LM, Singh KP. Susrutasamhita: Diagnostic Considerations in Ancient Indian Surgery. Allahabad; 1972.

CHAPTER THREE

14   Samuel G, Johnston J. Religion and the Subtle Body in Asia and the West: Between Mind and Body. Taylor & Francis; 2013.

15   Kwan SSM. Postcolonial Resistance and Asian Theology. Taylor & Francis; 2013.

16   Damasio AR. The Feeling of What Happens: Body and Emotion in the Making of Consciousness. Vintage; 2000.

17   Tzika E, Dreker T, Imhof A. Epigenetics and metabolism in health and disease. Frontiers in Genetics. 2018;9(361).

18   Maher M, Diesch J, Casquero R, Buschbeck M. Epigenetic-transcriptional regulation of fatty acid metabolism and its alterations in leukaemia. Frontiers in Genetics. 2018;9(405).

19   Sardon Puig L, Valera-Alberni M, Cantó C, Pillon NJ. Circadian rhythms and mitochondria: connecting the dots. Frontiers in Genetics. 2018;9(452).

20   Hunter R. Epigenetic effects of stress and corticosteroids in the brain. Frontiers in Cellular Neuroscience. 2012;6(18).

21   Gluckman PD, Hanson MA, Cooper C, Thornburg KL. Effect of in utero and early-life conditions on adult health and disease. The New England Journal of Medicine. 2008;359(1):61–73.

22   Whitman W. I Sing the Body Electric. Available at: https://interestingliterature. com/2018/11/i-sing-the-body-electric-a-poem-by-walt-whitman/

23   Wainwright SA. The Animal Axis. Integrative and Comparative Biology. 2000;40(1):19–27.

24   Swatmarama Muktibodhananda Saraswati Y. Hatha Yoga Pradipika. Bihar School of Yoga; 1450.

25   Kier WM. The diversity of hydrostatic skeletons. The Journal of Experimental Biology. 2012;215(8): 1247–57.

26   Khendkar Jayashree Chandrakant PJJ. Physiological and clinical significance of srotas. International Journal of Health Sciences and Research. 2016;6(9):451–7.

27   Vandana Verma GS. Review on concept of srotas. International Journal of Research in Ayurveda & Pharmacy. 2014;5(2).

28   Saatcioglu F. Regulation of gene expression by yoga, meditation and related practices: a review of recent studies. Asian Journal of Psychiatry. 2013;6(1):74–7.

29   Sullivan MB, Erb M, Schmalzl L, et al. Yoga therapy and polyvagal theory: the convergence of traditional wisdom and contemporary neuroscience for self-regulation and resilience. Frontiers in Human Neuroscience. 2018;12(67).

30   Bushell WC. Longevity: potential life span and health span enhancement through practice of the basic yoga meditation regimen. Annals of the New York Academy of Sciences. 2009;1172:20–7.

31   Mendioroz M, Puebla-Guedea M, Montero-Marín J, et al. Telomere length correlates with subtelomeric DNA methylation in long-term mindfulness practitioners. Scientific Reports. 2020;10(1):4564.

32   Bushell WC, Theise ND. Toward a unified field of study: longevity, regeneration, and protection of health through meditation and

related practices. Annals of the New York Academy of Sciences. 2009;1172:5–19.

33 Campbell AA, Wisco BE, Silvia PJ, Gay NG. Resting respiratory sinus arrhythmia and posttraumatic stress disorder: a meta-analysis. Biological Psychology. 2019;144:125–35.

34 Di Bello M, Carnevali L, Petrocchi N, et al. The compassionate vagus: a meta-analysis on the connection between compassion and heart rate variability. Neuroscience and Biobehavioral Reviews. 2020;116:21–30.

35 Kim JJ, Parker SL, Doty JR, et al. Neurophysiological and behavioural markers of compassion. Scientific Reports. 2020;10(1):6789.

36 Scarr G. Helical tensegrity as a structural mechanism in human anatomy. International Journal of Osteopathic Medicine. 2009;14(1):24–32.

37 Scarr G. Fascial hierarchies and the relevance of crossed-helical arrangements of collagen to changes in the shape of muscles. Journal of Bodywork and Movement Therapies. 2016;20(2):377–87.

38 Acland R. Acland's Video Atlas of Human Anatomy. Wolters Kluwer; 2020.

39 Singh HK. Brain enhancing ingredients from Āyurvedic medicine: quintessential example of Bacopa monniera, a narrative review. Nutrients. 2013;5(2):478–97.

40 Ten Upanishads with Notes and Commentary. Yoga-Vedanta Forest Academy; 1959.

41 Hareesh. The five koshas and the five-layered self: a comparison. 2015 Available at: https://hareesh.org/blog/2015/12/16/the-five-koshas-and-the-five-layered-self-a-comparison.

42 Datta PK. Tantra: Its Relevance to Modern Times. Punthi Pustak; 2010.

43 Mallinson J, Singleton M. Roots of Yoga. Penguin Books; 2017.

44 Charaka A. Charaka Samhita: Handbook on Ayurveda. Independently Published.

45 Rai Bahadur SCV. Siva Samhitā. 1915.

46 Venkatraman A, Nandy R, Rao S, et al. Tantra and modern neurosciences: is there any correlation? Neurology India. 2019;67(5):1188–93.

47 Skora KM. The hermeneutics of touch: uncovering Abhinavagupta's tactile terrain. Method and Theory in the Study of Religion. 2009; 21:87–106.

48 Loizzo JJ. The subtle body: an interoceptive map of central nervous system function and meditative mind-brain-body integration. Annals of the New York Academy of Sciences. 2016;1373(1):78–95.

49 Quadt L, Critchley HD, Garfinkel SN. The neurobiology of interoception in health and disease. Annals of the New York Academy of Sciences. 2018;1428(1):112–28.

50 Saraswati S. Asana Pranayama Mudra Bandha. Bihar Yoga Bharati; 1997.

51 Cowell EB. The Maitri Or Maitrāyanīya Upanishad: With the Commentary of Rámatírtha. W.M. Watts; 1870.

52 Cowell EB. The Maitri, Or Maitrāyanīya Upanishad: With Commentary of Rāmatīrtha (Classic Reprint). FB&C Limited; 2017.

CHAPTER THREE

53 Seth KN, Chaturvedi BK. Gods And Goddesses Of India. Diamond Pocket Books; 2000.

54 Garrigues D. Secrets of Yogic Breathing. Vayu Siddhi; 2016. Available from: https://davidgarrigues.com/shop/secrets-of-yogic-breathing-vayu-siddhi-book

55 Tirumular S. Tirumantiram. Open source; c. 5th century.

56 Huijing PA. Epimuscular myofascial force transmission: a historical review and implications for new research. International Society of Biomechanics Muybridge Award Lecture, Taipei, 2007. Journal of Biomechanics. 2009;42(1):9–21.

57 Ahmed A, Siddique JI, Mahmood A. Non-Newtonian flow-induced deformation from pressurized cavities in absorbing porous tissues. Computer Methods in Biomechanics and Biomedical Engineering. 2017;20(13):1464–73.

58 Udainiya N, Chandla A, Sharma N. A critical appraisal of Garbha Avkranti vis-a-vis modern embryology. Journal of Ayurveda and Holistic Medicine. 2017;V(IV):52–60.

4.1 Simplicity emerging   135

4.2 Aims and objectives   143

4.3 Samasthiti   144

4.4 Statement of constraints   147

4.5 The Five Filaments in postural yoga:
one example   148

- One: Shoulder Filament –
  the scapulohumeral rhythm (A, B)   148
- Two: Handstand Filament –
  pronation/supination (A, B)   150
- Three: Hip Filament –
  the pelvifemoral rhythm (A, B)   152
- Four: Footstand Filament –
  plantarflexion/dorsiflexion (A, B)   154
- Five: Axial Matrix Filament –
  twist/lateral flexion (A, B)   156

Kinematics come to life

4

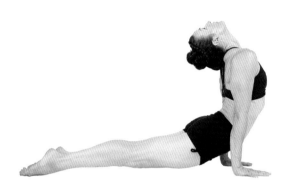

FIGURE 4.1

Upward Dog.

(Demonstrated by Sarah Hatcher)

Gheranda said:
There are eighty-four hundreds of thousands of asanas described by Siva. The postures are as many in number as there are numbers of species of living creatures in this universe.

The Gheranda Samhita[1]

4.1 Simplicity emerging

Although the spiral pattern in tissue organization and behavior is universal, it can be hard to talk about. Anatomy is much simpler to learn when we are cutting it into pieces! Linking everything together into one helical continuum is a lot easier with visuals that can show us the living patterns from micro to macro. The trouble is that these visuals can be hard to come by.

Developing this imagery often means independently surveying many fields and feeling it kinesthetically, since spiral patterns are generally not part of formal anatomy education. In fact, it is very *uncommon* to learn anatomy concerning the spiral nature of muscles, tissues and their organization in the living body. I aim to shine some light into this gap.

Yoga practitioners come to the study of anatomy from various stylistic backgrounds. The conversation (and translation of anatomy into motion) can become confusing because

of such variety, not only in yoga but also in the study of how we teach and learn anatomy. (Head to Appendix B for an enriched offering on nonlinear pedagogy for teachers and students.) I've learned as a researcher that confusion can be an invaluable phase of learning. Chaos is a catalyst for questioning, honing, and simplifying. There we can explore our curiosity, check biases and consider our choices of language.

Language (how we describe something) is different from nomenclature (the naming of it). Language affords us communication and insight, seeking to make continuous sense of our experience. Nomenclature, more of a cul-de-sac, offers tempting endpoints. In some ways, *naming* invites a sort of safety in universal agreement but in other ways, can reduce our experience to dead ends.

In this chapter, I get personal about what yoga means to me. There comes a time when years of experience converge with study; for each of us, this results in something unique.

CHAPTER FOUR

As teachers, we can develop language to share our findings, all interwoven with the classical pillars of nomenclature upon which we weave. Yoga practice is nothing if not compassionate reflection on a radically personal struggle.

Yoga is also a multifaceted field. My intent here is not to say which method, if any, is correct. Instead, as a lover and dedicated teacher of yoga in all its forms, I want to keep doing and exploring it for a long time. Working from a spiral-based curriculum keeps me teaching and practicing in a way that minimizes injury and supports my changing circumstances in education and practice, philosophy and lifestyle. As a mother, teacher, practitioner and seeker, studying spirality is a convergence of research in everything that keeps me evolving on all fronts. What I love about this work in spirality, which can quickly become cosmically abstract, is that it is also evidently practical.

The new language challenges some of the accepted classical nomenclatures. A spinal column, for example, as a stacked compression structure, would break or collapse under the most basic exploration on the yoga mat. Inversions challenge it entirely since the body stays organized and restores its shape. To date, in Warrior Pose, no one has been known to lose a hand off the end of an arm held out parallel to the ground. This may seem obvious. However, that might be where the key to the new paradigm we are in is hidden. There can be no such thing as a "spinal column" as a compression structure named as such would suggest. Embryologically and practically this ability to transfer weight and organize ground control upright and inverted suggests a calling for the biotensegrity model.

Joanne Avison

A rubric for the simplification of yoga anatomy

First, we started by looking at embryology to see the unfolding of our filamentous anatomy. Then, rotation was introduced and defined as (perhaps an underappreciated) characteristic of movement in general. This rotation can be harnessed as an approach for simplifying the nature of biomotion into a set of fundamental principles we can easily use on the mat. From this approach, I'm offering a method to streamline selected movement principles into five essential, biomotional flows: *Five Filaments*.

The previous chapters have distinguished "tubularity" as a structural basis for applying spiral action in movement. The story of the embryo shows us our toroidal topology, as the meso tissue twirls itself around the tubular network, integrating the wholeness in a spiral *modus operandi*. I've proposed the term srotas-kinematics for this integration, as it links the yogic idea of tubular fabric (gross and subtle) intimately with a name for interconnected movement (kinematics). Tubular movement!

Are you starting to imagine yourself more akin to the caterpillar and less like a plastic skeleton rigidly bolted together? If so, then we are on the right track. I intend to show how this integrated anatomy of spirals plays out at various levels, and how everything revolves around maintaining adequate spaciousness amongst (within and around) the tubularity of body fabric. In this chapter, we apply the Five Filaments (5F) as a rubric to a selection of asanas and look at the distinction of spirality defining each of them. We experience their counter-spirality (chirality) *as an expression of that distinction.*

Body geometry guides my perspective. We are here to study the closed nature of our kinematic

Kinematics come to life

chains, and to harness the biologic coupling across all sheaths of our experience from gross to subtle. Recall from Chapter 3: in the torus shape, we initially achieved the conditions for the advent of the gut tube. On a practical level, the cross-ply, tubular motif is illustrated in the knotwork of classical asana.

The fibrous fabric of the body *can* thread into and around itself, without tearing, like a reef knot or figure of eight. Further, our experience as a biologic form blends the inside and outside. As such, the lines and loops of our myofascial continuities pour into themselves as long as we are alive to integrate the experience. In particular, the Krishnamacharya-influenced yogasana seem to demonstrate – and celebrate – the interwoven time-bending, surface-permeating nature of our coupled 4D complexity.

What we consider the "formal" postures of yoga have emerged as part of the international physical culture over the last two centuries.[2] Postural yoga takes the body deep into its naturally spiraling kinematic expression. It becomes easy to see how rotation makes possible these shapes of ever-deepening complexity when you keep going with the arc of their narrative.

But let me be clear: in theory, these "yogahedra," or body shapes, could potentially be achieved by anybody with the morphological constraints particular to our species. In practice, of course, there is a wide range of factors that determine the personal outcome of possibilities where postural yoga is concerned. The body is nonlinear (see Appendix B for more about nonlinearity), the awareness is nonlinear, and so too is our pedagogy.

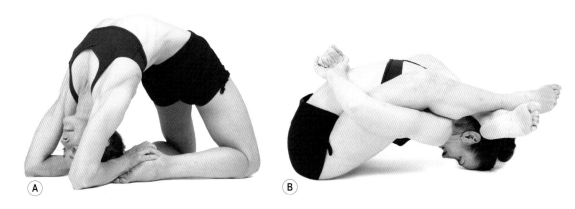

FIGURE 4.2

(A) Kapotasana and **(B)** Suptakurmasana. Comparing these two opposite postures shows the counterbalance of chiralities. In "Kapo," the shoulders are flexing/laterally rotating (Opening Spiral) while the hips are extending/medially rotating (Grounding Spiral). In Suptakurmasana, the arrangement is just the opposite: the shoulders are extending/medially rotating (Grounding Spiral) while the hips are flexing/laterally rotating (Opening Spiral).

(Demonstrated by Sarah Hatcher)

CHAPTER FOUR

This is a crucial distinction to make concerning getting one's own body into postures: just because anyone *could* potentially make a shape with their body doesn't mean that everyone *can*. Or that they should even try! The poses illustrated in this chapter are by no means a measuring stick for what I think anyone should be doing in their practice. The poses illustrated in this chapter are by no means a measuring stick for what I think anyone should be doing in their practice.

This question is one for self-reflection. Why would a practitioner work for years (decades) to get into these positions? There is no guarantee that we'll ever succeed, and indeed that we won't hurt ourselves by trying. So why bother? For me, it comes down to learning. As we gradually gain experience over time, the body learns more about itself. A practitioner develops their body wisdom with that time-bound care and guidance for the sake of learning.

I've chosen these presentations NOT because they're beautiful to behold or because I think they're suitable for everyone at every (or any) stage of their life. I have selected these postures to illustrate the geometry clearly and emphasize the core chirality we embody. Our ability to express it in this particular way is entirely personal. It comes with a clear warning to invest the time and seek professional guidance to establish the requisite safe practice parameters (see **Points to keep in mind**, and **4.4 Statement of constraints** on p. 147). Furthermore, in the formulation of the ideas behind the approach and method of this book, I am navigating around two loaded topics. The first of these is stretch science (see info box below), and is best dealt with elsewhere.[3,4]

> The term "stretch" is inextricably bound up in the popular definition of yoga. Many would still say that this simple equation holds true: yoga = stretching. I'm asking, can we retire that term and look for language that connects us to the nature of tissue? Living biologic form is a balance of stiffness and flow, whereas "stretching" keeps us thinking in linear terms that don't allow for that complementarity. Try using cues such as "reach" and "open" rather than "elongate" or "stretch."

The second topic is the teleological bias. This isn't so evident at first, but it is essential to understand why I state this clearly. **Teleology** gets us into language that implies a grand designer. Consider statements such as "our bodies were designed to spiral" or "the design of the such-and-such structure." These statements indicate that there is somebody up there doing the designing.

I catch myself out all the time with this one. I am careful to craft my language about the body *evolving*, and spirality *emerging*. What I mean to get across is that the spiral phenomenon influences all of nature, including our bodies. Nature self-assembles. It shows up in structure and function as rotation, guiding the movement that manifests in these shapes (what we call asanas) that illustrate so potently the power of the spiral as a natural motif. However, that is NOT to say that we were *designed* this way *in order* to make these shapes, and that the inability to do specific postures is somehow equivalent to a failure of an individual body to honor or express its inbuilt nature.

This faulty logic is understandable because the advancement of modern yoga is tied to the

Kinematics come to life

global transmission of images showing people doing fantastic things with their bodies. When we are inspired by postures and seek to emulate them, there can be a huge emotional attachment to the achievement.

Approaching yoga with the determination of an athlete can unlock potential. Still, I have seen the flip side of this attachment to achievement, breeding undue disappointment, unnecessary injury, and missed opportunities. I'm not here to push or decry what some understandably refer to as "extreme" postural yoga. I am here to say, "Please note: this is the geometry intrinsic to the form." We all have to decide for ourselves what to do with it, given our circumstances.

A false dichotomy?

In my experience, even this "extreme" yoga can be deeply therapeutic depending on one's approach, given the appropriate learning environment, timing, and guidance. To me, a progressive practice is one that is always guided by what is necessary to balance individual circumstances, and these circumstances are shifting all the time. Although the spiral patterns are universal to all humans, there is no one-size-fits-all approach to healing or revealing "ability" through yoga.

While I consider my practice as athletic, in the sense that it's effortful, it is also therapeutic in the sense that on whichever day or with whatever style I am seeking effortlessness and ease: *sthira-sukham* as appropriate that day. Years of experience and training reinforce what I can best describe as simple, common sense. I listen and tune in to that training to hear what it means in the moment, self-assembling from within. I only impose from without by using props and manual techniques that harmonize with my own body's natural constraints.

My choices as a teacher revolve not around taking a student beyond end range; quite the opposite – when I assist, I am always guiding a student back into their constraints. When we listen for the intrinsic chirality of the form, I have found that something already there waits to be heard. And we can learn to be midwives of that inner logic.

What are we birthing? Balance. Rhythm. Harmony with nature. My viewpoint is that daily movement in the *logos* of Five Filaments can lead to proficiency in more advanced awareness of body geometry. However, the outside appearance isn't in itself the goal. The goal is to harmonize effort with what's already happening in my body, and that is an ever-evolving process with implications for every stage of life.

As a practical example, take my tendency to over-pronate with my "soggy" arches. Because of my collapsing arches, in certain standing postures, I need to focus even more on the lateral rotation of distal lower limb, which for someone with an inherently stiffer/springier arch is not as crucial. Rotating your lower leg laterally (supination) has a subtle link to the activation of the arches, so I'm more interested in stabilizing my arches in standing postures to support my postural phenotype. I need to acknowledge my hypermobility and create protective awareness around regions such as these.

Supporting the tendency towards ligament laxity in my feet is a lifelong focus for me, so I modify poses to prioritize this work in my feet even though in standing postures this means I regularly have to let go of "deepenings" elsewhere. This "conscious sleeving" is a modification of priorities to make sure we're serving the system globally rather than sacrificing balance to "do the full posture" according to some pre-ordained aesthetic or stylistic measure.

CHAPTER FOUR

This conscious sleeving is about appropriate guidance over time. There is no point pushing "next level" postural yoga until we are steeped in the spirality of constraints and a deep understanding of the thixotropic nature of tissue discussed in the previous chapter. What we can do as teachers and practitioners is learn to expose our natural tendencies and nurture them gently towards biomotional integrity.

An evidence-based tool to account for the nonlinear nature of tissue in movement adragogy: VITAL for constraints-led physical practice

This **VITAL** tool is about maintaining a level of objectivity, or as we say in yoga, "cultivating the witness." It a practical method for yogis to manage tissue health long-term.

Here's how it works:

V - Variation

I - Iteration

T - Time

A - Approach

L - Logos

Variation

For me, *variation* is about doing different things whereas *variability* means doing the same things differently. Both are really important for maintaining the longevity of our joints. The joint spaces are an organ system unto themselves, a complex site of force transmission known as the **enthesis organ**.[5] The enthesis organ is a kind of distributed ecosystem of tissue densities around the interfaces of bones that are responsive to forces at various timescales.[6,7,8,9]

We need variation so we're not exposing these smart materials (they're constantly remodelling, for better or worse) to damaging repetitive forces at end ranges for extended periods. We need variability (practising consistent movement with variable intensity levels) so that our body can learn to move harmoniously as it adjusts to the loads required for that movement. To simplify: the helical filaments of collagen and associated proteins are strong and resilient as a result of their tight spiral configuration. Stretching the tissues is comparative to stretching the slinky beyond its ability to bounce back. When tissue is stretched beyond its capacity, the spirality of its particles can become permanently unwound and thus forever robbed of that elastic response upon which we depend for everyday functions.[10]

As leaders in functional movement are increasingly bringing their evidence-based approach to yoga, we are finally chipping away at the old "yoga = stretching" cliché. The evolving paradigm of yoga from the purely physical perspective has always been a bodyweight discipline with a focus on isometrics and end-range flexibility. Now, things are changing as stretching, and yoga as a biomechanical problem space, gets redefined. From the ground-breaking work of Jules Mitchell[11] to the Yoga Deconstructed method of Trina Altman,[12] varying load (adding external load!) and intensity relative to capacity is a promising route for the continuing evolution of yoga in our generation and beyond.

In short: sometimes we need to do different kinds of movement, and sometimes we need to do the same kinds of movement at different levels of load/intensity. That's how we can increase capacity and even play in the end ranges with the best chance of keeping the enthesis organ

Kinematics come to life

Iteration

I'm going to go back to my roots again to use Ashtanga as an example. In this practice, you go through the same set of postures first, known simply as "standing", and then into the "seated" postures. The seated postures are almost all based on deep rotations of the hip/knee during flexion. The methodology is linear, which is fundamentally problematic when we take linear *literally*. I'm saying we should take the linear nature of any activity as an *iterative,* not literal, project.

Many fitness programs are linear and sequential, and that's because we need some basis for organisation and progression. Historically, pedagogy is like that in every skills-based curriculum. You come to a lesson, study, get tested, pass the test, and move on to the next lesson. Fortunately, the conversation is evolving as practitioners embrace advances in our understanding of tissue. An iterative approach essentially means *innovate*. Do what you can. Do something else entirely if you need to. Don't force your body into a task just so you can pass the test and get to the next lesson.

Time

That brings us to the multi-dimensionality of tissue, sometimes oversimplified in terms of time. But it's a useful simplification nonetheless, one that gives us perspective about the cellular matrix. Because it's not just fascia, and it's not simply *extra*-cellular (meaning "outside" the cells)! We are living matrices of cellular force transmission that is constantly under the influence of earthly and organismic constraints and vectors in a nonlinear relationship.

Mechanical forces, chemical interactions, genetics, emotion, behaviour, the weather; all of these inform our present experience of having a body, and all will change over the course of a lifespan. We cannot assume that what feels good now is actually supporting our tissues in the most optimal way long term. Nor should we sell ourselves short and assume that just because a posture seems impossible means it will never be possible, or that it isn't worth doing.

Chronobiology informs our understanding of fascia by connecting our enquiry to the ubiquitous influence of circadian rhythms, Ayurvedic Prakriti, neuroendocrine balance, and all the other couplings in spatiotemporality that give rise to our experience of the body.[13] In short, we aren't built to live forever – in fact, we are sprouts of nature deploying herself through the elements in a momentary blast of multistability manifest in tissues that have a natural perishing arc. Rubber bands don't bounce back forever, neither do our waistlines or menisci.[14] The cellular matrix (including the fascia, cytoskeletal architecture, fluid matrix, and biofield) is a temporary crystallisation of all the concurrent processes we are going through simultaneously! Keep this in mind: **as your body matures, so too must your movement.**

Approach

Think about your approach to movement. Again, I'll use Ashtanga as an example. I would still consider myself an Ashtanga practitioner, but to look at my actual practice these days you might not think so! I'm approaching Ashtanga differently in light of all the previous points of the VITAL tool.

CHAPTER FOUR

After all, yoga is a science of mind. What we do with our bodies is always about supporting the bigger transformation happening within.

I've seen so many fellow students drop out of the practice for very understandable reasons. Six days per week is an enormous commitment over the years, and it can be selfish, self-defeating, and even self-harming when we don't take into account the points above about variation, iteration, and time. So, people quit. To me, that is often a wasted opportunity because all the reasons that make us want to quit something are the very same drivers of innovation. This aspect, Approach, is about feeling empowered to change the way you practice, to be creative and multidisciplinary. As Tiffany reminds us in her foreword, what is fascia but the ultimate multidisciplinary tissue?

Logos

Logos is the language of the body. In Ashtanga, we study yoga as an eight-limbed path of transformation as codified by Patanjali in the Yoga Sutras. *Svadhyaya*, self-study, is part of this path. To me, studying the inner logic of tissue is an important part of yoga, and over the years I've experienced the spirality of fascia as the fundamental logos of movement.

Having a logos practice means studying not just anatomy, but how anatomy is part of the continuum of life. Human anatomy is connected not only within itself in terms of fascia, but to the great tapestry of filamentous life from the mycelium of fungi to the subtle forces of nature manifest in plants and animals. When we study the philosophy behind yoga, **Samkhya**, it becomes easier to see that interconnectedness is fundamental to life and that Nature weaves a spiral web.

And that's the VITAL tool! We are waking up to the paradigm shift that is showing us the perils of lineage yoga. There is a concurrent and related paradigm shift in biology that talks more about how suffering anywhere results in suffering everywhere. I feel that for anyone interested in anatomy for yoga, waking up to this shifting paradigm is vital indeed.

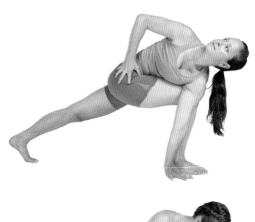

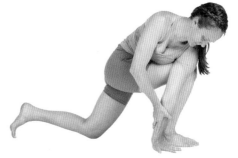

FIGURE 4.3

Overpronators can benefit from activating the windlass of the foot in lunge instead of choosing footwork that forces already overpronated arches to collapse further.

The Gheranda quote at the start of this chapter is sweet, as 84,000 species was considered a lot then

Kinematics come to life

(to date this figure is around 8.7 million, although that number is sadly on the decline). There is no doubt that a similar explosion of new postures is happening too, as functional movement and yoga create novel ways of exploring the what, why, and how of biologic shape-change. As we'll see in the images coming up, the classical postures are "old school" diagrams of posture "species" – rich with value but by no means the only animals in the zoo.

Micromovement, for me, is a way of using the breath to "cook up" the ingredients needed for more complex recipes. Whether I ever actually do the "big" posture itself is not the point. This laboratory is particular to my journey and forms the basis of my teaching the 5F as a method for methods. My **aims** are simple. I want to help fellow students and practitioners of yoga identify the imbalances interfering with sthira-sukham in their system and subsequently remodel from that clearing.

My **objectives** in teaching are all based on using a range of techniques to address each of the 5F. Using the VITAL tool, we can weave a responsive practice with posturality and movement where appropriate. Everyone is different, and among individuals, there is a vast range of shifting phases that correspond to people's actual lives.

During antenatal and postpartum phases, for example, a woman will experience her body changing in fundamental ways. Her apparent movement will often belie what she's managing and doing on the inside. I am so thankful for the vast lessons of my maternal years. Modifying my yoga practice to support the monumental tidal shifts of tissue integrity shows me that nothing about the body is permanent and there are no rules of movement that are true for *everybody* (or *anybody*) all the time. Instead, there are patterns

and rhythms and ways of dancing with them. Underneath all these, we find the periodicity of the spiral.

Pratipaksha-bhavanam: cultivate the opposite

Vitarka badhane pratipaksha bhavanam
Translation: Upon being harassed by negative thoughts, one should cultivate counteracting thoughts.

Patanjali, Yoga Sutras, 2.33[15]

Although most yogis talk about *pratipaksha-bhavanam* in the context of counteracting negative thinking, the principle applies to all practice. As teachers, we have to know that there is not a single correct recipe for adjusting asana because we are working with people (not just their poses). Every person has his or her particular (and changing) constitution. Each person will be calibrating their circumstances within the body geometry that guides us all into common patterns where we may rest comfortably. Your biomotional integrity and mine are distinct, unique to each of us and unique to the occasion. That might be the only thing that doesn't change!

4.2 Aims and objectives

We live and breathe in a net of tubes, both subtle and gross: a mandala of sorts. This heterarchical arrangement defines us as individuals, how we relate to each other, and how groups interact within the more extensive network. In the longer-term practice of yoga, there is no significant difference between teacher and student, in that each of us is a node with threads tying us into the mandala of yoga practice. When I talk about a yoga practitioner, I'm thinking about

CHAPTER FOUR

that person as both teacher and student, with aims and objectives that relate to both teaching professionalism and personal practice.

I do think it is essential to keep asking oneself: *why am I doing this*? The answer might be different each day, but it helps to have a focus. My aims and objectives today might be miles away from what I was working on in the years before I was pregnant. Yet, the work carries the same gentle curiosity. As I have learned from Dr Sarah Duvall's Pregnancy and Postpartum Corrective Exercise Specialist course, using the map of single muscle focus helps bring the joints back into optimal "roll and glide" function that supports the body's own healing chronology. We can use our education to set the body up for regaining its constraints, but when it comes to healing, tissue takes its own sweet time.

This postpartum work gets particularly technical, as we come to understand more about the way single muscle activation recalibrates at a faster timescale than the maternal tissues regain their elasticity after the almighty stretch (in this case an appropriate term!) of pregnancy and birth. This work of rebuilding stamina develops with appropriate bursts of intensity supported by proper rest. Your own goals will be relevant to your circumstances, and circumstances are always changing. The learning goals for a spiral-inspired anatomy practice are a lens through which to consider the following illustrations.

Aims:

- To organize the mind at will (nirodha).
- To rebalance the system as part of pratipaksha-bhavanam (opposition in balance).
- To experience sthira-sukham (steadiness and spaciousness).

Objectives:

1 Study the natural spiral rhythms of srotas-kinematics in personal practice.

2 Learn how to give and receive adjustments biomotionally in a level-appropriate way (contact, contactless, beginners, various ages, fitness and flexibility levels, etc.).

3 Make space for the mystery; contextualize the practice.

4 Practice and teach from the center outwards, using language that emphasizes:

- Breath-centric movement.
- Finding ease (that does not mean it has to be easy; challenges can be invited in a non-harming mode).
- Spiral/rotational instruction.

4.3 Samasthitiḥ

(Sah-mah Steet-ih-hee)
Equal standing

समस्थिति

Tāḍāsana and Samasthitiḥ refer to the same pose: equal standing, the void, or "zero state" of equilibrium. *Sama* translates to "same" and "sthitih" refers to steadiness. It is an asana unto itself, and simultaneously an archetypal moment to be found in every other asana. It is the experience of self-collection we look for in every pose. In it, we establish the steady state of relative equilibrium; stability characterized by conscious breathing coupled with bandha.

Kinematics come to life

I am suggesting that in equal standing posture, theoretically, all the directionalities of flow are in balance. In terms of the 5F rubric, they're either all "on" or all "off," depending on how you look at it. I've chosen to look at this as a neutral pose of potential when motion offsets itself.

Talking point

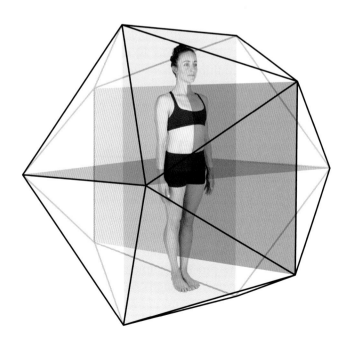

Counterspiral concept

As we look at the diagrams that follow, keep the counterspiral concept in mind: although the arrows indicate the active spirality of each posture, the body is always seated in counterspirality. The cross-ply of two opposing directionalities are always at play in the tissues, reflecting their inherent chirality and our body plan as bilaterally symmetrical. Adjusting/ cueing asana means that we always keep this counterspiral in mind as part of the project toward stabilization, especially toward end ranges.

We are looking at two vector spaces for considering movement in yoga:

- Postural (anatomical planes).
- Packing (closest-packing of spheres, expansion-retraction, convergence-divergence, breathing in and out as iterations of these principles).

We have organized the following asanas according to their planar orientation in traditional Euclidean 3-dimensional space. The sagittal plane is a natural place to start as it contains the continuity of the primary and secondary curves of our embryological origin. These are classically considered the first shapes of the body: flexion (primary curve) and extension (secondary curve). Urdhva Dhanurasana starts off the 5F asana profiles in this chapter as an iconic extension involving intense shoulder flexion.

Reflecting on the image of Simon attempting the same pose in Chapter 3 (see Fig. 3.4), notice

FIGURE 4.4

Samasthitiḥ. Equal standing within the intersection of planes brings the practitioner into a ready stillness, an equilibrium within the Icosahedron.

CHAPTER FOUR

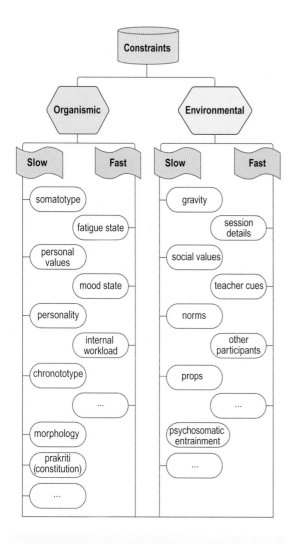

FIGURE 4.5

Classification of organismic and environmental constraints according its relatively faster or slower rate of change.

(Adapted for yoga from Balagué et al.[16] https://sportsmedicine-open.springeropen.com/articles/10.1186/s40798-019-0178-z/figures/3. https://creativecommons.org/licenses/by/4.0/)

served by exploring the filamentous flow within the constraints of its natural architecture as demonstrated elegantly by Fadzai (see Fig. 3.5). We till the soil and then dig the hole before planting the seeds to nourish growth.

With proper filamentous conditioning, movement can indeed grow from there. As the tissues become more resilient and reinforced in their constraints, it makes sense to increase and diversify the challenge accordingly. The posture becomes established in bandha and breath (see Chapter 5), with spiral patterns shown by the arrows. The directionality of the rotations corresponds to vayu, and the felt sense of transanatomical structure. First, figure out the shape of the asana in its planar orientation; then, deepen it through the expansion–retraction of breath.

This offering presents a selection of filamentous flows in postural anatomy. These are presented together with some techniques from the Five Filaments method developed to explore the associated range of motion. By "range" I mean the total package: flexibility and stability (see "fluxtability" in Appendix B) required to support the shape-shifting. These techniques are also defined by the use of breath and bandha and can slot into an appropriate time and place to keep a regular practice.

As you take in the pages that follow, let the feeling of the imagery inform your process of interpretation. Each of the Five Filaments represents a cascade of rotational flow, patterns of biomotion that influence movement at every level. Referring back to the anatomical ideas behind the 5F will help to fill in some of the gaps; however, much of the process of understanding postures is only possible through experience. It is the expression of a felt-sense conversation between the doing and the sensing of the process in progress.

that there is no point trying to push yourself into an asana if the micromovement for that filament is not first fully established. We are better

Kinematics come to life

Points to keep in mind:

- The rubric references the 5F as described in Chapter 2.
- Refer back to the full description of the 5F and make sure you're good with what rotation means before sinking your teeth into this section.
- This offering provides a focus on the spiral action of srotas-kinematics at the macro level.
- Inset images are suggestions for micromovement to activate the filament highlighted for that asana profile.
- This section is not intended for beginners to learn yoga.

4.4 Statement of constraints

The images presented in this chapter are for purposes of illustration and not intended as instructions. All bodies are different, and everyone carries their circumstances, each requiring a carefully considered approach to movement. In the demonstration of asana in this chapter, Sarah Hatcher displays what is possible for her particular body in a specific point in time, based on decades of experience.

Andragogy (as distinct from pedagogy) refers to our adult learning space. Here we can support our nonlinear nature with a constraints-led approach to teaching. I am especially interested in the nested approach described by Natàlia Balagué, professor of exercise physiology.[16] Balagué publishes on the psychobiology of exercise and complex systems in sport. I have adapted her infographic about the timescales at play within our constraints in this chapter, using terms more specific to yoga. In the next chapter, we'll develop these ideas to see what Balagué refers to as "nestedness" of task constraints to see

these as an emergent property of the body within its unique circumstances.[16]

In this chapter, the inset images show ideas for reinforcing constraints to illustrate how we can coax tissues into self-stabilization relating to the bigger picture. We can't assume that what is appropriate in one phase of a person's life will be valid for them at all stages. In the flow diagram of constraints in Figure 4.5, we are highlighting that organismic and environmental constraints come in different rates of speed. A person's chronotype represents their unique rhythmic signature, or how their daily rhythms come to bear on their constitution longer-term (known as dosha in Ayurveda). The factors listed in this diagram are simplified versions of an infinite number of influences at a range of timescales, never the same for everyone. We'll go into this more deeply in Chapter 5.

Is it evident that we should never co-opt someone else's practice as an example of what our bodies ought to do? By now, the broader yoga conversation has brought us into general agreement there. It may be less obvious, but the same is true, even within one person's body throughout its lifetime. What was good for you in your twenties will change over the decades. We can't dogmatically cling to what was right for our tissues in previous years! Likewise, what seemed possible or impossible in your twenties might not play out that way as the system matures: only time will tell.

There's no doubt about the multidimensional, nonlinear nature of our bodies. Our tissue *condition* changes with maturity, and yet the *morphologic constraints* of spirality remain the same. We urge you to respect your body's inner logos, and please seek out an experienced teacher to learn asana. Everywhere you see an * in this chapter, we suggest that you use that moment to reflect on this statement.

CHAPTER FOUR

4.5 The Five Filaments in postural yoga: one example

One: Shoulder Filament – the scapulohumeral rhythm (A, B)

A) Opening Shoulder Spiral

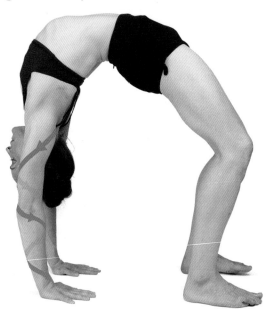

FIGURE 4.6 Ūrdhva Dhanurāsana
(Oord-vhah Danyoor-Asana)
Upward bow pose
ऊर्ध्व धनुरासन

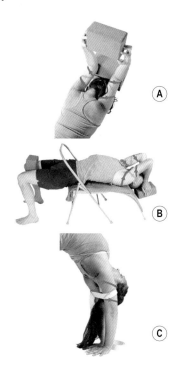

Urdhva Dhanurasana, sometimes Chakrasana or Wheel Pose, is the ultimate footstanding backbend. Resisting gravity requires spaciousness in the OSS for enough power to flow harmoniously. The key is to laterally rotate the shoulder spiral to align the tubular flow for keeping the subacromial space clear (refer to Figs 2.45 and 3.3). Filamentous rotation allows intensification of the shape without harming the tissues. Inset images offer key techniques for opening the OSS. This is required for developing the supine, tetrapodal family of backbend postures (applies to Kapotasana, Vrischikasana, and all associated postural variations).

Symmetrical	Grounding	Opening
Shoulder		●
Hand	●	
Hip	●	
Foot	●	
Axial	Extension	

Kinematics come to life

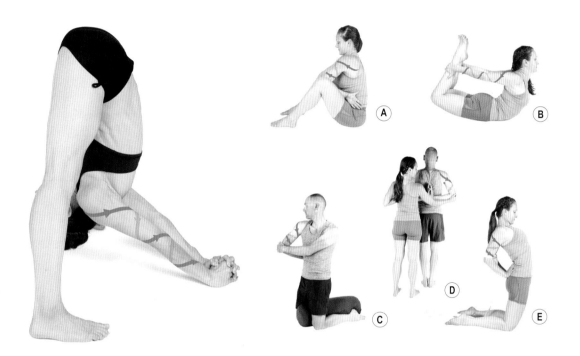

FIGURE 4.7 Prasārita Pādottānāsana C
(Prasa-rita Pado-Ton-Asana)
Wide-stance forward fold with shoulder extension
प्रसारति पादोत्तानासन

Prasarita Padottanasana C is a wide-legged forward bend that first calls for deep hip flexion before moving into increasing shoulder extension as shown in the 5F rubric. Notice the medial humeral rotation combined with scapular rotation and retraction. Collapsing the elbows in hyperextension is a common pitfall, especially in the female phenotype. A microbend of the elbow can help stabilize the arms and drive the rotation toward increasing the felt sense of space, or sukha.*

*See **Points to keep in mind**, and **4.4 Statement of constraints** on p. 147.

Symmetrical	Grounding	Opening
Shoulder	●	
Hand	●	
Hip		●
Foot	●	
Axial	Flexion	

149

CHAPTER FOUR

Two: Hand Filament – supination/pronation (A, B)

A) Opening Hand Spiral

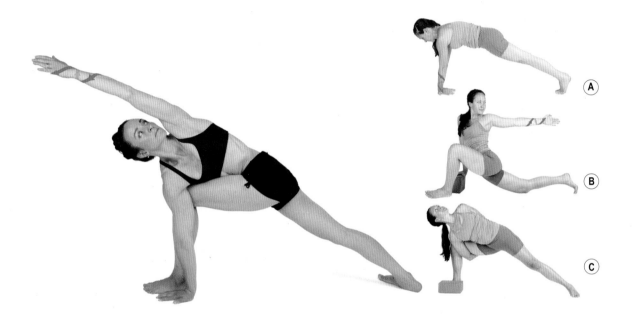

FIGURE 4.8 Parivrtta Parśvakoṇāsana
(Oot-hita Parshva-cone-Asana)
Extended Side Angle Pose
उत्थित पार्श्वकोणासन

Parivrtta Parsvakonasana, revolving side-angle pose, is
an elegant example of an opening mode in the forearm
and hand expression. The arm reaching overhead is
continuing the lateral rotation of the flexed shoulder,
flowing unopposed out through the fingertips. You can see
from the 5F rubric how the rest of the pose is working.
In this instance, we are looking at techniques for building
awareness of the uncrossed radio-ulnar spiral, known as
supination.

L ◦ R ●	Grounding	Opening
Shoulder	●	●
Hand	●	●
Hip	●	●
Foot	● ●	
Axial	Twist	

B) Grounding Hand Spiral

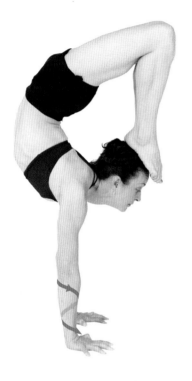

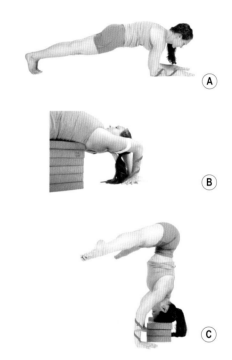

FIGURE 4.9 Vr̥ścikāsana
(Vrisch-cheek-Asana)
Scorpion pose
वृश्चिकासन

Vriscikasana, the Scorpion handstand, comes together on the hands through the pronated forearms. As a grounded handstand of great complexity, there is plenty to work on here! In this particular instance, we are looking at the pronation in the forearms paired with hasta bandha required for fine-tuning the balance. The techniques offered are designed to build confidence connecting bandha with the forearm pronation needed to explore the seemingly impossible.*

*See **Points to keep in mind**, and **4.4 Statement of constraints** on p. 147.

Symmetrical	Grounding	Opening
Shoulder		●
Hand	●	
Hip	●	
Foot	●	
Axial	Extension	

CHAPTER FOUR

Three: Hip Filament – the pelvifemoral rhythm (A, B)

A) Opening Hip Spiral

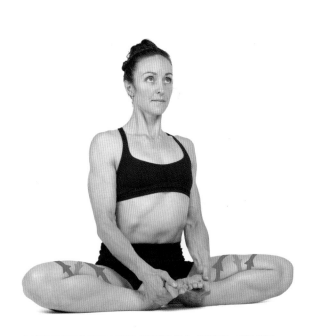

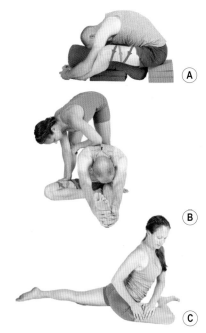

FIGURE 4.10 Baddhakoṇāsana
(Badd-ha-kone-Asana)
Cobbler's pose
बधकोणासन

Baddhakonasana offers a beautiful counterpoint to Urdhva Dhanurasana, and in it, we can see the opening hip spirals clearly expressed. This pose is known for opening the hip flexion with lateral rotation spiral required for building up toward increasing lateral rotation. Baddhakonasana is part of the legs-behind-head posture family (applies to Supta Kurmasana, Ekapada Sirsasana and other postures featuring deep ilio-sacro-femoral range).

Symmetrical	Grounding	Opening
Shoulder	●	
Hand		●
Hip		●
Foot		●
Axial	Flexion/extension	

Kinematics come to life

B) Grounding Hip Spiral

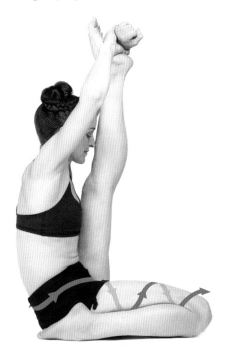

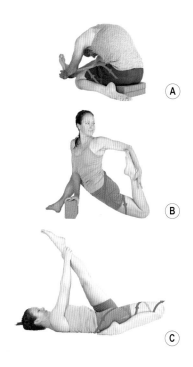

FIGURE 4.11 Krauñcāsana
(Krounch-Asana)
Heron pose
क्रौञ्चासन

Kounchasana is an intensely asymmetrical pose that most of us will never actually do in its full expression (nor do we need to).* This unique posture is presented here because it provides a beautiful illustration of how the grounding hip spiral is expressed when the legs adduct in hip flexion. In this upright, seated forward bend, the counterbalancing is possible under chiral conditions. Shoulders laterally rotate and harness the extended leg, drawing its chirality inward while simultaneously tensioning it. The Grounding Hip Spiral pairs with hip extension (in backbends) and hip flexion whenever the femurs are flexing at the hip (narrowing).

*See **Points to keep in mind**, and **4.4 Statement of constraints** on p. 147.

L ○ R ●	Grounding	Opening
Shoulder		○ ●
Hand	○ ●	
Hip	●	○
Foot	○ ●	
Axial	Flexion	

CHAPTER FOUR

Four: Foot Filament – supination/pronation

A) Opening Foot Spiral

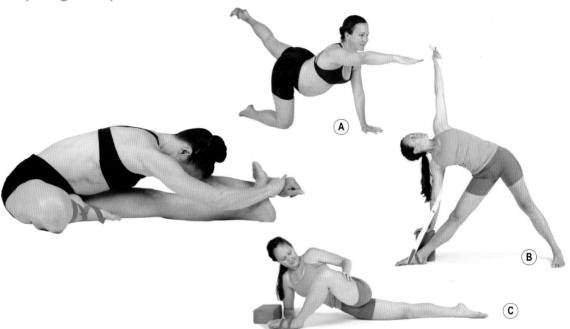

FIGURE 4.12 Janusirsasana A
Janu-sheer-shasana A
Head to knee pose
जानु शीर्षासन

Janusirsasana A is an asymmetrical pose that takes
the shoulders into opening mode and the hands into
grounding mode as they reach to find a bind. Both hips are
externally rotating, but the right leg is much further into
its opening hip spiral than the left straight leg. The right
ankle is carrying the external rotation into supination, a
continuous external rotation as the sole of the foot finds
its way around toward the sky. Bringing awareness to
supination is especially important for those who tend to
overpronate and need to reinforce their constraints as
shown in the inset images.

L ◐ R ●	Grounding	Opening
Shoulder		◐ ●
Hand	◐ ●	
Hip		◐ ●
Foot	◐	●
Axial	Flexion	

B) Grounding Foot Spiral

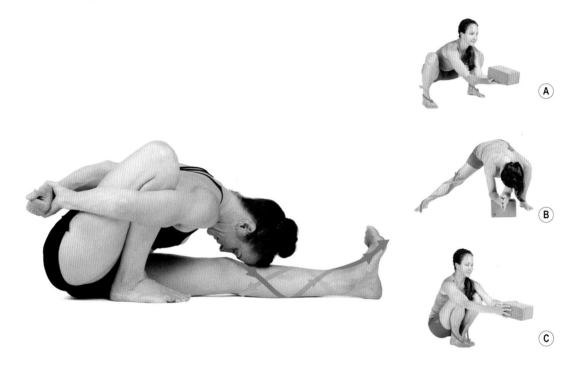

FIGURE 4.13 Marīcyāsana A
(Mary-chi-Asana)
After the sage, Marichy
मरीच्यासन

Marichyasana A, named for the sage Marichy, is an asymmetrical pose involving hip flexion paired with shoulder extension. This posture has been chosen to illustrate how both feet can be in a grounding mode footstand even if one is not actually standing on the ground. Both feet are balanced in the "stability stirrup" of dorsiflexion with the windlass mechanism. Featured here are some techniques for balancing and building in the grounding footstand.

L ○ R ●		Grounding	Opening
Shoulder		● ●	
Hand		● ●	
Hip			● ●
Foot		● ●	
Axial		Flexion	

Five: Axial Matrix Filament – twist/lateral flexion (A, B)

A) Twist

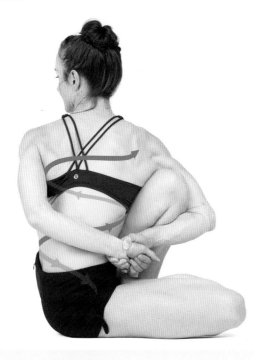

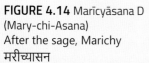

FIGURE 4.14 Marīcyāsana D
(Mary-chi-Asana)
After the sage, Marichy
मरीच्यासन

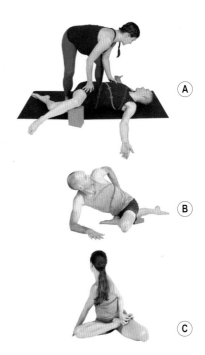

Marichyasana D, like the "A" version, is another asymmetrical pose involving hip flexion paired with shoulder extension. The difference is, of course, the deep twist as one shoulder is wrapped around the contralateral knee. Twist spirals are the key to unlocking range and integrity to support postures that seem to require more than our limbs can offer. Exploring the axial matrix, we invite and manage tensional range and offer expansion to the srotas-kinematics whole. The Twist spiral asks us to bring the humeral latissimus attachment in contact with the tibial attachment of the iliotibial band. Here the "X" of the TFL comes together onto and into itself (see TLFX from Chapter 2). For this reason, the techniques that deepen the Twist are universal and apply to the other spirals in every filamentous flow. *

*See **Points to keep in mind**, and **4.4 Statement of constraints** on p. 147.

L ● R ●	Grounding		Opening
Shoulder	●	●	
Hand	●	●	
Hip	●		●
Foot	●		●
Axial	Twist		

Kinematics come to life

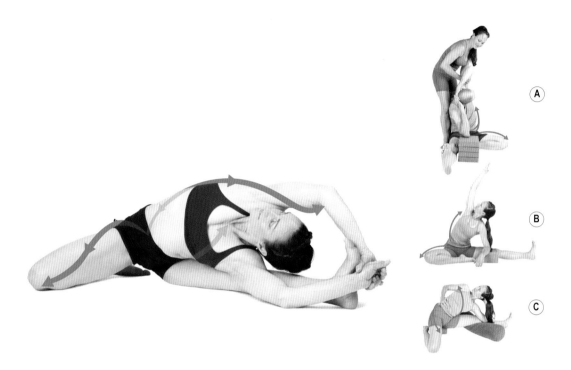

FIGURE 4.15 Parighāsana
(Par-ee-gHaa-sana)
Gate pose
परिघासन

Parighasana is an asymmetrical pose with nuanced filamentous flow. The flexed knee is medially rotated through the ankle, continuing the grounding spiral through that hip. Lateral flexion posturally animates the spinal engine (recall that a tube curved in one plane must rotate to bend in another plane). The Axial Matrix is the throuple, as the lordotic/kyphotic curves paired with any kind of flexion/extension consequently elicit rotation throughout the trunk, describing volume. Because our modern menu of movement simply doesn't include much lateral flexion paired with shoulder flexion, the side body is often "locked" into itself. Unpacking the lateral tissues that feed into the TLFX can empower the other spirals in every filamentous flow.

L ○ R ●		Grounding	Opening
Shoulder			○ ●
Hand		○ ●	
Hip		●	○
Foot		○ ●	
Axial		Lateral flexion	

157

CHAPTER FOUR

References

1   The Gheranda Samhita: A Treatise on Hatha Yoga. Adyar Library; 1933.

2   Mallinson J, Singleton M. Roots of Yoga. Penguin Books Limited; 2017.

3   Sharkey J. Stretching: the faux ami of yoga. In: Avison JS. Yoga, Fascia, Anatomy and Movement, 2nd Edition. Handspring Publishing; 2021.

4   Mitchell J. Yoga Biomechanics: Stretching Redefined. Handspring Publishing Limited; 2018.

5   Petty RE, Cassidy JT. Chapter 2 - STRUCTURE AND FUNCTION. In: Cassidy JT, Laxer RM, Petty RE, Lindsley CB, editors. Textbook of Pediatric Rheumatology (Sixth Edition). Philadelphia: W.B. Saunders; 2011. p. 6–15.

6   Waghray N, Jyothi GA, Imran M, Yaseen S, Chaudhary U. Enthesis: A Brief Review. Apollo Medicine. 2015;12(1):32–8.

7   Milella M, Cardoso FA, Assis S, Lopreno GP, Speith N. Exploring the relationship between entheseal changes and physical activity: a multivariate study. American Journal of Physical Anthropology. 2015;156(2):215–23.

8   Milella M, Giovanna Belcastro M, Zollikofer CP, Mariotti V. The effect of age, sex, and physical activity on entheseal morphology in a contemporary Italian skeletal collection. American Journal of Physical Anthropology. 2012;148(3):379–88.

9   Milella M, Cardoso FA, Assis S, Lopreno GP, Speith N. Exploring the relationship between entheseal changes and physical activity: A multivariate study. American Journal of Physical Anthropology. 2015;156(2):215–23.

10 Zitnay JL, Li Y, Qin Z, San BH, Depalle B, Reese SP, Buehler MJ, Yu SM, Weiss JA. Molecular level detection and localization of mechanical damage in collagen enabled by collagen hybridizing peptides. Nature Communications. 2017;8(1):14913.

11 Mitchell J. Yoga Biomechanics: Stretching Redefined: Handspring Publishing Limited; 2018.

12 Altman T. Yoga Deconstructed: Transitioning from Rehabilitation Back Into the Yoga Studio: Handspring Publishing Limited; 2020.

13 Bechtel W. From molecules to behavior and the clinic: Integration in chronobiology. Studies in History and Philosophy of Science Part C: Studies in History and Philosophy of Biological and Biomedical Sciences. 2013;44(4, Part A):493–502.

14 Nesbitt DQ, Siegel DN, Nelson SJ, Lujan TJ. Effect of age on the failure properties of human meniscus: High-speed strain mapping of tissue tears. Journal of Biomechanics. 2021;115:110126.

15 Bryant EF. The Yoga Sutras of Patanjali. North Point Press; 2009.

16 Balagué N, Pol R, Torrents C, et al. On the relatedness and nestedness of constraints. Sports Medicine – Open. 2019;5(1).

5.1 Self-directed transformation 162

5.2 Dvandva 163

5.3 Breath 166

5.4 Bandha: de facto structure 172

5.5 Dṛṣṭi 178

5.6 Seated in spirals 179

5.7 Resources for teachers 183

Acoustics of Self

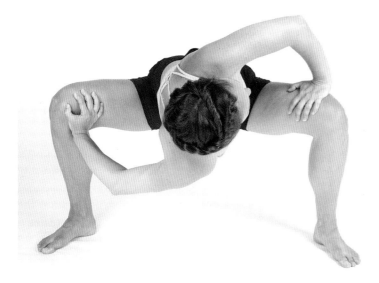

FIGURE 5.1

Standing spirality demonstrated by the author.

In this body infected with passions, anger, greed, delusion, fright, despondency, grudge, separation from what is dear and desirable, attachment to what is not desirable, hunger, thirst, old age, death, illness, sorrow and the rest – how can one experience only joy?

Maitrayaniya Upanishad, I.3 1

Key concepts

1   *Dvandvas* are pairs of opposing qualities that combine to make emergent properties.

2   Yoga can be a transformative psycho-physiological playground for balancing and unifying pairs of opposites (*dvandvas*) towards holistic balance and healing.

3   The oscillatory nature of breathing, via srotas-kinematics, links prana and apana together to form an internal "anchoring system" as part of biomotional integrity.

4   The breath brings volition to convergent-divergent movement in asana, balancing the coupled sympathetic and parasympathetic nervous systems.

5   *Pranayama* is the yogic practice of consciously introducing retentions to manipulate one's flow of breathing.

6   The breath is a rhythm that couples stiffness and suppleness with movement, giving rise to appropriate elastic compliance.

7   *Bandha* is the intentional coupling of stiffness and suppleness with movement and breath.

8   *Mudra/bandha* form an internal anchoring system within the body matrix for circulation as well as sensorimotor information.

9   *Vinyasa* is a movement practice incorporating *tristana:* breath, *bandha, drishti.*

10 Seated postures, an approach to stillness, are inherently spiral.

11 Variations on seated meditation positions are useful for learning to sit in equilibrium.

5.1 Self-directed transformation

At the very beginning of this book, I asked: *What makes the study of anatomy distinct from the study of yoga?* This is not a trivial question, as we learn the truth of our tissues emerging through pure experience. This question is with me all the time. Such gradual awakening to the geometry of our common constraints is transformative because it leads us from gross to subtle (and back again). Here we see that the jumping-off place at the end of the anatomy map lands us in the multidimensional territory of the ubiquitous fascia.

First of all, let's define "transformation". For a readership interested in well-being, transformation is a qualitative process that involves the upward spiral effect on all systems from gross to subtle, visible to invisible. Movement (intentional motion) can be a catalyst in that process. The power of movement relates to the unifying relationship amongst pairs of opposing qualities (such as gross and subtle, prana and apana, inhale and exhale, tension and compression, opening and grounding spirals) and how their relationship can bring about such transformation.

For a definition of fascia, we are coming to the moment when anatomists are recognizing fascia (or the Extracellular Matrix (ECM), together with the cellular matrix of cytoskeletal filaments) as the structural medium of anatomy as a whole. This chapter looks at how we can use movement to find stillness which, in turn, may allow the activation of

awareness of our inner nature. From the structural perspective of the Five Filaments (5F), the opposing forces of tension and compression (pranapana) form the operative pair, unifying to include the volume we animate. This dance of two creates a third, as we have seen in multiple examples.

The dance can start as an aesthetic or athletic performance (as the postures from the previous chapter illustrate) or indeed emerge as something much less obvious. With so many different styles out there, you have to wonder: what distinguishes "movement" generally (and yoga specifically) from exercise? I ask this question often, and there may not be a definitive answer.

Whatever it is we feel that yoga brings to us on a personal level, it can be interesting to look at what happens over time: how the practice changes us, and how we adapt the techniques in response to the process of maturation. Ultimately, a lasting relationship with yoga practice continues for its effect on the system as a whole. In a way, we could consider it as an empirical study of the Self, designed to bring us to a comfortable pause; the undefinable result of *sthira-suhkham.*

The study of Self is not *self-ish* in the egoist sense of being self-engrossed or self-oriented at the expense of other things. We are using the stuff of ourselves as a laboratory for the meeting, studying, and savoring of our spiral constraints, patterns that connect us all. On a practical level, the methods of yoga offer us various voluntary

Acoustics of Self

constraints that feed into the organismic constraints, both in stillness and in continuous movement. With enough practice, the body learns to sit quietly, comfortably, essentially listening to itself. This chapter deals with some ways of setting the stage for optimal acoustics.

> Upon entering the realm of consciousness, of the invisible forces that were divided somewhat from the visible, measurable forms in our historical study of anatomy, for example, we enter an arena that is difficult to describe and bravely navigated here. It is, as the ancient Vedic Sages say in many and various ways, beyond the reasoning mind, or the *citta vrtti* that runs a commentary alongside our vivid experience.
>
> There, the opposition of apparently complementary forces describe the "expansion and contraction" or the "up and the down" or the "inhale-exhale" of our innately reductionist view of anatomical forms and biomechanical explanations of movement; coupled as they are described in "antagonistic pairs" under laws of "coupled motions". That is *as if* those dualities represent "sides" or "balancing oppositions".
>
> However, no such thing limits the Self. That wisdom from ancient mystery schools honors the unifying result of a multidimensional, self-aware form; where Self (with a capital "S", much like Prana with a capital "P") – speaks of an aware, impersonal *state* of observation. There we learn about the "unstruck chord", a sound of stillness that is lost to the very language we have to describe it. It is invariably an experience in present time, harnessed by the experiencing experiencer.
>
> **Joanne Avison**

 Push–pull

1. The fabric of tissue is naturally prestressed and self-tethered as appropriately constrained to varying degrees.

2. That intrinsic tethering integrates tissue as animated by the co-creative forces of an outward push, constrained by that which it pushes, effectively pulling it back. That is the "push–pull".

3. These two opposing forces combine to continuously co-create one another – as a moving volume permeating itself; self-organizing as such.

5.2 Dvandva

Patanjali talks about the psycho-physiological power of paired opposites in the *Yoga Sutras*.[2] These pairs of opposite *qualities* are a kind of cross-ply, referred to as *dvandva* appearing throughout yogic literature.[3,4] Yadav's research shows five dvandvas about āsana in the PYS (Patanjali's *Yoga Sutras*), conflicts of opposition having a broad influence on the success of yoga techniques and our experience of the world in general (see Table 5.1).

tato dvandvānabhighāta
Through that [balanced yoga practice], pairs of disturbing elements/conflicts cease to attack.
Patanjali's *Yoga Sutras* II/48

These pairs of words relate directly to the human condition in Ayurvedic medicine. The basic tenet is that when one is caught up in choosing between so-called "dualistic opposites" then there is an inevitable imbalance that can be interpreted

CHAPTER FIVE

TABLE 5.1 Five dvandvas (pairs of opposites) pertaining to asana practice referred to by Patanjali in the *Yoga Sutras*.

Affected layer	Dvandva (pair of opposites)	Meaning
Physiological	śita-uṣṇa	Cold and heat
Psycho-physiological	sukha-duḥkha	Pleasure and pain
Psychological	māna-avamāna	Honor and dishonor
Psychological	kāma-krodha	Lust and anger
Physiological	kṣut-tṛṣṇā/pipāsā	Hunger and thirst

as more than just physical. In this context "disequilibrium" arises inevitably; not so much from either of the states, but from the conflict between the elements of these dvandvas if they cannot co-exist. They are thus misunderstood as co-creating the *average of their combination or unification*. This is central: each member of the pair maintains their integrity around a wholeness of the two, operating (co-creating) in balance: this is the essence of complementarity.

Complementarity is the principle from quantum physics that continues to shift the mechanistic view of bodies from collections of parts to amalgamations of wave/particles that defy measurement. Niels Bohr developed the notion that complementarity might be needed not just for the subatomic realm of physicists, but as a lens for biologists to study the natural world at all size scales. He proposed this view at a congress on light in Copenhagen in 1932, in a lecture titled *Light and Life*.[5]

A different theoretical framework is required that can embrace nonlinearity and complexity and that is open to admit the existence of higher levels of regulation...

Fulvio Mazzocchi[6]

Quantum biology is where science seeks to reconcile two ostensibly opposing (apparently paradoxical views) into balance. Here, the reductionist, molecular explanation for life processes co-exists with the holistic meta-view incorporating unquantifiable phenomena often referred to as waves. Here, we find space for the idea that biological systems are both open and closed at the same time.

We are open in a thermodynamic sense, as we interact with our environment, taking in materials and converting energy from one form to another in the process. In a biomechanical sense, our bodies are closed systems, as we have already established in the closed kinematic chains and

Acoustics of Self

coupled-to-throupledness of tissues. This open/closed dvandva is complementarity, expressed in the idea that both views are not only possible for life but simultaneously required.

The accomplished yogi, through the inward, not-so-interesting-to-watch process of reflection, can disentangle from the suffering of choosing between the polarities. We learn to allow these oscillations to self-regulate around an equilibrium, in the process of finding peace. By overcoming the "whole sense" of duality between one aspect or the other, s/he rises to the occasion in a multidimensional experience. There, we reside comfortably in the third element; the spacious volume created in balance of the whole.

Key concepts 1

Dvandvas are pairs of opposing qualities that combine to make emergent properties.

Maybe we can think about transformation as learning to sit with the opposition, to hold the paradoxical concepts of opposites at the same time. In other words, if we begin to see tension and compression, attraction and repulsion, good and bad, strength and flexibility, accessible and challenging (for example) as coordinated pairs rather than conflicting dualities, we can take a meaningful step towards understanding wholeness. There is joy in that step of feeling the third entity rising, as a combined state of wholeness. It becomes an emergent property of the whole combination.

 The Maitri

The *Maitrayaniya Upanishad* (Maitri) is a beautiful source text for its vivid discussion of the *vayu*. The Maitri, divided into seven *prapathakas* (chapters), also give us *dvandva*. It deals with the nature of the soul and asks the question we ask ourselves to this day: how is joy possible?

This chapter builds on the srotas-kinematics concept, linking together and incorporating the basics of yoga from a subtle and gross perspective, into practice. The tubular body is, essentially, a listening structure. Through yoga, we can improve what we might call the "acoustics of Self" by first tuning into the breath. In other words, we can, by listening to the breathing patterns within ourselves, tune and tune *into* ourselves to enhance self-regulation. What are we hearing?

 Śravaṇam

The ancient acharyas of Ayurveda were scholars who developed a valid method to study human health through full-body understanding. This method, the Vedic way, is not only the yogic way of understanding anatomy, but of life experience. Each experience is a fundamental unit of life, and life is described in the Vedas as a series of such incidents within the broad spectrum of health and disease.

In Ayurveda, meaning the "science of life," each experience has value, no matter how trivial it may seem. The idea is that

CHAPTER FIVE

understanding life as a whole is too ambitious a task for even the most erudite practitioner. However, by genuinely listening and integrating each experience, one can build a personal wealth of insight into the nature of life as a whole, as experienced by the individual. This listening/hearing, *sravanam* (shra-va-nam), becomes a rich whole-body experience humming along within each of us.

Key concepts 2

Yoga can be a transformative psycho-physiological playground for balancing and unifying pairs of opposites (*dvandvas*) towards holistic balance and healing.

5.3 Breath

The physiology of breathing is at the heart of *sravanam*. We use it in harnessing spiral anatomy for yoga. **Pulmonary ventilation** is the physiological term for breathing, which is, of course, crucial for gaseous transfer. Beyond respiration, the process of breathing offers a rich rhythmical key to our personal ability to experience the nature of inhabiting oneself. Breathing is well understood in yoga as an actuator of energy in the spectrum between stillness and movement. We could consider it as our gateway to an integrated approach to anatomy.

Breathing basics

The respiratory diaphragm (from the Latin, meaning "partition") is a double-dome-shaped sheet of tissue, invested with muscle protein and profoundly integrated with the fasciae of the deep costal surfaces, surrounding the bony framework across which it is tensioned. It is continuous with the inside edges of the lowermost ribs all the way around the rim of the thoracic cage. At the back, its crurae (legs) wrap around the aorta, arising from a spiral embryological origin, in complete continuity with the fasciae of the vertebrae and posterior abdominal wall as a de facto part of the thoracolumbar fascia.

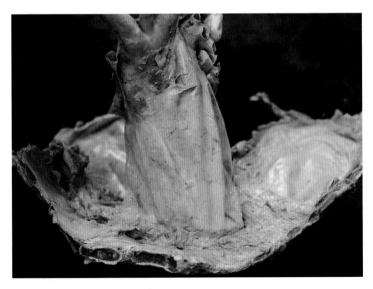

FIGURE 5.2

The diaphragm in continuity with the pericardial sac.

(Courtesy of Stecco C, Sharkey J, S chleip R. Fascia Net Plastination Project/von Hagens Plastinarium, 2018)

Acoustics of Self

When the diaphragm contracts, the central tendon (like the apex of a balloon) is drawn downwards towards the inner edges of the ribcage. The downward expansion of the diaphragm coordinates with omnidirectional expansion of the thoracic cavity in rhythm with unidirectional inward convergence. This constant, balloon-shape-change results in the changing volume/pressure gradients within the torso, driving breathing motion. The rotational power of coupled motion doesn't merely influence diaphragmatic biomotion. Our CKC architecture is bound up with the very essence of breathing: a motion we might usefully consider as a gentle spiral, especially during the orthograde forward momentum of gait.

 Trampoline – exercise in somatic awareness

N.B. This practical suggestion is not intended as a physical challenge for all; please observe and respect your own circumstances and only jump on the trampoline when and if it makes sense to do so.

The next time you have a chance, hop onto a trampoline and get bouncing. Tuning in to the amplified elastic recoil of the body as you jump, it becomes easy to feel that the rebound of your abdominal organs together with the CKC architecture pulls breath in and pushes it out. The same thing happens during gait and is amplified in running.

On the trampoline, we can emphasize the effect as bounce-breathing in a sense temporarily *overrides* the diaphragm, somewhat like a ventilator uses an outside mechanism to take over the rhythm of the breath. Bouncing rhythmically on the trampoline (where such is possible and advisable given your circumstances), you can feel the coupled CKCs integrated with the diaphragm as the shape-change coordinates with your bounce.

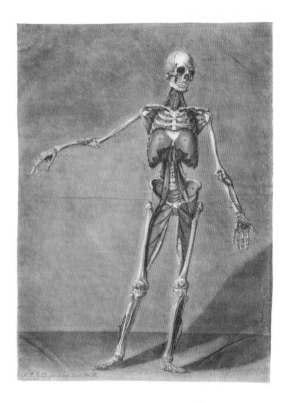

FIGURE 5.3

Anatomical illustration by Arnauld-Eloi Gautier-Dagoty (1741–1771) for the Royal College of Medicine of Nancy in Lorraine, France. Dagoty elegantly depicted muscles of the human body as perceived by scientists in the 18th century with precise details. His illustrations offer us a glimpse of medical practice in the age of enlightenment.

(The New York Public Library. Image public domain)

The coupled and throupledness we are now more familiar with, powers biomotional integrity in both our rhythmical gait and in the subtle tides within the stillness of posture. As we have seen, gait harnesses pelvic rotation in the pump-swing of contralateral propulsion involving angular momentum (continuous rotational falling) as we walk and run. Since the diaphragm is embedded in the TFLX, its contraction couples with the swing pump of gait for ultimate rhythmic efficiency in motion.

Studying the anatomy of breath integrated with yoga[7] leads to more clarity on the role of the diaphragm as a *postural* muscle intimately associated with the psoas and indeed the entire posterior abdominal wall. In yoga, we harness rhythm differently than we do in gait, but the principle of coupling movement with breath remains the same.

Breathing is a pivotal theme in yoga, and in its elegant complexity, we find a fascination in common with generations of enquiry. Ancient cultures investigated the role of breathing long before the discovery of oxygen. Aristotle believed that the function of breathing was to cool the heart.[6] But here we get to the crux of coupledness: whole anatomical systems are physiologically interconnected, and here we'll explore how breathing can be the actuator of systemic balance.

 Anahata

Skora comments: "the central act of salvation for Abhinavagupta was understood precisely as the 'body's recollection of Being', the touching or bodily felt awareness of the Pulsating Heart (of consciousness)."[8]

Human breathing is a sophisticated rhythmical system controlled autonomically, arising from a primitive complex in the brain stem.[9] Heart rate and breathing are intimately related. Reciprocal actions throughout our neurobiology are tied into breathing, in a multidimensional agency towards balance.[7,10] Clinical evidence is on the rise for the use of yoga breathing techniques in the treatment of various ailments, including (but not limited to) depression, anxiety and PTSD.[11]

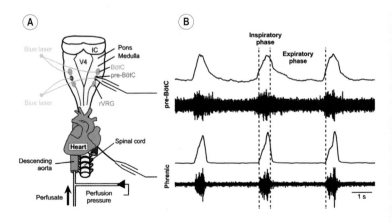

FIGURE 5.4

A Dorsal view of a mouse brain stem–spinal cord preparation. **B** Oscillations of neural activity during inhalation and exhalation in the brain stem (top) and phrenic nerve (bottom) that innervates the diaphragm, illustrating the neural involvement in the cardiorespiratory rhythm.

(Reproduced from: Ausborn J, Koizumi H, Barnett WH, et al. Organization of the core respiratory network: insights from optogenetic and modeling studies. PLOS Computational Biology. 2018;14(4): e1006148. https://doi.org/10.1371/journal.pcbi.1006148. https://creativecommons.org/publicdomain/zero/1.0/)

Acoustics of Self

Key concepts 3

The oscillatory nature of breathing, via srotas-kinematics, links prana and apana together to form an internal "anchoring system" as part of biomotional integrity.

Breathing patterns can be both voluntary and involuntary. Bringing volition to the breath is an option for "manually overriding" the prevailing autonomic rhythm. When we explore this rhythm voluntarily, we involve the sensorimotor cortex of the brain, bringing awareness to this multidimensionality. It is worth mentioning here that while it is useful to explore this voluntary override, the purpose is to restore autonomy to the subconscious rhythm in balance. These interventions are, as such, intended to be temporary and continuously adapting to the needs of the changing system. As ever, there is no one-size-fits-all for constraining from without until and unless we can constrain from within.

The result, in itself, is a whole-body demonstration of the behavior of **auxetic** materials.

 The body auxetic

Auxetics are materials that have a negative Poisson's ratio, which essentially means the material doesn't get thinner as it lengthens (see Table 1.2). Instead, auxetic materials expand omnidirectionally. Breathing in and out is an example of this (feel a model of this as you toss your Hoberman sphere up and gently catch it in your hands). Structurally this is achieved via the closed kinematic chain organization of the torso.

The so-called "breathing ball" or Hoberman sphere is a popular tool for teaching breath awareness as srotas-kinematic principles animate it (i.e., that illustrate *omnidirectional expansion* paired with *returning unidirectional retraction*). It further demonstrates that ventilation (as a whole) is coupled with respiration, which is in turn connected with cardiovascular rhythms. These link also into complex arrays of couplings at every level of detail in the system. These couplings give rise to the quality of a moving volume as a whole. This is what we call *throupling* – about whole body (at least 3D) experience. This integration is what happens naturally (autonomically) when coupled oscillators hum along together in time and unite to bring about the experience of equilibrium, whether or not we are conscious of it.

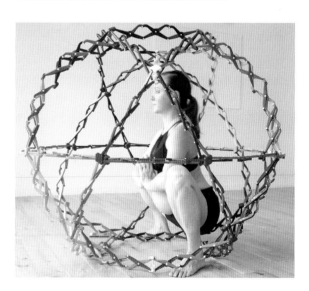

FIGURE 5.5

The breathing ball. This expanding spherical linkage is trademarked as the "Hoberman Sphere" and commonly known as the breathing ball in yoga culture.

CHAPTER FIVE

Volitional breathing

The simple act of paying attention to your breathing is, in itself, the first moment of tuning in. It can take years for a person to find that moment, so pregnant is the pause required to listen to one's breath. In philosophy and science, this voluntary aspect, or volition, connects beyond the physical to essential (psychosomatic) questions about the nature of consciousness. The act of intentional breathing, or prāṇāyāma (the 4th limb of Patanjali's 8-limbed yoga practice), is designed to enhance these oscillatory neural networks to integrate primal rhythms of breathing. Pranayama invites the potential for rebalancing the system at large; bringing conscious awareness to that which is usually unconscious or subconscious.

In mammals, breathing is the result of three phases:[12]

1. Inspiration (inhalation, or *puraka*)

2. Post-inspiration

3. Active expiration (exhalation, or *rechaka*).

In yoga, the breath is manipulated in various ways. Inhalation and exhalation are clipped, extended, paused and further managed to rebalance and condition the system. The retention of an inhalation or exhalation is called *kumbhaka*. The halt after inhaling is called *puraka*, or *abhyantara kumbhaka*, meaning internal retention. After exhaling, the retained breath is called *shunkaya*, also known as *bahya kumbhaka*, or external retention.

Key concepts 4

The breath brings volition to convergent-divergent movement in asana, balancing the coupled sympathetic and parasympathetic nervous systems.

 Sanskrit for breath and energy are the same: prāṇa. Through prāṇa (breath/energy) + ayāma (extension), we are given a system for consciously working with volition to the effect of improving concentration and self-regulation. This, then, contributes to a cascade of yogic effects.

Breath extension

The word *pranayama* is often translated into *prana*, breath and *yama*, control. However, there is another way to understand the Sanskrit word, given our growing appreciation of flow: Prāṇāyāma, Prāṇa + ayāma gives the long ā in the joining of the two terms. Ayāma, the negative of yama (to control or restrain) means to extend or draw out. So, perhaps we can look at pranayama as breath extension, the ability to develop our felt sense of breathing.

Key concepts 5

Pranayama is the yogic practice of consciously introducing retentions to manipulate one's flow of breathing.

The breath is not just a pressure-oriented function. It includes many elements, one of which is the rate. The speed of the breath changes based on context and can also be distinguished as

Acoustics of Self

three basic types, with associated effects on the nervous system:

1. Quiet breathing: the smooth, normal breathing that continues naturally without any effort.

2. Slow (deep) breathing: the protracted breathing achieved by deliberately slowing down the breath, sometimes referred to as "free breathing with sound" (a controlled form of *hypo*ventilation – lowering of the speed or breathing rate).

3. Fast breathing: the quick breathing that is caused by consciously increasing speed, such as in *Kapalabhati* (a controlled form of *hyper*ventilation) – raising of the speed or breathing rate.

The distinction between the three types of breath listed above and true pranayama can be considered as the use of specific techniques to punctuate the flow of breath in specific patterns. Intentional breathing (especially with kumbhaka) can help create an internal anchoring system that is intrinsically related to reversing intra-abdominal pressure, or part of what we call *bandha*.

The focus on slow, deep breathing in yoga was based on anecdotal evidence, but the research is starting to deliver a Western evidence base.[12–15] There is, invariably, an essential balance to be found between conscious/deliberate breathing rates and natural, spontaneous ones. The purpose of practicing the deliberate ones is only to tune the system. Once adjusted, unconscious or autonomic function self-regulates, *naturally* responding well to a particular demand at a given moment in time. Continued practice restores (and promotes) natural and efficient rhythm. This is the essential value of such conscious training in self-regulation; such that it becomes innate to the system.

Breathing is one of the fundamental life rhythms that pump the tubular system via the srotas-kinematics, guiding the energy available for movement. In movement-breath coordination, we find a new level of rhythmical linkage, for example, in recognizing heart rate variability.[16] Exhalation feeds into the compression of the torso whereby *Chaturanga Dandasana* (Four-Limbed Staff Pose) calls the body into a "stiffened" staff. This relates to the nonlinearity of speed-scale interactions: how we greet the ground.

This platform fires the *inhaling* (tensional) movement into Upward Dog. Conscious stiffening, via the breath and motion, can make the body more elastic, which fosters (and is facilitated by) purposeful breathing. As Avison put it back in 2015, "true elasticity is one of several fundamental principles of the fascial matrix profoundly enhanced by the practice of yoga."[17]

Key concepts 6

The breath is a rhythm that couples stiffness and suppleness with movement, giving rise to appropriate elastic compliance.

The dynamic action that the elastic body uses to "bounce" off the floor is usually coordinated with an exhalation. The squeeze of body materials (in exhalation) appropriately stiffens up the system to help the body spring, or bounce, using the ground, to capitalize on ground reaction force (GRF). However, it is also possible to stiffen and optimize GRF by hitting the ground on a sharp inhalation. And all of this can be experienced without ever having to perform Chaturanga – these principles apply for every moment our body greets the ground, however we do that.

CHAPTER FIVE

This coordination and exploration of the breathing rhythm-with-movement enhances the acoustics for self-listening and provides a path toward self-mastery. Such focus and virtuosity might look like mere strength from the outside. In actuality, it is better described as next-level, internal body-intelligence. If strength is the capacity for useful stiffness, then body-intelligence is the discernment for harnessing that stiffness at the appropriate moments for coordinated movement within spiral constraints.

We use voluntary/involuntary breathing to foster self-regulation. Like a flautist uses air to make music through holes in a tube, so the yogi learns to manipulate breath through the dexterous control of the in-and-out breath. Next, we'll look at breath's great ally – the intrinsic body "locks" known in yoga as *bandhas*.[18] Where breathing ends and bandha begins is a gradient with a dynamic overlap.

5.4 Bandha: de facto structure

Jalandhara bandha, uddiyana bandha and moola bandha are situated respectively, in the throat, abdomen and perineum.

If their duration can be increased then where is the fear of death?

Yoga Taravali (Sutra 5)[19]

Bandha is one of the more elusive subtle body concepts that we are faced with as beginners to the practice of yoga. In my early years, I did think that bandhas were elusive at best. Now I consider bandha as one of the essential practical differences between physical postural yoga and conventional exercise.

With continued practice, I experienced an increasingly potent inward/upwardness that I learned to evermore integrate with my breath and movement. That this intentional reversal of intra-abdominopelvic pressure can be attributed to the legendary bandha is one of the leaps that we make as modern yoga practitioners. From an anatomical point of view, bandha is certainly more *de facto* than *de jure*.

Looking at bandha as a transient anchoring system gives us a subtle physiological phenomenon that we can explore functionally and structurally. Going back to the embryology, anyone can see the toroidal shape formed by the root flowing "up itself." It is possible to imagine that first flow impulse as the lead of a polarity pattern at the essence of *mula bandha*. Continue the analogy of the flautist, gracefully covering and uncovering routes of flow in her instrument.

Bandha is treated traditionally in the many specialist books written by senior teachers of yoga,[20,21] having enormous significance as a kind of energetic lock or seal. The Sanskrit term bandha is usually translated as "bond" or "lock", or "to arrest." It refers to the body locks in Hatha Yoga that Krishnamacharya describes as a subset of mudra.[22]

There are 20 types of mudras described by Krishnamacharya; other texts interpret mudra in various ways. Krishnamacharya's mudras are energetic practices that focus attention in specific areas, prescribed by ancient texts as a means of promoting circulation of Prana through the nadis.

Out of Krishnamacharya's 20 mudras, he classifies four as bandhas:

1. Maha Mudra

2. Uddiyana Bandha Mudra

3. Jalandhara Bandha Mudra

4. Mulabandha Mudra

Acoustics of Self

Because of its transanatomical nature, bandha has been subject to interpretation and speculation. Simon Borg-Olivier outlines nine bandhas that oscillate between open and closed.[20] I am inclined to go with this idea of fluctuation between open and closed. As we consider bandha anatomically, it is a deployable internal anchoring system that can:

- Stabilize spiral action outward into the limbs from the center.

- Manipulate and promote circulation.

- Regulate the flow of postural information within the body.

In this way, I see bandha as a kind of valve that oscillates between open and closed. Just like the *yama* in pranayama can mean both closed and flowing, bandha in its locked form is one state of the valve. Bandha is sometimes translated as "fetter" like a leash on a dog, which in some ways is an unfortunate picture of how bandha might work. As all dog-walkers know, you can't just pull your dog toward you constantly and hope for a pleasant experience.

Truth be told, I don't have a dog, but I can relate because I have a toddler. Any leash, like bandha, functions optimally when it flows in a give-and-take relationship with movement. With practice, we can learn how to "lead" rather than "leash" our tissue-flow using the energetic valves of bandha and mudra harmoniously with vayu and breath. It is more a means of responsive listening than indiscriminate restriction, such as might be implied by the term "lock".

Gestures toward the center

Therefore the goddess sleeping at the entrance of Brahma's

door should be constantly aroused with all effort, by performing
mudra thoroughly.

Hatha Yoga Pradipika (3:5)[23]

Bandha has a prominent place in modern postural yoga practice, in part because beginners connect it with the Western idea of core strength. This is a lamentable oversimplification of its power, just as the concept of core strength is challenged by many a progressive exercise physiologist.[24] People often describe the bandhas as contractions of muscles, e.g., "contracting the pelvic floor to achieve mula bandha". A more accurate instruction is to "pull in," but this wording still implies that bandhas are bits of anatomy that you control with discrete muscle power.

Talking point

 Spectrum of bandha

When is it useful to cue hollowing versus firming? Are each of these a kind of bandha?

Prana-connected bandha: the reversal of intra-abdominal pressure resulting in the hollowing or "sucking in" of the navel.

Apana-connected bandha: the intentional firming of the abdominal membranes, such as when we cue "pull in the lower ribs" with posterior pelvic tilt.

Implications and instructions such as these are rooted in the linear idea that individual muscles are the be-all of anatomy. Many practitioners come to see bandha is an enhanced state of being that transcends the mere squeezing of muscles. Experiencing bandha starts with the intentional reversal of intra-abdominal pressure, using cues such as "hollowing" and "inward suction".

CHAPTER FIVE

Bandha *as a gesture* is elusive because it involves learning "to hollow," which might mean temporarily unlearning previous training. Developing bandha is a subtle journey of maintaining stability, so the body knows when to firm the abdominopelvic regions (as we do with corrective exercise postpartum) and when to intentionally hollow (experience the inverse of firming). What I'm saying is that bandha can be all that and much more. I'm pointing, once again, to the inherent stability of a dynamic reciprocity in something that is whole in motion. Our linear approaches do not tend to account for the multistability and multidimensional range of tissue. Calling it "bandha" might help us to embrace that subtlety in context.

Key concepts 7

Bandha is the intentional coupling of stiffness and suppleness with movement and breath.

Mudra and bandha are gestures that foster linkages between and among the gross and subtle srotas-kinematics. Bandha has a significant place in tensegral body awareness as a de facto element of an anatomical structure. Intimately related to the breathing/postural practice of pranayama, bandha results in the sense of "appropriate stiffness" that facilitates the internal anchoring mentioned earlier. This anchorage is often attributed to the psoas and pelvic floor, but bandha as a practice takes us way beyond the parts list and includes much more subtle access to conscious awareness of the body.

Primary bandhas:

- Mula bandha, corresponding to the pelvic floor (as the pelvic tissues tether into the surrounding bony substrate; they anchor the lower torso).

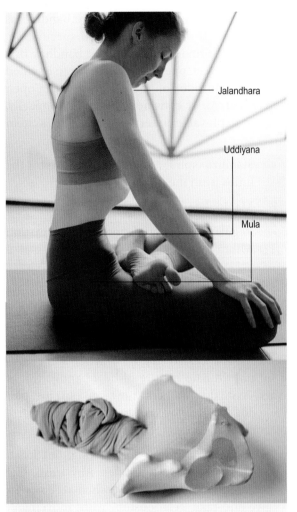

FIGURE 5.6

Bandhas breakdown: Mula bandha, corresponding to the pelvic floor; Uddiyana bandha, corresponding to the lower abdominal membrane; and Jalandhara bandha, corresponding to the jugular notch. Prestress, the body's intrinsic tension draws the fascial matrix into itself like the membrane of a drum. This pelvis model is compressed by the fabric, its bone pushing outwards into the fabric membrane. The result shows us the areas where the tensioned fabric is "drawing inwards" shaped by the outward push of the bones.

(Demonstration by Emma Isokivi)

- Uddiyana bandha, corresponding to the lower abdomen (the abdominal mesh; drawing into the ventral cavity)

- Jalandhara bandha, corresponding to the jugular notch (the vocal diaphragm; anchoring the upper thorax and base of the throat)

- Maha bandha, a practice working with all three that invites balance in all the cavities and coordinates of the form.

Then there are the secondary bandhas. Including them invites us to fulfil the relationship between the ground and the innermost body, via the palms of the hands and the soles of the feet, in a profound reciprocal relationship. As Joanne reminds us, this also takes us beyond the parts list as it incorporates *the ground* as part of the form.

 ### Secondary bandhas

- Palmar arches (drawing into the palmar/hand space)

- Metatarsal arches (drawing into the hollow of the plantar/midfoot space)

In the membrane

Bandha is a function of intensified prestress (pre-existing tension/compression balance). Membranous bandha holds something of universal application in yoga. From a biotensegrity perspective, bandha can be seen to orchestrate the relationship of tension/compression behavior of membranous tissues. Take the zipper as an analogy: you have to tension the fabric for the structure of the zipper to work. A floppy zipper is useless but stiffen up the material, and suddenly it works.

In the ventral cavities, bandha is linked to the temporary and intentional reversal of intra-abdominal pressure. The respiratory diaphragm does not just manipulate pressure in the thoracic cavity for breathing. It also contributes posturally in harmony with other diaphragmatic regions such as the pharynx and perineum. Breath-movement practice thus brings conscious awareness to these subtle relationships. Such voluntary reversals of pressure deliberately create an occasional, internal, at-will anchoring system that forms a basis for further exploring and fine-tuning breath-and-movement.

 ### Experiencing Bandha

If you're new to bandha, keep that practical trampoline experience in mind here, with the same gentle guidance asking yourself if the exercise is appropriate for your circumstances before trying it. Please consider that the following exercise must be approached with care if at all.

First, take a deep breath. Then, while blowing out the breath slowly and firmly, squeeze your lower abdominal membrane. Empty the lungs, hold the breath out, and seal the external retention with Jalandhara bandha. If you can safely further retain your exhalation, do so by sealing the vocal diaphragm (tissues regulating airflow in the throat). Simultaneously activate the respiratory diaphragm as if to take the next breath in, the result will be the ability to powerfully "suck up" the lower abdominal membrane.

Taking up the slack and tensioning this region gives it a kind of stiffened quality, transforming it temporarily into an anchor that makes other micromovement possible in that moment. Release the seal, inhale, and the de facto structure becomes something else in readiness for the moment.

CHAPTER FIVE

Key concepts 8

Mudra/bandha form an internal anchoring system within the body matrix for the circulation of power, flow, and sensory information.

Bandha isn't just a postural effect. The power of bandhas to promote circulation and tension-compression emphasis within body intelligence, can transform personal health if used wisely and learned incrementally. Bandha can be an intentional practice that acts as a component of the circulation of information, both subtle and material.

(i) *Tadagi Mudra*

Figure 5.7 shows a version of the classic Tādāgi Mudrā, Pond (or Tank) Seal described in the *Gheranda Samhita*.[25] Also called "gesture of the pond," Tadagi Mudra is about the experience of the abdominal region hollowing, creating a concavity in the shape of a pond applicable to all forward bends and upright sitting postures. Bandha characteristics are, as such, not at all limited to the three classics: *Mula*, *Uddiyana*, and *Jalandara*.

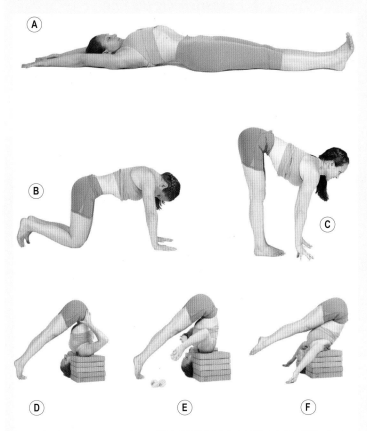

FIGURE 5.7

Pond (or Tank) Seal. Also called "gesture of the pond," Tādāgi Mudrā can be expressed in a number of different postures to heighten the experience of both prana and apana-connected bandha. At the end of the exhalation, seal the lips and instead of allowing the next diaphragmatic action to draw the next inhalation, direct the effort towards drawing in the lower abdomen and pelvic tissues. (A) The classic reclining version; (B, C) versions on all fours and upright movement; (D–F) the inverted version which couples with the effects of gravity to intensify the experience of in-drawing, especially as the pelvic tissues and viscera of the abdominopelvic cavities are drawn in by their own weight. Using blocks to relax in the inversion can help you tune into the space, and the tennis ball game offers a way to connect with the space in a playful way.

Acoustics of Self

Bandha is related to:

- the interplay of stabilization and mobility
- promoting circulation
- optimizing the work of the heart
- regulating body temperature
- protecting the joints
- massaging the organs
- creating a flow state
- optimizing the structural balance of breath-and-movement.

Taking the body-wide fabric into account, the entire bodily response is not limited to the primary bandhas (e.g., Mula, Uddiyana, and Jalandara), or even the *upa* bandhas in the hands and feet (e.g., Hasta and Pada bandhas). For example, the pose *Purvattonasana* induces tension and compression forces along the entire front of the body. We immediately experience this pose as a sense of activation throughout the whole back and core, simultaneously. With intention and awareness, it is possible to magnify the front/back balance to refine the pose further.

Indeed, yoga is not all about flexibility, or in a mechanical sense, the compliance needed to get into a "deformation". Posture practice asks us to fortify our elastic recoil capacity, which is the degree to which we bounce back or reform *after* a deformation. Enhancing one's experience of this recoil is a crucial aspect of practicing bandha.

Krishnamacharya emphasized the benefits of yoga to circulation, tying in the optimum state of ligaments with blood circulation. Vinyasa with bandha produces "good nadi granthi, healthy body and good health".[22] Bandha is an intrinsic feature of asana. Asanas are the shapes possible for human body tissues; bandha and breath enhance the flow of circulation, concentration and eventually, global integration, within and for those shapes. This is vinyasa.

 (i) *Vinyasa*

From the Sanskrit *nyasa*, to place,
+ *vi*, in a special way.

Vinyasa offers certain advantages to more conventional exercise. It is a practice built for playing with the srotas-kinematics. Breathing through the nose with a pharyngeal squeeze, the breath takes on a heightened pneumatic dimension that opens up a rhythmic experience of expansion and retraction, tension and compression.

Combined with the bandha and visual focus (dṛṣṭi/drishti), flowing movement in coordination with the breath can eventually become more like a moving meditation. As the proficient musician's hands dance with the wind over and through her instrument, movement and breath join seamlessly to make music. Similar to the cochlea of the ear, specialized tissues in the eye convert external inputs into neural signals for higher processing by the brain. This song becomes so much more than the sum of its notes, just as the body itself is more significant than its individually named anatomical sections, systems or sites.

CHAPTER FIVE

5.5 Dṛṣṭi

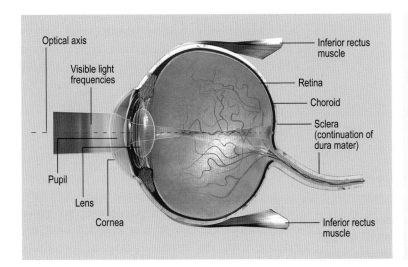

Optical axis
Visible light frequencies
Pupil
Lens
Cornea
Inferior rectus muscle
Retina
Choroid
Sclera (continuation of dura mater)
Inferior rectus muscle

FIGURE 5.8

Basic anatomy of the eye showing visible light frequencies refracting through to the retina where light is transduced into neural information for higher processing in the brain. The meninges, connective tissue coverings of the brain and spinal cord, are continuous through the optic nerve and wrap around the eyes.

(Christoph Burgstedt/Science Photo Library)

Intentionally gazing at a prescribed point is known in yoga as dṛṣṭi (pronounced *drishti*). Drishti gives the practitioner a means of harnessing physiological attention. Looking where you're going in some way is a basic instruction for most skills-based practice, because we all know that where you look can determine your direction of travel. The anatomical basis for drishti tells a lot of the story: the tissue that covers the eyes is continuous with the optic nerves, which are in turn continuous with the central nervous system (CNS). The CNS is interconnected with the fascial matrix and all the systems nested therein. Like volitional breathing, volitional *looking* is another means of directing the orchestra of oscillations within.

I like to think of my eyes as grasping structures, in that I can gaze with intensity and "get a hold" of the point (of view). Like an ice climber uses the ice axe to seize the substrate and pull herself closer to it, we can use drishti as a point of energetic fixation. Through the srotas-kinematics, the drishti harness connects with all the other sheaths and harnesses them. With practice, the drishti

TABLE 5.2 Drishti	
Aṅguṣṭhamadhye	Toward the thumb
Nāsāgre	Toward the nose
Bhrūmadhye	Toward the eyebrow centre (third eye)
Nābhicakre	Toward the navel
Hastagrahe	Toward the hand
Pādayoragre	Toward toes
Pārśva Drishti	Distant right
Pārśva Drishti	Distant left
Ūrdhva	Upward

changes in rhythm with the breath, as each breath coordinates with bandha and movement; so goes the dance of vinyasa.

Acoustics of Self

Key concepts 9

Vinyasa is a movement practice incorporating *tristana*: breath, *bandha, drishti.*

The spiral-bound ideas integrate any breath-based practice for safe tissue reconditioning. As the tissues become more appropriately constrained, so can personal perspective. As an approach to living, vinyasa is a poetic way of applying the progressive awareness of yoga to all the rhythms of life, including;

- creativity
- healing
- self-care
- relationships
- work
- pregnancy and postpartum recovery
- personal growth.

5.6 Seated in spirals

The challenge of the living body is not to move...
the challenge is to stop.

Leonid Blyum

Movement and stillness together form another pair of seemingly opposite modes. If we see movement as a result of oscillation around an equilibrium, the opposition in balance can make stillness more comfortable. In yoga, we use posture to prepare the self for repose; and in stillness, we experience and appreciate the constant movement of a changing universe through increasing proficiency in concentration. The positional basis for practicing the more in-depth work of yoga is classically described as seated.

 Disclaimer

As we get into the description of asana, please be advised that yoga is always best learned with a teacher in real-time. Any attempts to perform the techniques described (asana, pranayama, bandha) will come with associated risks, and we advise our readers to seek out individual instruction to learn proper technique.

There are several traditional variations of yogic sitting, such as:

- Sukhasana/Svastikasana
- Siddhasana
- Padmasana
- Vajrasana

Key concepts 10

Seated postures, an approach to stillness, are inherently spiral.

Seated meditation positions

All three of the classic seated meditation positions can be enhanced by elevating the pelvis. Sit on a folded mat or a block to foster the natural expression of comfortable sitting, with the pelvis gently tilted forward (anterior pelvic tilt).

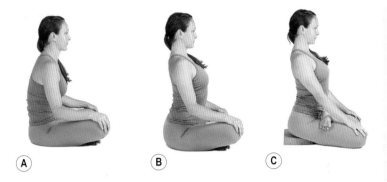

(A)   (B)   (C)

FIGURE 5.9

Pelvic tilt: no matter your choice of asana for seated practice, seek an upright posture. (A) Posterior pelvic tilt. (B) Work toward sitting upright with a (gently) anteriorly tilted pelvis, but avoid overly extending the lumbar as pictured here. (C) Sitting on props will elevate the pelvis and allow tighter bodies greater ease in tilting the pelvis forward without strain.

Sukhasana/Svastikasana

This is "easy cross-legged" sitting pose. The crucial difference between the two is that the ankles, while passive in Sukhasana, are actively dorsiflexed in Svastikasana (sometimes *Agnistambhasana*).

Sukhasana is aptly named after the idea that it should be pleasing, or natural, thus known in English as "easy pose." Simply sit cross-legged and use blocks or bolsters to prop up the knees for comfort if necessary.

Svastikasana is the embodiment of the auspicious symbol from ancient Indian culture, approximating a spiral. To achieve the pose, start in Sukhasana and then dorsiflex your ankles. This subtle but powerful action activates the external rotation from the distal aspect of the lower limb spirals and substantially increases the intensity of the pose.

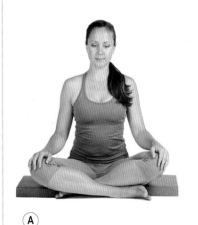

(A)

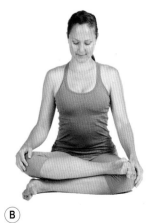

(B)

FIGURE 5.10

Winding up the spirals. (A) Sukhā-sana, easy pose; and a little more intense: (B) Svastikāsana, "double pigeon" or "Agnistambhasana" – dorsiflex the ankles and increase the acuity of the lateral rotation.

Siddhasana

This is "the accomplished pose": cross-legged sitting with feet tucked between thighs and calves.

In Sanskrit, *Siddha* means "accomplished" or "adept". *Siddhasana* is more complex than Sukhasana and Svastikasana as the spirals "wind up" and become more acute. Start in Sukhasana and then bring your right heel to rest against the perineum (there are different gender-based versions you can learn from a teacher). Sit upon that foot and press the sole of that foot along the inner thigh. Place the opposite ankle on top of the first, so the top heel presses the pubic joint directly.

The toes and the outer edge of the feet nestle between the calf and inner thigh. It is possible to find comfort in Siddhasana with practice, when the hips are more open, and in turn, it can help open the hips even more than sitting cross-legged.

Padmasana

This is the classic Lotus position: cross-legged sitting with feet tucked into the hip creases. Note: Padmasana should not be approached casually.

Padmasana, lotus pose, is the most challenging of the seated meditation poses. The knees are brought closer together with the increasing spiral winding as the feet

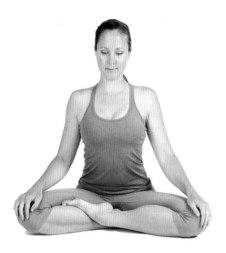

FIGURE 5.11

Siddhāsana (Pose of the Adept). Progressing further into knee flexion and hip rotation: for a ladies' version, place the right heel gently against the yoni. Then place your left heel on top of your right heel, left foot crossing over the right. Both heels are thus drawn inward and eventually contacting the body. The toes move toward the ground, as do the knees.

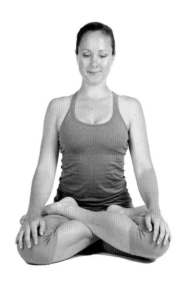

FIGURE 5.12

Padmāsana (Lotus Pose). "Full Lotus" has chirality in that the right leg is pulled in first to nestle into the left hip crease, then the left leg is woven on top to rest in the right crease.

are both drawn over the thighs deeper into the abdominopelvic cavity. Winding the leg spirals into Padmasana requires very open hips to protect the knees from potentially dangerous oblique forces.

Contraindications for Padmasana include any injury and instability in the hips and knees. The best way to incorporate Padmasana into practice is to build up to it slowly and gradually and only as part of regular practice, with guidance. It is not a casual pose and should be approached with care.

 Be where you are

Adjust your seat to a comfortable setting given your personal constraints! Celebrate the journey. Life is hard enough without feeling pressured to tie yourself in knots. You can use a chair with or without back support, lean against a wall or a tree, sit on a balance ball, or recline.

Key concepts 11

Variations on seated meditation positions are useful for learning to sit in equilibrium.

Vajrasana

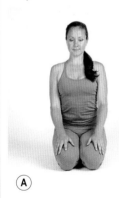

(A)

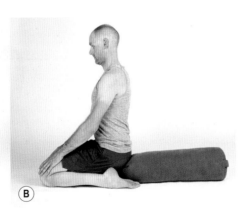

(B)

FIGURE 5.13

Alternatives: (A) Vajrāsana, "Lightning bolt pose" provides an alternative to lateral hip rotation and is a good place to start for beginners working on knee flexion. Either kneel sitting squarely on the heels, sit supported on blocks; or as in (B) Vīrāsana, "Hero Pose", progress further to sit on the floor between the feet. In this pose, we can feel the medial spiral of the lower limbs with intensifying plantarflexion and full flexion of the knees.

The kneeling pose is an alternative to all of the external hip rotations above. As with all seated poses, Vajrasana can be propped to provide maximum support. Being seated on the heels or a higher substrate, the practitioner can control the degree to which knees modulate the appropriate spiral during flexion. This elevation allows the student to experience a seated position while minimizing discomfort and is a good option for beginners or those with specific injuries/conditions.

Acoustics of Self

These ancient seated meditation positions advance in complexity as the leg spirals draw further inward toward the convergence of limbs within the trunk. The activity of vinyasa is designed to bring comfort to the body for sitting "still" in equilibrium. It can bring us into the kind of dynamic stillness characterizing a body that is the living convergence of countless oscillations in rhythm. As our ears have evolved to transform waves into mechanical vibration and again into neural signals for higher processing, our bodies also convert mechanical signals into flowing charge. Hearing and feeling become the double doors of perception that we can explore further as practice takes us deeper into the house of Self.

Here we come back to the notion of self-transformation through self-*regulation*.[26] In learning to sit still for more extended periods, perhaps our listening can be refined. As a stage of this process, we may hone the learned skill of concentration, cultivating the seedbed for spiritual practice. For many reasons, sitting still is a particular challenge for most yoga beginners to enjoy; it can be much more challenging than staying in motion. Learning to press pause, look inward, and listen brings us to the feet of (our inner) nature.

5.7 Resources for teachers

If you've made it with me this far, you are well steeped in spirals, tubes, and waves. But what good is a theory, spiral or otherwise, if it doesn't find a permanent place in our lives as practicing educators? Further, how can our anatomy pedagogy support a safer and more transparent learning experience for teachers and students of yoga? This is where we circle back into the

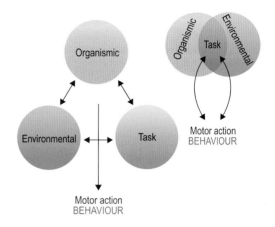

FIGURE 5.14

Left: organismic, environmental, and task constraints as independently defined interacting entities. Right: organismic and environmental constraints as independently defined interacting entities, and task constraints as emergent properties of the organism–environment system.

(Redrawn and adapted from Balagué N, Pol R, Torrents C, et al. On the relatedness and nestedness of constraints. Sports Medicine - Open. 2019;5:1. https://sportsmedicine-open. springeropen.com/articles/ 10.1186/s40798-019-0178-z/ figures/1. https://creativecommons.org/ licenses/by/4.0/)

constraints-led pedagogy that underpins the practical message of this book, explicitly presented in Chapter 4 (4.4 Statement of constraints).

Given that we have established ourselves biologically as nonlinear systems, it makes sense that we teach and practice movement in such a way that honors the constraints of our self-assembly. As technical as it sounds, the concept is so straightforward: our best chance of non-harming comes with moving – and living – within the reasonable limits.

CHAPTER FIVE

The notion that all these fragments are separately existent is evidently an illusion, and this illusion cannot do other than lead to endless conflict and confusion.

– David Bohm, Wholeness and the Implicate Order[27]

References

1   Cowell EB. The Maitri Or Maitráyaníya Upanishad: With the Commentary of Rámatírtha. W.M. Watts; 1870.

2   Yadav SR. Study of the concept of dvandva in the Pātañjala Yogasūtra from a philosophical and psycho-physiological perspective. Yoga Mimamsa. 2014;46(3):76–80.

3   Nemec J. The Ubiquitous Siva: Somananda's Sivadrsti and His Tantric Interlocutors. Oxford University Press; 2011.

4   Oliphant SG. The Vedic Dual: Part VI, The Elliptic Dual; Part VII, The Dual Dvandva. Journal of the American Oriental Society. 1912;32(1):33–57.

5   Bohr N. Light and Life. Nature Publishing Group; 1933.

6   Mazzocchi F. Complementarity in biology. EMBO Reports. 2010;11(5):339–44.

7   Kaminoff L. What Yoga Therapists Should Know About the Anatomy of Breathing. The Breathing Project; 2005.

8   Skora KM. The pulsating heart and its divine sense energies: body and touch in Abhinavagupta's Trika Śaivism. Numen. 2007;54(4):420-58.

9   Ausborn J, Koizumi H, Barnett WH, et al. Organization of the core respiratory network: insights from optogenetic and modeling studies. PLoS Computational Biology. 2018;14(4):e1006148.

10 Avison JS. Yoga: Fascia, Anatomy and Movement. Handspring Publishing; 2015.

11 Sengupta P. Health impacts of yoga and pranayama: a state-of-the-art review. International Journal of Preventive Medicine. 2012;3(7):444–58.

12 Ramirez J-M, Anderson TM, Garcia AJ, 3rd. The ins and outs of breathing. eLife, 2014;3:e03375–e03375.

13 Nivethitha L, Mooventhan A, Manjunath NNK. Effects of various prāṇāyāma on cardiovascular and autonomic variables. Ancient Science of Life. 2016;36(2):72–7.

14 Russo MA, Santarelli DM, O'Rourke D. The physiological effects of slow breathing in the healthy human. Breathe (Sheff). 2017;13(4):298–309.

15 Zaccaro A, Piarulli A, Laurino M, et al. How breath-control can change your life: a systematic review on psycho-physiological correlates of slow breathing. Frontiers in Human Neuroscience. 2018;12:353.

16 Novaes MM, Palhano-Fontes F, Onias H, et al. Effects of yoga respiratory practice (Bhastrika pranayama) on anxiety, affect, and brain functional connectivity and activity: a randomized controlled trial. Frontiers in Psychiatry. 2020;11:467.

17 Kim JJ, Parker S, Henderson T, Kirby JN. Physiological fractals: visual and statistical evidence across timescales and experimental states. Journal of the Royal Society, Interface. 2020;17(167):20200334.

18 Avison JS. Fascial form in yoga. In: Schleip R (editor). Fascia: The Tensional Network of the Human Body. Churchill Livingstone; 2012.

19 Saraswati S. Asana Pranayama Mudra Bandha, 12th edition. Bihar School of Yoga (first published 1969); 2002. p. 544.

20 Shankaracharya. Yoga Taravali.

21 Borg-Olivier S, Machliss B. Applied Anatomy and Physiology of Yoga. Yoga Synergy; 2005.

22 Maehle G. Ashtanga Yoga: Practice and Philosophy. New World Library; 2007. p. 320.

23 Krishnamacharya T. Yoga Makaranda. Mysore: Madurai C.M.V. Press; 1934 (translation published 2006).

24 Swatmarama Muktibodhananda Saraswati Y. Hatha Yoga Pradipika. Bihar School of Yoga; 1450.

25 Lederman E. The myth of core stability. Journal of Bodywork and Movement Therapies. 2010;14(1):84–98.

26 The Gheranda Samhita: A Treatise on Hatha Yoga. Adyar Library; 1933.

27 Dorjee D. Defining contemplative science: the metacognitive self-regulatory capacity of the mind, context of meditation practice and modes of existential awareness. Frontiers in Psychology. 2016;7:1788. Bohm D. Wholeness and the Implicate Order. Routledge; 2002.

28 Bohm D. Wholeness and the Implicate Order. Routledge; 2002.

A.1 Modeling movement 188

A.2 Tensegrity 189

A.3 On the value of models by Susan Lowell 190
de Solórzano

A.4 The tensegrity icosahedron (T–icosa) 192

A.5 In the wild 192

A.6 Biotensegrity 195

A.7 Heterarchy: simultaneity and circularity 195

A.8 Modularity 200

A.9 Expansion and contraction: outward-
push and inward pull 202

A.10 The body: a home for configurations 203

A.11 Biotensegrity in yoga practice by Chris
Clancy 211

Yoga's missing link

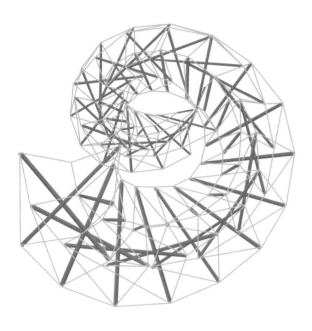

FIGURE A.1

Vector schematic redrawn after the sculpture, *Pavilion*, by Marcelo Pars.

Nature uses only the longest threads to weave her patterns, so each small piece of her fabric reveals the organization of the entire tapestry.

Richard P. Feynman

Key concepts

1 Tensegrity is a useful model for the balance of opposing forces in any structure, and it has a place in the shared curriculum for students of the living body.

2 T-icosa is a tensegrity model of the icosahedron, often used to illustrate some of the principles of biotensegrity.

3 Tensegrity has roots in art and architecture and now informs biology and body culture as a nonlinear, alternative model of biomechanics.

4 In a heterarchy, everything in the system is always influencing and under the influence of everything else.

5 As complex adaptive systems (CAS), organisms are structurally hierarchical and behaviorally heterarchical.

6 Bodily experience arises from the integration of modularity (self-contained, quasi-autonomous units) at all size scales.

7   The vayus of prana and apana (pranapana) together form the stability and flexibility of body shape.

8   In yoga, we are working with a sphere-based (60 degrees, triangulated) vector space in addition to the conventional anatomical planes (90 degrees, cubic).

9   The fascial continuum, including the bones, contains body elements of oscillating push and pull.

10 A biotensegral approach to functional anatomy based on spirality is an appropriate framework for yogis studying the body in asana.

A.1 Modeling movement

Working in the new paradigm is going to require more than a few deep breaths. As much as the felt sense of biotensegrity is natural for yoga practitioners (and anyone inhabiting a living body, for that matter), the words can be confusing for everyone involved. I will always touch back on the first principles established at the outset: nomenclature, while useful, is fundamentally incomplete at best, flawed (and potentially dangerous) at worst.

First of all, it is challenging enough to gain expertise in any one field. Worse, we tend to silo ourselves inside that expertise. So how can a person possibly work with confidence in the languages of the anatomical sciences *and* soft matter physics *and* biology *and* materials engineering *and* the art of movement? How in the world will an interdisciplinary language evolve into something on which we can all agree?

Maybe we don't have to. Surely, we aren't here just to observe, reference and regurgitate. I've come to see that this emerging paradigm is the ultimate playground where highly experienced scholars, bodywork practitioners, and the genuinely curious get together. Since nobody can be an expert in every field simultaneously, the vibrance of the community depends on... *play*. It requires participation as we venture out of our comfortable corners to contribute to its development with strong opinions loosely held. While we can accept that no model accounts entirely for the mystery of wholeness in motion, we can all be inspired by the model of biotensegrity to augment and update the conversation.

Yoga, in all its rich sociocultural evolutionary history, benefits from the same open-source status as practitioners continue to innovate. Many of us who tread tentatively in our teachings do so out of respect, and perhaps a kind of "imposter guilt" in our awareness that we are now rapidly transfiguring yoga exponentially faster in the shift to online teaching *en masse*.

It has taken me years in yoga and my academic work to fall in line with the art of referencing and the required deference to establish credibility. Ashtanga yoga instils deference. Only recently has it dawned on me that, at some point, the pastiche of deference eventually reduces to a missed opportunity if we can't emerge from it, to own our truth. As yoga teachers and researchers, I hope we can *all* come to a moment of confidence, reflecting in our teachings that which we can feel in our bodies from repeated and established experience.

Yoga's missing link

The Five Filaments (5F) for yoga I have proposed in this book are emerging out of many years of personal experience and study. Spiral movement is not new, and as I've mentioned often, I think it is something most teachers and students of yoga will come to independently, in their own time. The theoretical structure underlying this practical way of modelling movement, srotas-kinematics, is not new either. Rather, it is new, but I didn't make it up. In this book, I am simply spotlighting connections between concepts from different fields and applying some new terms to help link us and our nature, together.

A.2 Tensegrity

I was recently discussing anatomy with a fellow yoga teacher. I find it hard to talk about my research in moments like these because it can sound pretty bonkers. On this particular occasion, she seemed genuinely interested, so before I knew it, the word "tensegrity" came out of my mouth. She smiled politely but bristled at the term in a way that implied a yawn mixed with a rolling of the eyes. I pressed on, asking if she had the experience of tensegrity. Her response was refreshingly honest; she flashed me a knowing smile and said, "Well, the term *does* get bandied about." I had to laugh because it's true: tensegrity *does* get thrown around the physical culture scene. But what does it mean for yoga anatomy educators?

Reflecting on that perspective, I can see why many of us hear the term and dismiss it as somebody trying to sound clever (or just bonkers). If you're studying anatomy to be a better yoga teacher (complicated enough), why on earth would kinetic sculpture or mid-twentieth century architecture be in the curriculum? I first got into tensegrity as an art student, but only later saw its relevance to tissue.

I came back into the tensegrity conversation when I started 3D printing anatomical models because the mesh underlying the "anatomy" of a 3D print is built on triangulated spheres. But it wasn't until I began making sticks and string models of tensegrity that it all came together for me as essential for understanding the interconnectedness and functionality of body materials, movement, and, essentially for this narrative, *spirals*.

Key concepts 1

Tensegrity is a useful model for the balance of opposing forces in any structure, and it has a place in the shared curriculum for students of the living body.

In a yogic context, the body is balanced between prana and apana (pull and push, respectively) within the web of tissue architecture. The interconnectedness of this architecture is *prāṇāpāna*, a state in which the forces of outward push and inward pull are dynamically balanced. Now we move into an exploration of biotensegrity concepts from a yogic perspective, which for many of us can be as intimidating as it is compelling. For those of you already wincing, take a deep breath and make yourself a cup of tea. Better yet, why not make yourself a model? My online course, Anatomy Inspired, walks you through a DIY approach.

Appendix A

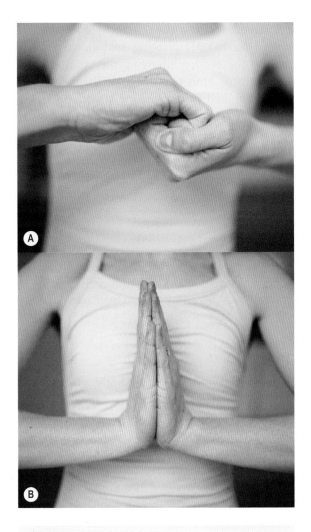

FIGURE A.2

Tension and compression: terms from a mechanical world need a little wiggle room to fit biologic materials. (A) Tension considered as a pulling apart, or stretching. In the round, a tensioned or "pulled apart" matrix will actually result in the squeezing of the tissues inward, like the skin of a balloon. (B) The result of tensioned tissues squeezing inward is compression, or a kind of "pushing together and inward" that resists the squeeze, pushing outward.

A.3 On the value of models by Susan Lowell de Solórzano

How can we fathom the nature of our structure? As spherical single-celled organisms, we begin. After a time in this state, we replicate our cells into more and smaller spheres within us, while still maintaining our one spherical body. Eventually, we form heads and tails and arms and legs and spines and hearts and hands, but even after our more familiar forms emerge, a spherical aspect remains in different ways and at varying levels of our being. How can we get a sense of this?

The push of our spherical selves is omnidirectionally outward, but we are also and always pulling ourselves together. The pulling forces, including pulls in the webbing we spin and thread sphere-to-sphere within us, are always along straight lines. The push is also always along straight lines, and it allows us to respond to and resist deformation from external forces, protecting our space in the world. But what can help us discern this experientially?

The forces between us and our home planet (also, and not coincidentally, spherical) move in straight lines. Here again, there is push and pull. The force of pull we know well: gravity drawing our centers straight to the center of the Earth. The push we may feel less familiar with intellectually, but our bodies are intimate with it. Our bodies do not need a name for the ground reaction force that pushes back up at us from the ground below, just as our bodies do not need a name for the push of electromagnetic repulsion: even my one-year-old grandson has learned that his hand cannot go through the chair.

But within our organismic bodies of pulsing, intelligent fluidic spherical volume and lines of force, we are dynamically balancing our constantly changing pushes and pulls, and

Yoga's missing link

neither push nor pull acts alone, nor could they. Each creates the other, and together they can do far more than either could by itself.

This collaboration of push and pull in our unique tensegral arrangement is what we want to grasp. It is nested, heterarchical, and constantly transmuting. It creates our inner spirality and our ability to respond omnidirectionally to incoming forces. It allows us to condense and expand in different internal zones as needed, to come together or differentiate through densifications and alliances that continuously take shape and evanesce across all scale levels of our systems.

How can we comprehend nature's talent for distributing forces so immediately and thoroughly, or for reconfiguring so dramatically with such a small demand of effort? We need models. They help us to crack open the door to the unfathomably vast marvel that life is. They are the physical constructs that help us connect concretely with otherwise untethered abstractions.

We can understand our physical systems better by applying conscious awareness and our powers of observation, particularly of the natural world, of which we are an interlinked part. We can accelerate our understanding by working with models to inform our views and experiences, and then continue to cycle between observation, experience and reflection. Improved understanding will be the natural result.

And so, we study spheres, and we examine lines of force. We study tensegrity models and other models related to biological phenomena. Our irreducible necessary model is a six-strut spherical tensegrity made with non-extendible cables, but we don't stop there. Eventually, we may end up with boxes and bags and shelves filled with magnetic building sets, Jacob's ladders, paper finger traps, marshmallows and paper clips, Superballs and Silly Putty, and cornstarch and string and sticks and whatnots galore for models yet to come.

Models deliver a direct physical experience, conveying information that bypasses linguistic and conceptual frameworks that can limit us. We can ground our study in our physical experience and then integrate it with the more theoretical framework. Experiencing models tactilely and visually does not rely on the constructions of language, which is useful because the study of biotensegrity is so new that we do not yet have an agreed-upon set of needed technical terms to describe all we are seeing and sensing. Look to metaphor. Look at poetry. Look to cooking. These can offer relevant and complementary models.

I have lost count of the number of exchanges I have had with people who want to study biotensegrity but who "do not have the time" to build and work with models, or who feel that working with virtual models on the computer is sufficient, or that watching videos of others who are handling models is enough.

If someone were to tell you they knew about yoga because, although they had never actually taken a class or done any of the movements, they had read several books about yoga and seen a number of videos, what would your response be?

Just as a person who has read all the best books on swimming, but who has never actually been in the water would not be prepared to jump in over her head, there are some things that must be experienced to be understood. In the same way, biotensegrity is in part a physical practice, and without its physical component, the study of biotensegrity cannot be complete. Here I am reminded of an observation from Mark Twain's

Tom Sawyer that (paraphrasing here) there are things one can learn by attempting to carry a cat home by the tail that would not be soon forgotten and that some might not learn any other way.

When we work with models, it clarifies our thinking. What is structurally sound? What comes together effortlessly? Build your models, and the relationship of tensegrity to things such as force vectors, spheres and spirals becomes ever more apparent. As your first tetrahelix emerges in your hands, for example, it becomes stunningly obvious: spirals are not a fancy of nature, but a structural inevitability.

The study of biotensegrity is less than half a century old. We are still at the very beginning of this science – still early enough for anyone to become a pioneer. Build your models. Work with them. Put in the necessary time. The science of biotensegrity needs your informed voice.

A.4 The tensegrity icosahedron (T-icosa)

The T-icosa model is enjoying increasing popularity in body culture media, but how many of us in the yoga community could talk about why that might be? It is tempting to reduce it to the explanation that the struts are bones and strings represent muscles and tendons. This oversimplification is a good start, but it comes at the cost of seeing wholeness in motion. The tensegrity icosahedron (T-icosa) is ultimately a symbol of balance, which is why we see the icon so often in the media related to body culture. Its "perfect" regularity illustrates the state of equilibrium in flux.

In a living system, where things are always in flux, the T-icosa would be hustling as part of a symphony in time with the rest of the network of *srotas* (tubes) and *nada* (waves). Like the *tattva*, the elemental polyhedra are never found in their pure state as uniform in nature; they're always found in flux, oscillating around that perfect state of equilibrium. T-icosa is an asana unto itself, a heterarchical module of interlinked sub-units, ever-changing and adapting within themselves. It is our ideal visualization for the srotas-kinematics.

Key concepts 2

T-icosa is a tensegrity model of the polygon icosahedron, often used to illustrate some of the principles of biotensegrity.

The T-icosa is a model for helping us to understand how the srotas connect and animate body materials in and among the subtle and gross sheaths of volumetric anatomy (recall koshas from Chapter 3). One crucial aspect to understanding anatomical structure is that the entire system gets stiffer as it is loaded. Levin states that this self-limiting response is a *sine qua non* of tensegrity.[1] Loading causes the tensegrity to spiral down into itself; unloading allows the structure to spiral back out. Now is an excellent time to have one in your hands.

A.5 In the wild

The T-icosa is a diagram of tension and compression force vectors that shows up

Yoga's missing link

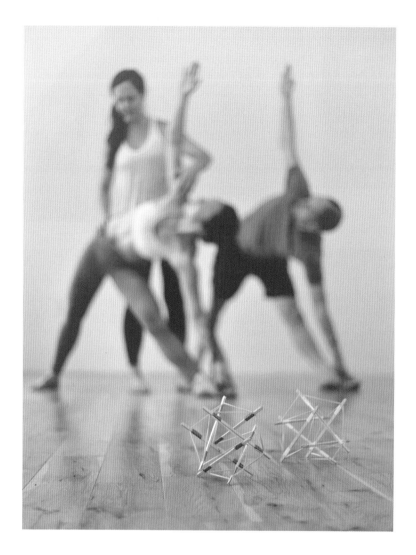

FIGURE A.3

Teaching yoga with biotensegrity principles in mind.

(Photo by Charlene Lim)

everywhere in nature, including our bodies. As Guimberteau has shared with his endoscopic exploration of living tissue (see Fig. A.4), the gooey polyhedral fibrils of the fascia world are continually lengthening, dividing, and migrating.[2] The visual evidence he provided with fluoroscopic imaging showed what he calls a **vacuolar** system capable of supporting blood vessels within the fascia. These vacuoles, microscopic fluid-interspersed channels, glide adaptively and independently of muscle contraction.

The continuous adaptation of fibrils along energy-minimizing paths (geodesics) gives rise

Appendix A

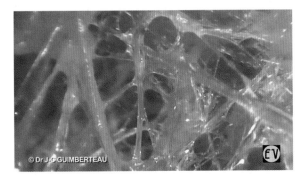

FIGURE A.4

Microvacuoles: the intersection of fibrils in three dimensions that form an irregular polyhedral unit of volume.

(Image by Jean-Claude Guimberteau, courtesy of Handspring)

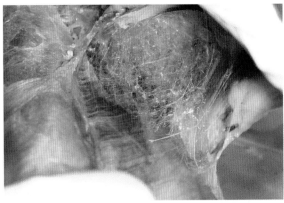

FIGURE A.5

Image by clinical anatomist John Sharkey demonstrating the moist, fractal, multifibular, omnidirectional, chaotic nature of fascia.

(Courtesy of John Sharkey)

to the fractal-like nature of cellular structure and secretions, evident even from the outside texture visible on the surface of the skin.[3] It is well known that living beings embody fractal geometry[4] and this factors into the essence of anatomy. Fractals explain self-similar structures and also have applications in the dynamic processes that have fluctuations over multiple time scales such as those found in physiology.[5] (The relationship between fractality and spirality comes alive in the online chapter.)

Moving further into the web, observers meet with the seemingly chaotic entanglement of filamentous fibers that define, connect, differentiate, and permeate the fabric of our inner world. This network of threads is tied into the *meso* as described in the first chapter. Recall that the related Ayurvedic tissue principle is *mamsa vaha srotas*, which is linked with the srotamsi shareera (tubular body) at all levels from gross to subtle via srotas-kinematics. This fractal inner world is home to the T-icosa, and perhaps we are coming to see that we are intra- and inter-connected through its subtle manifestations.

It is at this level we can observe the network of an interconnected, dynamic, fractal-like architecture of fibers in constant communication to preserve our shape without rupture by moving responsively according to tensegral architecture. This architectural activity can be approximately modelled in a state of stillness using the sticks-and-string or elastic band method. The chimerical nature of tissues in flux is another story because as yet there is no better method of modelling (outside of the computer) the oscillations inherent in the body architecture of living organisms. The best way to study it functionally is still to feel it for yourself.

A.6 Biotensegrity

A tensegrity structure is (among other things) one in which tension and compression balance through a particular arrangement. This arrangement is unique in part because it can handle being turned upside down, on its side and thrown into any of an infinite number of relationships to the ground. It can expand omnidirectionally and retract into itself, its movement is self-limiting, and it spirals.

Can your house do that? Have you seen a column that breathes or a post-box that squeezes? Pause here and have a play with your model. As Lowell de Solórzano reminds us, the best way to explore tensegrity is to have it in your actual hands, to appreciate the *qualitative nature* of its resistance to deformation and agency towards balance, from the co-creative forces of tension and compression.

The term *tensegrity* was coined by Buckminster Fuller, who was inspired by a novel 20th century architectural principle originating in the work of the sculptor, Kenneth Snelson, one of his students. Snelson first referred to the principle as "floating compression",[6] whereas Fuller created a syntactic of "tension" and "integrity" (or, *tensegrity*). The term tensegrity stuck. Structurally, tensegrity is a celebrated arrangement emerging from nature; the embodiment of natural forces interacting within a biologic form.

Key concepts 3

Tensegrity has roots in art and architecture and now informs biology and body culture as a nonlinear, alternative model for biomechanics.

So how is biotensegrity different from a regular tensegrity? Simply put, a *biotensegrity* refers to a living system; a wet, breathing organization of multiple types of tissue expressions. From the BIG point of view, *you* are a biotensegrity. Considering how living things might work as tensegrities offers powerful insight into physical practice. In this chapter, we'll get a bit more perspective on biotensegrity and look at the features of heterarchy, modularity, and a bit of vector space.

The word *bio*tensegrity originated in the work of American orthopedic surgeon, Dr Stephen M. Levin. He proposed a structural model for living organisms that incorporates the same physical laws that also relate to triangulated structural forms, "closest packing", and foams.[7] We saw the same principle in Chapter 1 with the section on prestress in the structure of cells, and we'll expand on that here.

In a tensegrity, when you move one element, all the other components are affected. When you adjust a student by pulling their hand skyward in Trikonasana, the response can be felt not just in their hand, but globally throughout their body as well as integrated with your own. We have previously looked at structure through the lens of hierarchy. Now, the lens of *heterarchy* puts a soft focus on the picture of anatomy so we can see that everything blends into the whole; both *hier-* and *hetero-* are evident ruling principles in the study of living anatomy.

A.7 Heterarchy: simultaneity and circularity

A heterarchy is a flexible organizational structure. The term heterarchy comes from *heteros* (another, or other) and *archai* (ruling principle) and represents a flexible structure composed of unranked, modular units "ruled" by an intrinsic self-order. In a heterarchy, all components are of influential significance to the whole system, regardless of size. This is in contrast to a **hierarchy** (from the Greek, "sacred ruler"). Functionally, a hierarchy is a top-down organization based on importance, in which an arrangement is "ruled" by a prominent entity *independent of feedback.*

Like a set of Russian dolls, a collection of things can look like a hierarchy from the outside due to the noticeable size difference. However, living systems are characterized by the importance of feedback. They can thus also be considered as *structurally hierarchical* while embedded communication is *organized heterarchically.*[8] The body is multistable and works simultaneously in both modes, as a "fluxtable entity" (see Appendix B for more on **fluxtability**).

Such an arrangement amounts to continuity, in that the body itself is a **continuum**, a complex adaptive system (CAS). CASs are characterized by the property of emergence, which means that qualities arising from the network are not qualities of any single component of that system.[9] Emergent properties are another way we see the throuple occurring in nature.

In the classical anatomical dissection paradigm, one bit of anatomy gets hard focus through a lens that forces specific delineations at the exclusion of other areas. Such attention is valuable for rote memorization but tends to exclude phenomena that are intrinsic to the wholeness of the living system. It gets easier to feel the body as a CAS with both hierarchical and heterarchical qualities when we consider the broader context of communication and appreciate the various needs for both.

Systems science literature points to the *heterarchical embeddedness*[8] of layered causal links in something that device communication people call the "3 Cs": consistent, continuous complementarity.[10] Is it kind of sad to look at

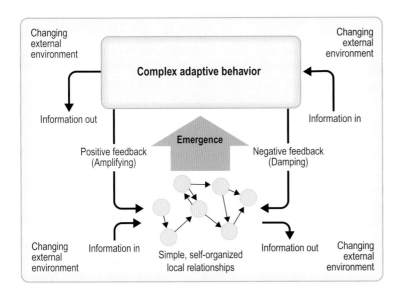

FIGURE A.6

Complex adaptive behavior of complex adaptive systems (CAS).

Yoga's missing link

device users as an example of heterarchy in yoga anatomy? In 2021, we are more integrated with our devices than ever before, for better or worse. For those of us straddling Gen X and Millennial generations, there are still memories of what life was like before devices.

Heterarchy addresses the diversity of relationships among elements in a system and offers a way to think about a change in spatial, temporal, and cognitive dimensions.[11] – Crumley

Accepting that most of us are now under the influence of several devices at once, with their "clouds" hovering over each and all of us at any single moment, there is probably no better means of exploring the idea of embedded communication. We have our desktop computer, laptop, pad, iPhone, watch, and other devices continually talking to each other via cloud platform interconnectivity and associated apps and algorithms. If you line them all up, the desktop computer appears largest, and as such the array would look like a hierarchy, but functionally they're all influencing one another via invisible routes of interconnectedness (digital srotas-kinematics?).

> If the cloud is the chariot, then a new view of anatomy is essential for us to adapt to understanding networks at the same time as we appreciate our "haptic perception" in interacting with the messages we store there and deliver – to ourselves and each other.
>
> **Joanne Avison**

Key concepts 4

In a heterarchy, everything in the system is always influencing and under the influence of everything else.

Device people talk about designing the user experience as an "ecosystem" within which the user is embedded. The successful design of user experience creates a sort of "auto-regulating" influence space that provides users with a sense of familiarity.[12] The dynamics of circularity pervade top-down, bottom-up, and peer-to-peer relationships.[13]

The point is this: we no longer have to control each device individually to keep them current with our chosen content (remember having to transfer your contacts?!). For better or worse, that function is now managed to various degrees through algorithms and distributed simultaneously amongst the devices, all of which talk to each other (so we can get on with creating and consuming content).

This kind of interconnectedness fails when there is a fault in simultaneity and circularity, like when you've just taken a video on your iPhone and expect it to load in your photo cloud for instant viewing on your desktop. If it doesn't load due to a fault somewhere (forgot password?), how frustrating is *that*? When immediate availability is blocked, either in our device-based experience or in our personal bodily experience, there is a disruption in the ecosystem. A CAS is a system that finds workarounds for these disruptions toward the ultimate immediacy.

Another analogy comes in the phenomenon of confirmation bias. Social media apps decide very quickly who we are and what we want to see based on our initial online activity. We are then presented with content that reflects our bias, and we see only what we want to see, or what the marketing elite think will make us buy stuff. There is something of this in our srotas-kinematics too: as we get used to the conditioning of assumed patterns, these patterns tend to stay "dyed in the wool."

Appendix A

 The yogic idea of "blockages" is a good description for disruptions in the flow of biological information.

In this era of neural networks and network thinking, the old understanding of top-down power arrangement is rapidly evolving into something more like a mesh. This paradigm shift is happening across disciplines in contemporary cultural and scientific discourse. Self-organization in biological systems is well documented as a means of understanding the "robustness and evolvability" of natural systems.[8,14]

Nothing operates in isolation

The balance of forces in anatomy is not controlled exclusively by large-scale structures such as the trunk, arms, and legs. Everything within the body is linked to everything else. The nervous system is an excellent example of simultaneity, whereby hierarchical and heterarchical principles are in continuous co-influence via voluntary movement, autonomic function, and reflex arcs nested within the sensory matrix, the largest organ of which is the fascia.

The way we experience our bodies is a balancing act from the macro end scaled to the molecules and everything in between. Cell biologist Donald Ingber has demonstrated that the contribution of the cytoskeleton is as relevant as postural alignment in the anatomical heterarchy of a living organism.[15] The global information exchange within individual bodies and between individuals within a community arises from a heterarchy and hierarchy in balance. The point is that we are not one or the other, but both in *multi*stability.

Key concepts 5

As complex adaptive systems (CAS), organisms are structurally hierarchical and behaviorally heterarchical.

Cellular tensegrity

As previously mentioned, the principles of intrinsic stress are modelled in our anatomy through the balance of push and pull with regions of density held in a matrix of continuous tension. The constant low level of muscle activity and tension generated by the cytoskeleton creates this inherent tension. The same tensegral arrangement appears in cells and molecules.

The molecular structural framework of the cell, its cytoskeleton, mechanically stabilizes the cell through tensegrity. Working independently of Levin, Donald Ingber has published his research on tensegrity in the cell, his work appearing extensively in the literature.[15-18] This section offers a tip-of-the-iceberg glimpse at cellular tensegrity, which of course follows the same principles as the rest of the body architecture.

Cytoskeleton

The cytoskeleton (CSK) rigidity gives cells their structural integrity. Recall prestress inherent in our bodies as explained in Chapter 1. This inherent tensional matrix allows for cell migration, communication, regulation, and just about every other functional attribute that brings the cell to life. The cytoskeleton of almost every cell (apart from mature **erythrocytes**) consists of three basic types of proteins (biopolymers):

- microfilaments
- microtubules
- intermediate filaments (thinnest).

Yoga's missing link

Adhesions in the extracellular matrix (ECM) are where transmembranous proteins such as integrins, cadherins, etc., cross the cell membrane and link the inner CSK with the outer ECM. This means that tensional forces can be transferred between them.[16] Consider these transmembranous proteins within a more extensive network: body, fascia, ECM, cell, CSK and nucleus. Both the CSK and ECM can generate tension and influence each other.

The **intermediate filaments** (**IFs**) are tensional; they integrate the cytoskeleton and hold it in place. The IFs connect the **microfilaments, microtubules**, the cell membrane, and the cell nucleus to one another. This dynamic molecular network of nano-scale struts and cables is continuously adapting the balance of tension and compression throughout the cell. Without this intrinsic force attenuation, cellular function would be impossible. Cells have to move, adapt, respond, manufacture, regenerate, and communicate, in addition to withstanding the imposition of outside forces, none of which would be possible without a resilient structure.

A central feature of tensegrity structures is that they stiffen when loaded. When cells are loaded, they behave as the T-icosa model does: they stiffen up and preserve their original shape by self-limiting further deformation. This happens as an essential response to any loading, for instance, the interlinked proteins of the cell adjust their firmness in response to prodding.[17]

Strictly speaking, the cellular tensegrity model is an example of the prestressed, or "intrinsically stressed" variety of tensegrity (as opposed to geodesic). However, the same fundamental mathematical rules underpin the different geodesic forms as they do the closest packing

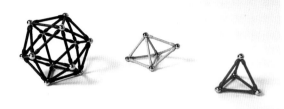

FIGURE A.7

Icosahedron, octahedron, and tetrahedron: the archetypal polyhedra that are composed of triangles.

of cells within the ECM.[18] (For an approachable discussion on close packing, head to Lowell de Solórzano's book, *Everything Moves*.[19])

The interplay of tension and compression is a motif that has many avatars on a molecular level in nature. Hexagonal arrangements (a hallmark of triangulated spheres) can be found in:

- basement membrane proteins
- polyhedral enzymes
- viral capsides
- lipid micelles
- RNA and DNA molecules.

From molecules to cells, into tissues, through whole organ systems, and finally into the shapes the body makes, tensegrity describes the formation of living things as a diagram of forces. Tensegrity models and anatomical structures are visible representations of the invisible forces of tension and compression within them. Living tissues self-organize in a heterarchical way with the CKCs describing the underlying interactions.

Appendix A

The fibrous matrix moves responsively, and out of this vast sea of auto-tuning linkages, we find a sense of self.

> Many prestressed architectures in engineering are fraught with linear logic of straight things. We humanoids are prestressed because the bone-tubes in the middle of the limb tubes (guided by the circulatory tubes, orchestrated by the heart tubes), grow considerably faster than the tissues surrounding them. Take our outer covering – the "neoprene wetsuit" that we can't unzip: we already fill it, like a baby-grow that is slightly too small for us (as it is supposed to be, or we would be too soggy to walk around). If you race your hand into a surgical glove, your fingers will be held in a curled position, predisposed to "cup" in flexion. Laws of round things (not straight things) are governing this world of nonlinear biologic forms, and it is amplified and honored by exploring these Five Filament themes.
>
> **Joanne Avison**

 Prestressed and nonlinear

The literature shows current efforts to reconcile traditional hierarchical assumptions about motor control in the body with updated models to incorporate the role of fascia and resting tonus.[20] This is an exciting area of research, as the notion of motor control is revised to consolidate disparate levels that have been studied independently in the 70 years since Bernstein introduced his essay in Russian, *Levels of Construction of Movements*.

Considered by many to be the founder of biomechanics, motor control, and physiology of activity, Nicholai Aleksandrovich Bernstein shaped long-standing views of voluntary movements and dexterity. The English translation of Bernstein's hierarchical neural model was published in 1996.[21] Bernstein's anatomical model addressed the coordination of neural levels to produce voluntary movement, without integrating the influence of connective tissue in the maintenance of basal tension in the body.

Basal tension has replaced the vague term "tonus" in contemporary biomechanics. As hierarchical models morph into embedded heterarchies to better explain biologic structure, the tensegrity model is rising to the forefront as an illustration of how basal tension works. As demonstrated by Souza et al.,[22] this basal tension functions as *prestress*, or intrinsic tension, that accounts for the anticipatory characteristics of the body's default status first mentioned in Chapter 1.[23] Primed for movement, tissue densities exhibit the multifractality observed in fluctuation patterns across timescales.[24] These fractal fluctuations integrate with sensory experience to produce coordination of haptic perception.[25]

A.8 Modularity

Modularity is a foundational principle of integrated anatomy. Wagner suggested in 1996 that the body is composed of locally integrated, quasi-autonomous units.[26] A module is like a part in the sense that the integration of many modules creates a whole. But unlike a mere part, modules are self-contained and quasi-autonomous (they have intrinsic completeness, like a modular unit of storage).[27]

Yoga's missing link

Tensegrity models exhibit modularity, composed of units that are complete within themselves into assemblies of "higher-order" complexity that can be disassembled without disrupting the inherent balance. As we have seen in our spiral-bound survey of anatomy, the appendages can be functionally segmented into movements that have a kind of symmetry.

These movements are powered by relatively autonomous, interconnected components. Recall our look at the arms and legs in the first few chapters. We saw that the arms can be like the legs of the upper body and vice versa. These modules share similar traits that have been influenced selectively for development into "arms" and "legs" as we now know and love them. The somites self-organize into a metameric array of tissue that gives rise to the segmented nature of our spine. Vertebrates are then, by definition, inherently modular.

Plants and animals are anatomically modular in the sense that they are organized in developmentally and anatomically distinct units. These units are often repeating in body segments such as petals, fingers, and compartments.[28] Modularity has applications in mathematics, design, biochemistry, behavioral science, neuroscience and many other fields. A network of interactions can also be modular.[29]

Modularity in organisms is observed during the development of the embryo (ontogeny) and is thought to facilitate evolutionary development (phylogeny).[30] In so-called "evo-devo", the emergence of modularity in the developing organism refers to sets of traits that are closely linked. From these, patterns of anatomical modularity in adult forms are better understood.[31]

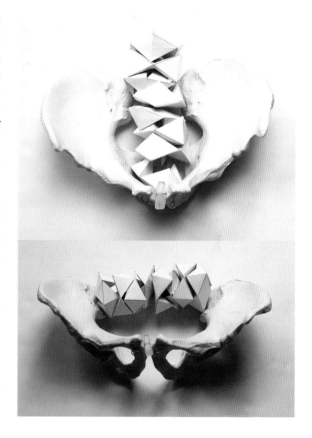

FIGURE A.8

Flexagons as anatomical regions demonstrating modularity.

Human beings can experience the loss of a module and still function perfectly well. Although losing a limb is unquestionably more than a little disruptive, it is common for amputees to develop workarounds for lost "modules" like arms and legs. There is a profound built-in predisposition to adaptability and auto-responding workarounds at play in the new paradigm.

Appendix A

Key concepts 6

Bodily experience arises from the integration of modularity (self-contained, quasi-autonomous units) at all size scales.

A.9 Expansion and contraction: outward push and inward pull

Complexity in human movement arises from the coupled interplay of balanced opposing forces (*dvandvas*) as we have explored in earlier chapters. These combinations of push and pull, attraction and repulsion, tension and compression create *dynamic reciprocity*; from which a third state arises – that which we have termed throupled. At the very least, it is an unpredictable result, emerging from the sum of the individual qualities and structures at play; especially when they are so-called oppositions.

 Reciprocity

Dynamic reciprocity is a term for the intimacy of relationships within anatomy. Ida and Pingala, when in balance, allow Sushumna to arise spontaneously. We are making a case for anatomy to be taught in the same way.

In the study of tissue, dynamic reciprocity refers to a continuous and bidirectional relationship between cells and the matrix.[32,33] The literature growing around fascia and the extracellular matrix (ECM) abounds with the critical importance of *dynamic reciprocity* (relationship between the living cell and its 'non-living' secretions). This is because it describes the relationship that gives living tissue the properties required for essential life functions such as structure, balance, healing, reproduction, communication, and coordinated movement.[34] Flow and transport have also been formally shown to contribute to dynamic reciprocity.[35]

Yoga practitioners are already familiar with the concept as we use it in every movement we make. A push needs the pull and vice versa, Ida needs Pingala and vice versa. Students need teachers as much as the teacher needs students. Our living cells require their fibrous and gel substrate as much as the substrate needs the cells to exist in the first place (cells secrete the matrix).

Pranapana

In my evolving understanding, prana is the energetic flow, or movement wind (vayu), that leads us into our source, inwards. The in-drawing action of prana that leads us into ourselves would be impossible without the outward push of apana (or there wouldn't be anything to pull into!). The outward-moving energy of apana is al dente, it takes us energetically out into the world, and could not do so without the pranic flow that keeps the body entity together as a whole.

Key concepts 7

The vayus of prana and apana (pranapana) are the stability and flexibility of body shape.

The yogic concept of this energetic directionality is embodied in our tissues anatomically – we saw it in the vayu of Chapter 3. By playing with tensegrity in the models of tension and compression, we can get a feel for aspects of this directionality in our hands. Models and bodies both show how the dynamic reciprocity of the two critical forces of push and pull (structurally experienced as tension and compression) unite in co-creative force transmission. The tension makes the compression compress; the compression struts make the tension tensioned. Together they make the constraints of multidimensional, volumetric shape-change.

A.10 The body: a home for configurations

In the spiral-bound view of anatomy, the body is a playground of vectors like the push and pull of the previous section. Put simply, a vector is a force: think of an arrow, it has magnitude and direction. In linear algebra, vector *fields* allow us to visualize the magnitude and direction of forces.

The human body itself is a vector field. As a biologic organism, the human body obeys the same physical laws of triangulation and closest packing that also govern space-filling spherical vector spaces such dandelions, seafoam, bee larvae, chia seed pudding, and caviar.[36]

In traditional anatomy, the student works toward memorizing origins and insertions, etc., concerning length, width, and depth as the anatomical planes. The classical anatomical terms of movement and position came out of this three-dimensional, planar orientation that puts everything at 90 degrees to everything else. In the conventional Cartesian vector space of the anatomical planes, we can talk about points in the same three dimensions to find locations of

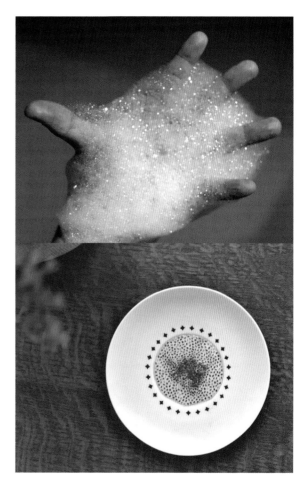

FIGURE A.9

Fractal-like: bubbles on the polyhedral texture of your skin tell the story of how things continue into the deeper layers. In the bottom image, a saucer of hydrophilic chia seeds demonstrates the way round things coalesce geodesically in the most minimal-energy configurations.

(Photo by Charlene Lim)

Appendix A

parts in cubic relationships. Since we are not made of Lego bricks, why stick with the right angles for describing movement?

Talking point

In body geometry, vector space starts in the 90 degrees of Legoland when we learn about the so-called anatomical planes. Flat planes are great for describing groups of postures along a single axis like forward bends, backbends, side bends, and twists. But what about the constant in-and-out movement of breath? There is no such thing as a cubic plane that can describe breathing. So, what is the body geometry for movement that breathes? How we do we talk about the anatomical position of continuous tubular fabric in the round?

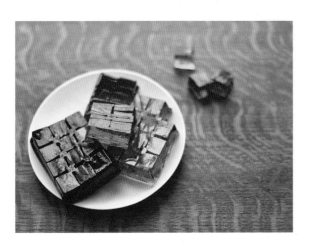

FIGURE A.10

Soft matter: all things squishy, including you, me, and this modular presentation of gelatin.

(Photo by Charlene Lim)

Although it is not featured in traditional anatomy textbooks (yet), there is an alternative to the cubic vector space, one that describes the omnidirectional in-and-out of biologic movement. This alternative is the srotas-kinematics, the Sriyantra (see the Online Chapter for much more on the sacred geometry!)  expressed in the "synergetic" coordinates of Buckminster Fuller's explorations[37] that have so inspired the new paradigm in biology.

This alternative body geometry is just as important as the planes (if not more so) for understanding anatomy because it allows for the consideration of movement within a mesh in the round. The sphere-based vector space offers a triangulated playing field, a perspective that makes sense of our physical experience of how the body moves. Integrated anatomy in balance is the home of srotas-kinematics, the geometry of biomotion.

 The spiral-bound anatomy space for yoga is framed in the closest packing of spheres. This geodesic mesh forms a structural heterarchy while remaining directed by and responsive to its hierarchical connectivity. From molecules to joint systems, forces play out the same way through the tissues because, at each level, nature works the same minimal-energy way, adapting optimally to changes in circumstances (whether these are related to a new day on the mat, or a new way in the metropolis).

Key concepts 8

In yoga, we are working with a sphere-based (60 degrees, triangulated) vector space in addition to the conventional anatomical planes (90 degrees, cubic).

Yoga's missing link

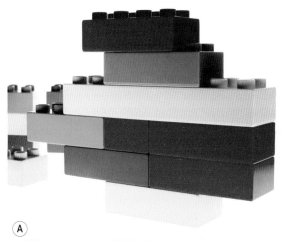

(A)

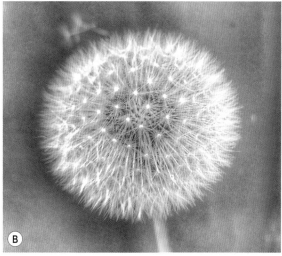

(B)

FIGURE A.11

Vector spaces for placing the body. (A) Duplo demonstrating the Euclidean vector space of the anatomical planes in 90 degrees: length, width, and depth. (B) The dandelion exemplifies a sphere-based vector space for convergent-divergent shape change (breathing).

Interconnectedness

Continued study of yoga reveals interconnectedness at increasingly high definition, not only among parts within the body but between our bodies and the rest of the world. In asana, we can quickly feel that wherever the body meets a surface, that surface becomes part of the shape and informs it. The geometry is innate and continuous, incorporating both.

This interconnectedness of the tubular mesh balances within the push–pull of the forming, responsive fascial arrangement. In a practical sense, the modularity of one body fits together with the modules of adjacent bodies when we give and receive adjustments. In the next sections, we explore how interconnected body elements self-stabilize, move, and continuously autoregulate.

 ### Tension and compression: a dynamic reciprocity

What exactly do tension and compression look like? Without tension (stress along a given force) compression cannot exist, and vice versa. Prana and apana are the subtle body cognates of tension and compression. Pranapana is a *dvandva* that describes a tensegral balance of push and pull, inwardness and outwardness, stiffness and softness in appropriate proportion.

A tensional force flows along the length of a medium. The word *tendon* arises from tension, a force associated with flexible materials. Kenneth Snelson referred to the body as a "sea of tension."[6] In such a 3D arrangement, the tensional force draws body elements

Appendix A

inwards. This in-drawing comes from the state of intrinsic stress, particular to body architecture.

...Islands of compression floating in a sea of continuous tension

Kenneth Snelson[6]

TABLE A.1 The dvandva of push and pull: making sense of tension and compression in a yogic context	Tension/prana	Compression/apana
Player	Cable/string	Strut/stick
Force	Pull	Push
Direction	Inward	Outward
Qualities	Stiffness/flexibility	Frame, integrity
Everyday example	Wheel/spokes	Hub/rim
In yoga anatomy	Bandha/prana	Turgor/bone/apana
Physiology	Inhale/ingest	Exhale/excrete
Allegory	The sea	Islands
Divine principle	Feminine	Masculine
Tantric orientation	Nivritti	Pravritti

 Bouncing bones, breathing tendon

Feeling integrated anatomy in yoga is easy, we do it with the breath all the time. Next time you're on the mat, take your attention to the idea of tendons. A tendon is classically known as the bit of connective tissue that holds muscles onto bones. Visualize the Achilles tendon and its continuities expanding outwards in all directions with each inhalation and contracting down with each exhalation. The fasciae, mesentery, ligaments, fibrocartilage, bursae; all breathe in time with the whole.

Once you've got the hang of breathing with your connective tissues, then tune into the bounce of the bones by emphasizing recoil each time you step, jump, or otherwise meet your mat with either hands or feet. Just as much as the so-called "soft tissues" can be loaded with recoil, bones also have the propensity for elastic energy. Bones, like all fascia, are part of the fascial continuum whose job it is to respond to the forces of being alive.[38]

Key concepts 9

The fascial continuum, including the bones, contains body elements of oscillating push and pull.

Kinematic dynamism

If you are reading this book, you've invested in making sense of anatomy as integral to (instead of separate from) lived experience. We all study and memorize anatomical "facts" to increase our knowledge, right? It can be very daunting when we realize that all the facts we spent years memorizing are part of the reductionist thinking that interferes with understanding how it all fits together in a live body in motion. But take heart, fellow yogi. Unlearning it is part of transcending its linear hold on us nonlinear, soft matter creatures – while it can simultaneously act as a useful constraint!

As Avison reminds us, we *are* mystery manifest. There is nothing in your body that can be copyrighted or reduced to memorable parts. Titles for individual muscles are like postal codes; we learn them to communicate about the more extensive network of places. But when you're on the ground exploring the neighborhoods, cities, countries, and continents, it is easy to see that there are no clear boundaries or labels drawn on the Earth. Those boundaries are the training

wheels of learning; at some point, it is necessary to trust your balance.

What we are accustomed to thinking of as "the muscles" are in reality contractile elements of omnidirectional tension. The biotensegrity view describes these as defaulting to the isometric, isotonic state in which directionality has evolved to produce the most efficient movement. Rather than either/or states of muscle contraction, they are simultaneous features of elements within the tensegral balance of living systems, animated through their srotas-kinematics. The muscles "tune" the acoustics of each movement; they are not the sole orchestrators.

Tensegrity as a model for biological architecture applies across the whole size spectrum, from molecules up to joint systems. Recall the cellular networks from Chapter 2, in which isometric tension (cytoskeletal prestress!) gives the body is propensity for bounce, elasticity, and integrity.[15,39] In vertebrates, the interconnected joint systems will optimally manage forces by amplifying or attenuating them in service to the organism. Whether the forces are self-generated or environmental in origin, and whether or not the response is voluntary, the network of srotas-kinematics responds.

One magnificent illustration of this concept in kinematic sculpture is the *Strandbeest* of Theo Jansen (Fig. A.12). These "beach animals" are animated by the wind, and once they get going, require no further contractile or motor power to ambulate. Jansen describes them as "skeletons that walk on the wind, so they don't have to eat."[40] The wind animates Jansen's sculpture like the vayus of the subtle yogic body. Add tension and compression, *et voilà* – we happen!

Although we do still have to eat for our fuel (unlike the wind-powered Strandbeest),

Appendix A

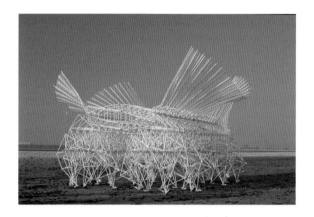

FIGURE A.12

Strandbeest by the artist Theo Jansen. No muscles are contracting, and yet it moves!

(Animaris Currens Ventosa Oostvoorne, 1993)

 Dancing with gravity

The living spine can flow functionally in all the various gravity-independent postures of yoga. Stephen Levin makes an interesting observation of yoga, that in fact "Yoga may be an attempt to reproduce a gravity-free environment for body and mind while on the earth's surface".[42]

vertebrates benefit from this same kinematic architecture where forces are managed within the system to work in the most efficient way possible. Like the vayus, the srotas organization moves with a minimum of contractile effort required to "pump up" the system to progressively higher energetic activity levels.

Steven Levin's paper, "Muscles at rest",[41] describes this process from the biotensegrity point of view, offering the analogy of a swing. Once you get the rhythm going, it doesn't take much additional effort to maintain the action. Here we see resonance finding resonance! The vinyasa method and srotas-kinematics show us much the same idea but from a yogic whole-body perspective.

This intrinsically stressed resting state is oscillating with the vibrations of the heart, respiration, eyes, GI tract, and cellular activity. The whole system is further animated to harness tension to increasing levels for purposeful activity. In dynamic yoga, the body in motion propels itself through a continuous rebounding dynamism fueled by the "pranapanic" breath, rather than relying on the work of many individual muscle actions working in isolation.

Nature uses srotas-kinematics to couple multiple tissues and thus endow the entire system with higher overall efficiency. These nested, modular units form an integrated movement system. The evolutionary conservation of this concept has maximized energetic efficiency through a regulatory system embedded into the morphological structure itself.[43] This self-regulating heterarchy is more like a web of influence and less like a chain of command. The shift toward complex network thinking can be observed in all kinds of systems, from biology to politics and into biomechanics and sports science.[44]

Yoga's missing link

TABLE A.2 Training or synergizing? Contrast of theoretical principles		
Approach	**Training (traditional)**	**Synergising (complex systems)**
Conception of practitioners	Machines	Complex adaptive systems
Conception of yoga practice	Static entity	Dynamic entity
Scientific approach	Cybernetic Control Theory	Dynamic Systems Theory
Relations among components	Linear cause-effect	Nonlinear dynamic interactions
Integrating mechanisms	Control loops	Circular causality
Control	Internal/external programs	Spontaneous synergies
Organization	Externally designed	Self-organized
Adaptive properties	Homeostasis	Homeodynamics, synergetic reorganization, degeneracy, pleiotropy
Training goal	Maximizing performance attributes	Satisfying diversity/ unpredictability potential
Training periodization	Pre-programmed	Co-adapted

Adapted for yoga from Pol R, Balagué N, Ric A, et al. Training or synergizing? Complex systems principles change the understanding of sport processes. Sports Med – Open. 2020;6:28. https://doi.org/10.1186/s40798-020-00256-9. https://creative-commons.org/licenses/by/4.0/

 Asana aboard

Asana isn't limited to the parts of your body involved in a traditional anatomical breakdown of a particular pose. The asana requires ground reaction force from the Earth. Anything and everything we touch becomes a genuine part of the pose. This includes the ground, the wall, any prop, block, belt, or another person.

Key concepts 10

A biotensegral approach to functional anatomy based on spirality is an appropriate framework for yogis studying the body in asana.

In this Appendix, we compared the srotas-kinematics of integrated anatomy with ideas from biotensegrity, an elegant structural theory

Appendix A

TABLE A.3 Training or synergizing? Contrast of methodological principles		
Approach	Training (traditional)	Synergising (complex systems)
Programs	Fixed training programs	Contextually sensitive methodological criteria
Practitioners	Executors	Co-designers of the process
Periodization	Fixed, decontextualized	Contextually sensitive
Conditioning, skill acquisition, motor abilities	Prescription-based	Based on nested dependence and circular causality of constraints
Training unit	Practitioners and their components, community	Practitioner-environment system, community
Short-term training plan	Based on stereotyped performance solutions and movement templates	Based on exploration of representative performance contexts
Training tasks	Non-representative (through task decomposition)	High level of representativeness (through task simplification) and beyond
Practice criteria	Right/wrong	Contextually (un)functional
Evaluation	Fragmented	Holistic
Role of the teacher	Prescribing solutions	Co-discovering with the practitioner

Adapted for yoga from Pol R, Balagué N, Ric A, et al. Training or synergizing? Complex systems principles change the understanding of sport processes. Sports Med – Open. 2020;6:28. https://doi.org/10.1186/s40798-020-00256-9. https://creative-commons.org/licenses/by/4.0/

that offers rich metaphor and visuals. In it, we see elements balanced within a tensional network of push–pull oscillating in coupled modules forming a self-regulating body mesh situated within a spherical coordinate system.

The significance of this spherical system is further developed elsewhere in the literature of biophysics.[45,46] The closest packing of spheres has application in the divergent-convergent movement of spirality and is well worth exploring. After all, we are made of soft matter, not hard matter. As such, the new paradigm goes for 60-degree angles that describe spheres and close packing – not the 90-degree angled forces described in classical biomechanics and anatomy.

Yoga's missing link

Panning out from the cubic thinking of linear biomechanics is probably easier for yogis. Since our entire curriculum is based on breathing, we *get* the idea of a tubular body mesh animated by flowing expansion-retraction. Breathe-in, breathe-out, find confidence in personal experience. You are a subtle set of self-listening acoustics. Together in yoga, we are adding resonance to the paradigm shift in biology through connecting some of the patterns we all see emerging in nature.

A.11 Biotensegrity in yoga practice by Chris Clancy

Bringing an understanding of biotensegrity to the practice and teaching of yoga, we are encouraged to let go of standards that evolved under a strict biomechanical model. We let go of outer ideals based on visual or proprioceptive cues and attune to the inner sensations of the body. The waves of the thinking mind grow calm, judgement fades, and we rest in the seat of the observer. Biotensegrity is nature's design; thus, with this deep inner listening, we discover the tensegral properties that already and always exist in the body.

Teaching yoga through the lens of biotensegrity can be as simple as drawing awareness to one or more tensegral properties that exist within the body. Since biotensegrity is scalar and heterarchical, the possibilities are endless. We are invited to imagine the vertebrae, and indeed all of the bones, floating in a tensional web of soft tissue. Consequently, there is a felt sense of fluidity, space and ease.

Knowing that the body is continuously connected by a dynamic tensional matrix from molecules, through cells and into the body as a whole, we can refine our ability to perceive the sensations within. We might notice the movement of the breath reflected on the gross level of the lungs or belly, to the fingers and toes, to the surface of the skin and beyond. We might have the sensation that the cells themselves are breathing. Then, we can focus on a tiny point and feel a whole-body response.

Seeing that a tensegrity icosahedron spirals as it expands or contracts omnidirectionally, we can ask if this same possibility exists in the body. Finding that it does, we can allow the torso to grow and spiral into a pose as if on its own, merely by watching the breath.

We might choose to introduce techniques that help balance and integrate the relationship of tension and compression throughout the body to optimize tensegral properties. For example, by tapping into an energetic connection from "tips to tips (fingertips, toes, tongue) and crown to tail" through to center and back, we feel better balance, lightness and ease.

References

1   Levin SM. Shear or not to Shear. 2003. Available at: http://www.biotensegrity.com/resources/shear-or-not-shear.pages.pdf

2   Guimberteau J-C. Fibre world. In: Guimberteau J-C (editor). Dundee Biotensegrity Dissection. 2017.

3   Sharkey J. Concise Book of Neuromuscular Therapy: A Trigger Point Manual. Chichester, UK: Lotus Publishing; 2008.

4   Paar V, Pavin N, Rosandic M. Link between truncated fractals and coupled oscillators in biological systems. Journal of Theoretical Biology. 2001;212(1):47–56.

Appendix A

5   Goldberger AL, West BJ. Fractals in physiology and medicine. The Yale Journal of Biology and Medicine. 1987;60(5):421–35.

6   Snelson K. Continuous tension, discontinuous compression structures. US Patent No. 3169611A, 1965. Available at: https://patents.google.com/patent/US3169611A/en

7   Levin SM (editor). The icosahedron as a biologic support system. 34th Annual Conference of Engineering in Medicine and Biology, 1981; Houston, TX.

8   Bruni LE, Giorgi F. Towards a heterarchical approach to biology and cognition. Progress in Biophysics and Molecular Biology. 2015;119(3):481–92.

9   Ridder DD, Stöckl T, To WT, et al. Noninvasive transcranial magnetic and electrical stimulation: working mechanisms. In: Evans JR, Turner RP (editors). Rhythmic Stimulation Procedures in Neuromodulation. Academic Press; 2017. pp. 193–223.

10 Levin SM. Designing Multi-Device Experiences: An Ecosystem Approach to User Experiences Across Devices. O'Reilly Media; 2014.

11 Crumley CL. Heterarchy. Emerging Trends in the Social and Behavioral Sciences. John Wiley & Sons, Inc.; 2015.

12 Liao I-C, Deng Y-S, You H-C. The emotion and personality user perception in multi-screen interaction. In: Marcus A (editor). Design, User Experience, and Usability: Novel User Experiences. Springer; 2016.

13 Cumming GS. Heterarchies: reconciling networks and hierarchies. Trends in Ecology & Evolution. 2016;31(8):622–32.

14 Gunji Y-P, Sasai K, Wakisaka S. Abstract heterarchy: time/state-scale re-entrant form. Biosystems. 2008;91(1):13–33.

15 Ingber DE. Cellular tensegrity: defining new rules of biological design that govern the cytoskeleton. Journal of Cell Science. 1993;104 (Pt 3):613–27.

16 Ingber DE. Integrins, tensegrity, and mechanotransduction. Gravitational and Space Biology Bulletin. 1997;10(2):49–55.

17 Ingber DE. Mechanochemical basis of cell and tissue regulation. National Academy of Engineering. 2004;34(3).

18 Ingber DE. Tensegrity II. How structural networks influence cellular information processing networks. Journal of Cell Science. 2003;116(8):1397–408.

19 Lowell de Solórzano S. Everything Moves: How Biotensegrity Informs Human Movement. Handspring Publishing Limited; 2020.

20 Profeta VLS, Turvey MT. Bernstein's levels of movement construction: a contemporary perspective. Human Movement Science. 2018;57:111–33.

21 Latash ML. Dexterity and its development. In: Latash ML, Turvey MT, Bernsteĭn NA (editors). Dexterity and Its Development – Resources for Ecological Psychology. Taylor & Francis; 1996.

22 Souza TR, Fonseca ST, Gonçalves GG, et al. Prestress revealed by passive co-tension at the ankle joint. Journal of Biomechanics. 2009;42(14):2374–80.

23 Turvey MT, Fonseca ST. The medium of haptic perception: a tensegrity hypothesis.

Journal of Motor Behavior. 2014;46(3): 143–87.

24 Cavanaugh JT, Kelty-Stephen DG, Stergiou N. Multifractality, interactivity, and the adaptive capacity of the human movement system: a perspective for advancing the conceptual basis of neurologic physical therapy. Journal of Neurologic Physical Therapy. 2017;41(4):245–51.

25 Schleip R, Mechsner F, Zorn A, Klingler W. The bodywide fascial network as a sensory organ for haptic perception. Journal of Motor Behavior. 2014;46(3):191–3.

26 Wagner GP. Homologues, Natural kinds and the evolution of modularity. American Zoologist. 1996;36(1):36–43.

27 Stewart D, Wilson-Kanamori JR. Modular modelling in synthetic biology: light-based communication in E. coli. Electronic Notes in Theoretical Computer Science. 2011;277: 77–87.

28 Rosslenbroich B. On the Origin of Autonomy: A New Look at the Major Transitions in Evolution. Springer International Publishing; 2014.

29 Wagner GP, Pavlicev M, Cheverud JM. The road to modularity. Nature Reviews Genetics. 2007;8:921.

30 Schlosser G, Wagner GP. Modularity in Development and Evolution. University of Chicago Press; 2004.

31 Kavanagh KD. Modularity and Integration in Evo-Devo. In: Kliman RM (editor). Encyclopedia of Evolutionary Biology. Oxford: Academic Press; 2016. pp. 41–3.

32 Schultz GS, Davidson JM, Kirsner RS, et al. Dynamic reciprocity in the wound

microenvironment. Wound Repair and Regeneration. 2011;19(2):134–48.

33 Gjorevski N, Nelson CM. Bidirectional extracellular matrix signaling during tissue morphogenesis. Cytokine & Growth Factor Reviews. 2009;20(5-6):459–65.

34 Thorne JT, Segal TR, Chang S, et al. Dynamic reciprocity between cells and their microenvironment in reproduction. Biology of Reproduction. 2015;92(1):25.

35 Kaul H, Ventikos Y. Dynamic reciprocity revisited. Journal of Theoretical Biology. 2015;370:205–8.

36 Levin SM. Tensegrity: the new biomechanics. In: Hutson M, Ellis R (editors). Textbook of Musculoskeletal Medicine. Oxford; 2006. pp.69–80.

37 Fuller RB, Applewhite EJ. Synergetics: Explorations in the Geometry of Thinking. New York: Macmillan Publishing Co., Inc.; 1975.

38 Levin SM. Bone is fascia. 2018. Available at: https://www.researchgate.net/publication/ 327142198_Bone_is_fascia

39 Labouesse C, Verkhovsky AB, Meister JJ, et al. Cell shape dynamics reveal balance of elasticity and contractility in peripheral arcs. Biophysical Journal. 2015;108(10):2437–47.

40 Jansen T. Strandbeest. Available from: http:// www.strandbeest.com/.

41 Levin SM. Muscles at rest. Available from: http://www.biotensegrity.com/resources/ muscles-at-rest.pdf.

42 Levin SM. Personal correspondence. 2018.

43 Levin SM, Lowell de Solórzano S, Scarr G. Kinematic chains: tensegrity in biology.

2017. Journal of Bodywork and Movement Therapies. 2017; 21:664–72.

44 Pol R, Balagué N, Ric A, et al. Training or synergizing? Complex systems principles change the understanding of sport processes. Sports Medicine – Open. 2020;6(1):28.

45 Rashevsky N. An approach to the mathematical biophysics of biological self-regulation and of cell polarity. The Bulletin of Mathematical Biophysics. 1940;2(1):15–25.

46 Jansen KA, Donato DM, Balcioglu HE, et al. A guide to mechanobiology: where biology and physics meet. Biochimica et Biophysica Acta (BBA) [Molecular Cell Research]. 2015;1853(11, Part B):3043–52.

B.1 Nonlinear pedagogy   218

B.2 Non-proportionality   219

B.3 Fluxtability   221

B.4 Noise   223

B.5 Creativity and empowerment: the
         rewards   224

Nonlinear teaching

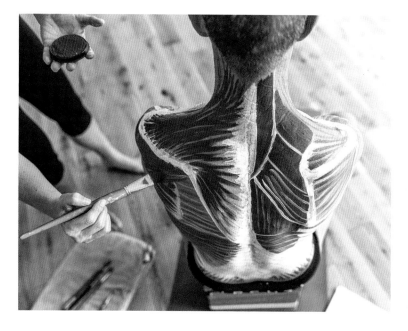

FIGURE B.1

Body painting anatomy is a tool for experiencing the gap between what we think we know and the nonlinear, ungraspable reality of tissue.

(Demonstrated by Stu Girling, loveyogaanatomy.com)

There is a vitality, a life force, an energy, a quickening that is translated through you into action, and because there is only one of you in all of time, this expression is unique. And if you block it, it will never exist through any other medium and it will be lost.

Martha Graham[1]

Key concepts

1 Nonlinearity is a word that is used to describe the behavior of complex systems such as a biologic structure.

2 Yoga andragogy and anatomy are nonlinear systems.

3 Pedagogy is teaching and learning in education; andragogy is the same but for adults, especially in the realm of self-directed learning.

4 Linear systems are proportional; nonlinear systems are non-proportional.

5 Nonlinear systems are multistable.

6 The yoga space is nonlinear in that systems are manipulated through parametric control to produce progressive states of self-organization.

7 Noise has a functional role in the progression of learning systems.

8 As teachers, we choose constraints that set our students up for self-discovering empowerment in "Aha!" moments.

9 Empowerment can lead to creativity and joy.

Appendix B

B.1 Nonlinear pedagogy

From a grasp of biotensegrity, we get a glimpse of the nonlinear behavior that is characteristic of biological systems. Recall that nonlinearity describes the behavior of complex systems such as biologic structure. In such multistable systems, the boundary between hierarchy and heterarchy bends and blends. Instead of one or the other, we have both states at the same time, as in the quality of complementarity we saw in Chapter 5.

Nonlinear behavior characterizes not only our bodies but also our ways of learning about the body. We can break down linear systems analytically into direct relationships.[2] In contrast, nonlinear systems (like you, your dog, the weather, a flock of seagulls, etc.) describe networks that exist as complex expressions of their interconnectedness (recall the complex adaptive systems (CASs) mentioned previously).

Nonlinearity is a keyword finding its way into many fields across the hard and soft sciences. In the anatomy for yoga context, the term is of great significance as it describes both biologic tissue and the learning space. It also works through the broader context of coupled functions as introduced in Chapter 2.

Research in biology points to the nonlinear nature of our tissues, showing that our bodies often defy account.[3,4] There are countless variables at play depending on the context. These range from organismic variations (species, age, gender, genetics) to activity-specific variables in the movement context. What we do, how intensely, how often, and for how long we do it are factors that inform tissue along intersections of immeasurably complex vectors. Accounting for all these calls for more than "linear" allows.

Here, we may come to experience the inscrutable *quality* of body habitation where the linear rules of theoretical biomechanics get bent. We can measure individual direct relationships in linear terms, and this data is valuable for its insight, but biologic organisms are inherently nonlinear. As such, anatomy for yoga as an andragogical subject exhibits many of the same qualifiers.

Key concepts 1

Nonlinearity is a word that is used to describe the behavior of complex systems such as a biologic structure.

Nonlinear pedagogy is a theory about how people learn and has been explored by Chow[5] and recently, Button et al.[6] in physical education for its role in skill acquisition. In this Appendix, we'll look at the differences between linear and nonlinear systems, then check out Chow's four characteristics of nonlinear learning behavior,[7] and finally explore how this relates to the body as a teaching and learning space in yoga. Nonlinearity gets us closer to appreciating the movement of biologic structure for what it is. Here, yogi, we can get barefoot and comfortable inside our chariot, despite the academic nature of the enquiry.

In linear dynamics, a substantial change in a system's behavior is initiated by a substantial shift in its cause(s). For example, linear systems are used to:

- Convert from one currency to another.

- Describe the data relationship between things (e.g., femur length and overall height).

Nonlinear teaching

- Calculate rates (how fast do you have to count the closing sequence to finish your class on time?).

Linear relationships are easily quantifiable, which makes for a desirable quantitative experiment. Everyone loves a tidy equation and problems that resolve under measurable controls. These are essentially linear systems.

In nonlinear dynamics, we are talking about the so-called "butterfly effect". This effect describes how a tiny shift in the dynamics of a system or group of systems dynamics may also generate massive, essentially *qualitative* shifts in its behavior, including unpredictable and disproportionate differences. The expression of a linear system is always proportional to its causes, whereas nonlinear systems often exhibit proportional and disproportional sets of properties simultaneously. Stress-strain curves in human tissue are a perfect example.

Key concepts 2

Yoga andragogy and anatomy are nonlinear systems.

As we are coming to realize, the biological systems studied in science are nonlinear, and yet have been traditionally examined with the linear lens because it makes things much easier to grasp. For example, in Chapter 2, I codified a system of spiral movement based on linear models like the pelvifemoral and scapulohumeral rhythms. Like everyone in the movement world, I'm doing my best to put the linear bits together using the (essentially linear) language currently available to describe them!

Indeed, in anatomy, things are a lot easier to study when we focus on tiny bits and look at simple, direct (linear) relationships of cause-and-effect. Looking at anatomy linearly is the only way to memorize parts, so it's the natural starting point. However, such cause–effect proportionality is the hallmark of linear behavior, so its recipe only gets us as far as the ingredients list. Once we've got the ingredients measured, the nonlinear space takes into account everything that we know makes an actual loaf of bread. Likewise, a macro-system such as the human body requires a nonlinear approach to see the conceptual adjacency of our andragogy and our*selves*. Where yoga and anatomy are concerned, our bodies form the curriculum and the assessment.

B.2 Non-proportionality

Nonlinear systems are characterized by **non-proportionality**. Continuing the cooking metaphor, consider bread making. A pinch of yeast makes the bread rise but adding two pinches won't double the size of the loaf. In fact, adding too much yeast is likely to make the dough go flat by releasing the gas before the flour is ready to expand. These are emergent properties of nonlinear compositions – the unpredictable sum of the balance of the parts!

This idea is key to my entire understanding of yoga practice in general, in that it sheds light on how my body can feel so different during practice one day to the next or at other times on the same day. Small changes lead to large differences or vice versa on an unquantifiable timescale. The implications are that tiny factors can conspire to produce significantly different outcomes.

Appendix B

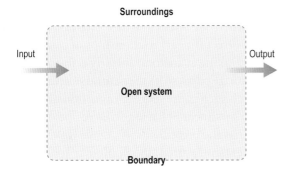

FIGURE B.2

Open systems.

(Image by Krauss. https://creativecommons.org/licenses/
by-sa/4.0/)

Key concepts 3

Linear systems are proportional; nonlinear
systems are non-proportional.

In terms of living tissue, non-proportionality
describes how biomotion stands aside from
the realm of biomechanics. Systems scientists
acknowledge that what makes something different
from its parts list are the non-proportional
interactions amongst those parts.[8] It sounds
really complicated, but the principle is super
easy. Let's say you're in a forward bend applying
a tensile load along the back body. If you were
to double that load, for example, your hamstrings
would not get twice as long! They do something
very different from that as part of their evolved
response to stress (constraints!).

Most processes in biology are understood to be
non-proportional,[9,10] and biomechanical models
have only recently innovated their methodologies
to account for the non-proportionality of (for
example) tendons concerning the wider problem
of data analysis.[11,12] Research in continuum
biomechanics (CB) has been accumulating a
literature base around non-proportionality[13]
in looking at the non-Newtonian behavior of
tissue.[14–17] CB, as a subfield, seems to resonate
with the biotensegrity curriculum in the research
of tissue as multistable, soft matter.

(i) Just when you think you've got
a straightforward proportional
outcome (like thinking that the
surgery you had on your knee was what fixed
it), somebody publishes a study showing it
might all be an artefact of expectation. In
2013, Finnish researchers demonstrated
that outcomes after arthroscopic partial
meniscectomy were not any better than those
following a sham procedure.[18]

Their trial involved patients with symptoms
of a degenerative medial meniscus tear. Out
of a total of 146 randomized patients, 70
underwent arthroscopic partial meniscus
removal and 76 had a sham surgery.
Although both groups reported a remarkable
improvement up to 12 months after the
procedures, the researchers found no
significant differences between the groups in
the change from baseline to 12 months in any
of their outcome measurements.

This famous study raises plenty of relevant
discussion points. For us, I think it is enough
to see the results as an example of the
nonlinearity in our experience of pathology. In
another study, arthroscopic lavage (washing

Nonlinear teaching

out of the interior of the knee with saline) or debridement (lavage with the removal of bits of loose tissue) was administered to patients with established knee osteoarthritis.[19] The treatment "did not result in better outcomes than a sham procedure involving skin incisions only."

I'm not suggesting that we say, "to hell with knee surgery." My own knees seemed to respond instantly to the two partial meniscectomies I had in 2013 when both knees failed to heal on their own after much time and nonsurgical therapy. The point is that studies like those involving sham surgery point to the difficulty of accurately measuring up the unintended consequences of life against those we like to think are under our control. *This is the essence of nonlinearity.*

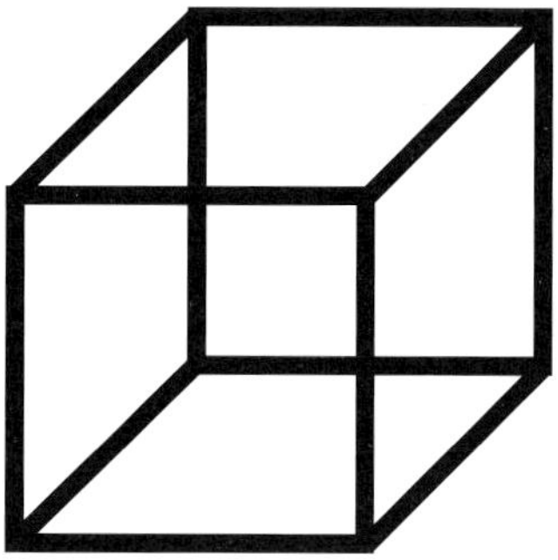

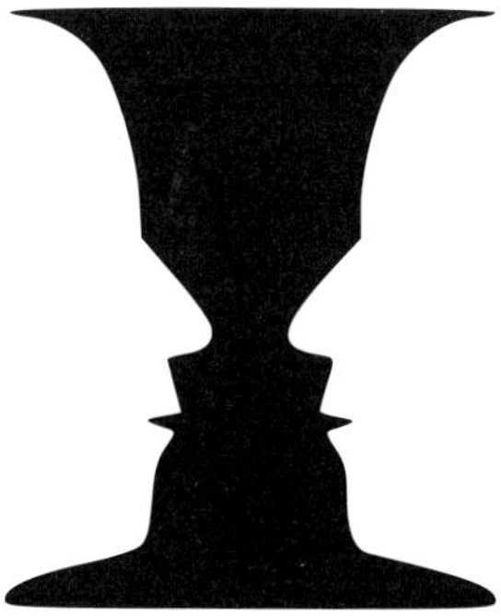

B.3 Fluxtability

That brings us to a second (significant) difference between linear and nonlinear systems; **multistability**. We can see multistability is applied naturally everywhere – both literally (in molecular arrangements of living things) and symbolically (in the meanings of words and images).[20] We could consider our entire nervous system as an example of "co-ordination dynamics of multistable states",[21] in terms of both action (re-action) and perception. Linear systems can be "mono-stable". We are "multistable" as we are nonlinear; or we are nonlinear, so we are multistable. We do not display one behavior as a result of one cause. As multistable systems, we may have multiple performance effects from a cause.[22]

FIGURE B.3

Multistability is the property of nonlinear systems that gives them the ability to function well in different states. The images above can be perceived as different constructs equally well.

Nonlinear systems (such as living organisms) can be both mono- *and* multistable.[23] Multistability is a generic, default phenomenon of dynamic systems like our bodies. In systems biology, scientists are interested in fluctuating states (oscillations) being an intrinsic part of that system's overall integrity. Take, for example, a school of fish, moving collectively in response to stimuli without the need for a central command. These individual fish are all agents, collaborating

Appendix B

as a unified force,[24] much in the way of the integrated neurofascial elements of our bodies.

In my view, multistability is also a way of understanding the "asymptomatic" experience of those whose tissues are clinically damaged. In a 2015 study, cervical spine imaging revealed that in 1,211 adults between the ages of 20 and 70 years, 87.6% had bulging discs; for those in their 20s, the incidence of disc pathology was 37%.[25] Mitchell reviews the literature in her book and makes the point that this is "good news" because people can function pain-free despite the large-scale prevalence of so-called abnormalities.[26]

A 2003 study found that asymptomatic damaged knees are as common as symptomatic ones.[27] A more recent study by Horga shows that 97% of the 230 knees of the 115 uninjured, sedentary, asymptomatic adults showed abnormalities in at least one knee structure.[28] Multistability explains how, despite the idiosyncratic nature of tissue, the body figures out how to get on with the show.

Key concepts 4

Nonlinear systems are multistable

Multistability is a conserved strategy in biology that also shows up in large-scale neural circuitry in humans.[29] Gracovetsky refers to it as "controlled instability"[30] when he describes the lumbosacral region. Within the tensioned body fabric, the sacrum is suspended akin to a hub within a bicycle wheel. During gait, the region is dynamically stable, or "manageably" (and rhythmically) unstable. The engine has to be turning if it is to drive the chariot!

Adaptive properties of our structure, such as the multistability of the lumbosacral region, are at

work at all size and time scales.[31] As is any complex adaptive system (CAS), we are *stable in flux*. Like schools of fish or murmurations of starlings, our tensioned fascial matrix oscillates in various states as it attenuates forces in constant "fluxtability" (my own term). This fluxtability is tissue-specific, and it operates on every scale from self-organizing cell structures to self-aware postures.

Talking point

Quirks in our experience of capacity and pain mean that some people with damage feel no pain and maintain their capacity. In contrast, others with no apparent damage are afflicted with pain that profoundly reduces their capacity and quality of life. Research shows the incidence of idiopathic lower back pain and inflammation arises in patients who appear perfectly healthy.[32,33] As a yoga teacher, how do we account for the "absence of pain with injury" and the "pain with the absence of injury" in our scope of practice?

In our bodies, this fluxtability is always at work. The fascial matrix can deform, spring back, and instantly relay positional information that contributes to the stability of the system, as a whole, over time. Stiffness and flexibility could be described as simultaneous states of this fluxtability.

In teaching and practice, by changing specific learning outcomes, or parameters, yoga teachers can intentionally lead a learning session to foster or craft experiences of appropriate progression. Chow et al.[7] refer to "**parametric controls**"; which means "manipulating system parameters", the third of Chow's four characteristics of nonlinear systems. Parameters like the tristana of

Nonlinear teaching

vinyasa yoga (breath, bandha, drishti as described in Chapter 5), for example, run wide and deep in skills-based practices. Different systems teach using various parameters, with a wide range of outcomes.

Regardless of what you're trying to teach, parametric controls are how we can design teaching and learning activities with specific constraints that allow the task to evolve as a nested emerging property. Through trial and error, teachers and students can co-create constraints by agreeing on acceptable parametric controls. These are the features of a practice space within which we all have some agency. For example, there are at least ten different ways of teaching headstand. Choosing a set of parameters to suit the circumstances is what teaching yoga is all about. First, you have to decide if headstand is even worth teaching! Each of us can come to our own pedagogical constraints, rather than conclusions as such.

Key concepts 5

The yoga space is nonlinear in that systems are manipulated through parametric control to produce progressive states of self-organization.

B.4 Noise

The fourth characteristic is my favorite, as it brings us back to the mystery: **noise**. Conventionally, noise represents the uncontrollable factors acting within system dynamics: unpredictable, unruly, and, therefore, often unwanted (especially in linear system measurement). Linear systems often either ignore noise or make up new rules and exceptions to account for it. In multistable nonlinear, dynamical systems, Chow indicates that "noise can play a functional role by enhancing the probability of system transition between multiple states."[7]

In yoga, teaching and learning new postures means accepting all the noise to embrace spontaneity. The intricacies of a teacher's tone of voice, pre-existing trauma how crowded the room is, temperature, what you had for dinner last night, the stories you have established as doctrine in your mind about particular postures; all of these and many more will expose our systems to noise. These factors have a significant physiological impact on both the tissues *and* the nonlinear model of movement learning (a great example of the embedded andragogy). I have experienced some of my most meaningful teaching and learning moments as a result of noise factors that, to this day, defy explanation. The tick of a clock or someone sneezing can be enough to knock me out of concentration if I'm not fully established.

Vaughan et al. talk about how "creative moments, skill and more generally talent in sport, are not traits possessed by individuals alone, but rather can be conceived as properties of the athlete-environment system shaped by changing constraints."[34] There is an exciting literature base emerging around creativity in nonlinear pedagogy for sports groups, one that might guide our changing understanding as we adapt to a compassionate curriculum.

As teachers, we can benefit from being tuned into all four factors of nonlinearity in the yoga space, and in particular, the element of noise. Think of your student who is utterly terrified of trying a headstand, and yet half a dozen other people in the room are doing it with ease. There are a lot of parameters at work here that inform the teaching scape. For some, seeing others do the seemingly impossible will inspire. Another student will be intimidated, angry, and at worst, triggered.

Key concepts 6

Noise has a functional role in the progression of learning systems.

It isn't just the tentative student trying headstand who will be "noised up" with countless uncontrollable factors coming to bear simultaneously and on longer-term strata. There is an infinite number of psychosomatic cues at play on the systems of everyone in the room, some contradictory, others unconscious, gross, subtle, and unquantifiable. This "signal variability" will be simultaneously creating challenges all while contributing to the students' exploration of potential solutions. Noisy situations like these can enhance the flexibility of learning[35] and offer spontaneous constraints.[36] All of this vibrates in the web of srotas-kinematics.

 Constraining to set free

Balagué et al.[37] discuss the relatedness and nestedness of constraints based on four claims:

1) Task constraints are distributed between the person and the environment and hence are relational variables,

2) Being relational, task constraints are also emergent properties of the organism/environment system,

3) Constraints are nested in timescales, and

4) A vast set of constraints are correlated through circular causality.

Key concepts 7

As teachers, we choose constraints that set our students up for self-discovering empowerment in "Aha!" moments.

B.5 Creativity and empowerment: the rewards

Constraints and creativity are a hot topic in cognition and skills acquisition literature.[38] Orth et al. talk about how innovation happens in moments of confusion.[39] During times of uncertainty, people often discover creative solutions and apply them in nonlinear ways. Solutions can occur spontaneously in the face of fear with appropriate constraints. It appears that constraints foster spontaneity: in such moments, the practitioner allows solutions to emerge, rather than developing a solution first and subsequently "forcing" it, or conforming to a received method and rigidly adhering to it.

Constraining our class planning and teaching methodology to honor human patterns not only improves our chances of doing less harm, but it also fosters creativity and empowerment. The Martha Graham quote at the beginning of this Appendix is a reminder that each of us contains a unique spark, and I consider it our role as educators to foster its discovery.

Nonlinear teaching

 Nonlinear teaching

How can you extend your teaching awareness to adjust the noise in the room to create a supportive set of constraints for your students to experience their own "Aha!" moments? How do you shift the idealization from people looking to you as the teacher for all the answers? Do you frame noise to highlight the constraints of spontaneous learning that empowers your students?

 Sculpting constraints for self and others

To recap, these four significant characteristics of nonlinear behavior inform learning in the yoga space:

1. Non-proportionality
2. Multistability (fluxtability)
3. Parametric controls
4. The functional role of noise

Chow's four characteristics of nonlinear pedagogy can be applied to our work as yoga teachers in adult learning. Nonlinear andragogy honors the infinite vectors at play, all coupled together to inform the individual learning journey. They point to a structure that self-regulates and encourages emerging properties, constraints within which individuals can experience creativity in-the-moment.[40,41] Mennin talks about knowledge co-creation as an "authentic recursive transactive process" that is inherently nonlinear.[42]

The inhale creates an inner spiral, the feminine force. With the inhale you release, let the pubic bone drop back and the sitting bones ground. With the exhale, you bring the tail in and create an outer spiral, the masculine force.

Richard Freeman[43]

In yoga, seeing everything as interconnected is kind of the whole point. Doesn't it make sense that we are singing from the same hymn sheet when it comes to anatomy? That our bodies could afford us tools for creative moments of personal empowerment? That there might be some inbuilt sense of knowing when we're on the right track? Recall the VITAL tool outlined in Chapter 4. Variation is vital on every level. As we apply variation to intensity, we are also encompassing the need for changes in pace to harness the stimuli of various inputs to the system.

Moving slowly deploys one set of constraints, and a faster pace offers another. Varying intervals of practice and duration will change response and recovery rates. Using periodicity is another way to bring variation to your intensity of practice; for example, try building up to different kinds of peak intensities and then easing off.

Key concepts 8

Empowerment can lead to creativity and joy.

Appendix B

This balancing act is one of discernment. The Five Filaments rubric is but a starting point, a catalyst for your creative spiral-bound flow in the moment. Movement and breath coordination can put us in touch with powerful self-healing mechanisms that amount to transformative healing. And, yes, joy.

Just as objects are not revealed without the presence of light, Self Knowledge does not occur by any means other than Inquiry.

Sankaracharya[44]

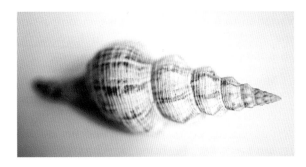

FIGURE B.4

Filifusus filamentosus, in the family Fasciolariidae, commonly called the tulip or spindle shells.

References

1 De Mille A. Martha: The Life and Work of Martha Graham. Vintage Books; 1992.

2 Strogatz SH. Nonlinear Dynamics and Chaos: With Applications to Physics, Biology, Chemistry, and Engineering. Avalon Publishing; 2014.

3 Kahn CJ, Wang X, Rahouadj R. Nonlinear model for viscoelastic behavior of Achilles tendon. Journal of Biomechanical Engineering. 2010;132(11):111002.

4 Andriotis OG, Desissaire S, Thurner PJ. Collagen fibrils: nature's highly tunable nonlinear springs. ACS Nano. 2018;12(4):3671–80.

5 Chow JY, Davids K, Button C, et al. Nonlinear pedagogy: a constraints-led framework for understanding emergence of game play and movement skills. Nonlinear Dynamics, Psychology, and Life Sciences. 2006;10:71–103.

6 Button C, Seifert L, Chow JY, et al. Dynamics of Skill Acquisition: An Ecological Dynamics Approach. Human Kinetics, Incorporated; 2020.

7 Chow JY, Davids K, Hristovski R, et al. Nonlinear pedagogy: learning design for self-organizing neurobiological systems. New Ideas in Psychology. 2011;29(2):189–200.

8 Boogerd F, Bruggeman FJ, Hofmeyr JHS, Westerhoff HV. Systems Biology: Philosophical Foundations. Elsevier Science; 2007.

9 Donze A, Clermont G, Langmead CJ. Parameter synthesis in nonlinear dynamical systems: application to systems biology. Journal of Computational Biology. 2010;17(3):325–36.

10 Qian H. Hill's small systems nanothermodynamics: a simple macromolecular partition problem with a

statistical perspective. Journal of Biological Physics. 2012;38(2):201–7.

11 Jachno K, Heritier S, Wolfe R. Are non-constant rates and non-proportional treatment effects accounted for in the design and analysis of randomised controlled trials? A review of current practice. BMC Medical Research Methodology. 2019;19(1):103.

12 Durandau G, Farina D, Sartori M. Robust real-time musculoskeletal modeling driven by electromyograms. IEEE Transactions on Biomedical Engineering. 2018;65(3):556–64.

13 Epstein M. The Elements of Continuum Biomechanics. Wiley; 2012.

14 Holmes MH, Mow VC. The nonlinear characteristics of soft gels and hydrated connective tissues in ultrafiltration. Journal of Biomechanics. 1990;23(11):1145–56.

15 Almeida ES, Spilker RL. Mixed and penalty finite element models for the nonlinear behavior of biphasic soft tissues in finite deformation: Part I – Alternate formulations. Computer Methods in Biomechanics and Biomedical Engineering. 1997;1(1):25–46.

16 Ahmed A, Siddique JI, Mahmood A. Non-Newtonian flow-induced deformation from pressurized cavities in absorbing porous tissues. Computer Methods in Biomechanics and Biomedical Engineering. 2017;20(13):1464–73.

17 Atzeni F, Lanfranconi F, Aegerter CM. Disentangling geometrical, viscoelastic and hyperelastic effects in force-displacement relationships of folded biological tissues. The European Physical Journal: E, Soft Matter. 2019;42(4):47.

18 Sihvonen R, Paavola M, Malmivaara A, et al. Arthroscopic partial meniscectomy versus sham surgery for a degenerative meniscal tear. New England Journal of Medicine. 2013;369(26):2515–24.

19 Moseley JB, O'Malley K, Petersen NJ, et al. A controlled trial of arthroscopic surgery for osteoarthritis of the knee. New England Journal of Medicine. 2002;347(2):81–8.

20 Kruse P, Stadler M. Ambiguity in Mind and Nature: Multistable Cognitive Phenomena. Springer; 2012.

21 Kelso JAS. Multistability and metastability: understanding dynamic coordination in the brain. Philosophical Transactions of the Royal Society of London Series B, Biological Sciences. 2012;367(1591):906–18.

22 Ribeiro J, Davids K, Araújo D, et al. Exploiting bi-directional self-organizing tendencies in team sports: the role of the game model and tactical principles of play. Frontiers in Psychology. 2019;10:2213.

23 Laurent M, Kellershohn N. Multistability: a major means of differentiation and evolution in biological systems. Trends in Biochemical Sciences. 1999;24(11):418–22.

24 Pratt SC. Collective intelligence. In: Breed MD, Moore J (editors). Encyclopedia of Animal Behavior. Oxford: Academic Press; 2010. pp. 303–9.

25 Nakashima H, Yukawa Y, Suda K, et al. Abnormal findings on magnetic resonance images of the cervical spines

in 1211 asymptomatic subjects. Spine. 2015;40(6):392–8.

26 Mitchell J. Yoga Biomechanics: Stretching Redefined. Handspring Publishing Limited; 2018.

27 Asymptomatic meniscal tears are as common as symptomatic ones. British Medical Journal. 2003;326(7394).

28 Horga LM, Hirschmann AC, Henckel J, et al. Prevalence of abnormal findings in 230 knees of asymptomatic adults using 3.0 T MRI. Skeletal Radiology. 2020;49(7):1099–107.

29 Kelso JAS. Multistability and metastability: understanding dynamic coordination in the brain. Philosophical Transactions of the Royal Society B: Biological Sciences. 2012;367(1591):906–18.

30 Gracovetsky S. Stability or controlled instability? Movement, Stability & Lumbopelvic Pain. 2007;279–94.

31 Etkin D. Disasters and complexity. In: Etkin D (editor). Disaster Theory. Boston: Butterworth-Heinemann; 2016. pp. 151–92.

32 Lassiter W, Allam AE. Inflammatory Back Pain. In: StatPearls (online). Treasure Island (FL): StatPearls Publishing; 2020. Available at: https://www.statpearls.com/articlelibrary/viewarticle/23508/

33 Yap KS, Ye JY, Li S, et al. Back pain in psoriatic arthritis: defining prevalence, characteristics and performance of inflammatory back pain criteria in psoriatic arthritis. Annals of the Rheumatic Diseases. 2018;77(11):1573–7.

34 Vaughan J, Mallett CJ, Davids K, et al. Developing creativity to enhance human potential in sport: a wicked transdisciplinary challenge. Frontiers in Psychology. 2019;10:2090.

35 Schöllhorn WI, Beckmann H, Michelbrink M, et al. Does noise provide a basis for the unification of motor learning theories? International Journal of Sport Psychology. 2006;37:1–21.

36 Newell K. Constraints on the development of coordination. In: Wade MG, Whiting HTA (editors). Motor Development in Children: Aspects of Coordination and Control. Martinus Nijhoff Publishers; 1986.

37 Balagué N, Pol R, Torrents C, et al. On the relatedness and nestedness of constraints. Sports Medicine – Open. 2019;5.

38 Torrents C, Balagué N, Ric Á, Hristovski R. The motor creativity paradox: constraining to release degrees of freedom. Psychology of Aesthetics, Creativity, and the Arts. 2020. Available at: https://doi.apa.org/doiLanding? doi=10.1037%2Faca0000291

39 Orth D, van der Kamp J, Memmert D, Savelsbergh GJP. Creative motor actions as emerging from movement variability. Frontiers in Psychology. 2017;8:1903.

40 Hristovski R, Davids K, Araujo D, Passos P. Constraints-induced emergence of functional novelty in complex neurobiological systems: a basis for creativity in sport. Nonlinear Dynamics, Psychology, and Life Sciences. 2011;15(2):175–206.

Nonlinear teaching

41 Coste A, Bardy BG, Marin L. Towards an embodied signature of improvisation skills. Frontiers in Psychology. 2019;10:2441.

42 Mennin S. Self-organisation, integration and curriculum in the complex world of medical education. Medical Education. 2010;44(1):20–30.

43 Freeman R. Workshop in Evanston, Illinois, 2001. Available at: http://www.yogachicago.com/2014/03/the-physiology-of-enlightenment-exploring-the-essence-of-ashtanga-yoga-with-richard-freeman/.

44 Sankaracharya A. Aparokshanubhuti (Direct [Self] Experience).

Permissions

Preface

Engraving from 1872 featuring the muscles of the human body.

www.thegraphicsfairy.com

FIGURE 1.1

Photo by Charlene Lim

FIGURE 1.2

Levers and loads. Drawing from an 1872 physiology textbook demonstrating traditional anatomical lever mechanics: the rigid lever (radius and ulna) pivots about a fulcrum (elbow joint).

thegraphicsfairy.com

FIGURE 1.4

Human embryo in development.

apokusay at www.vectorstock.com, with modifications by the author.

FIGURE 1.8

Brightfield photomicrograph of chick (*Gallus gallus domesticus*) embryo development at 60 hours; 29–32 somites.

Scenics & Science/Alamy Stock Photo

FIGURE 1.11

This diagram of the anatomy of spinal nerve segmentation shows the early elements of the developing peripheral nervous system including the migrating neural crest cells and outgrowing motor and sensory axons. These are shown with reference to the somite derivatives (dermomyotome and sclerotome). Most of the dermomyotome has been peeled back from the somite on the left, revealing the sclerotome as subdivided into anterior (A) and posterior (P) aspects.

Redrawn from Kelly Kuan CY, Tannahill D, Cook GMW, Keynes RJ. Somite polarity and segmental patterning of the peripheral nervous system. Mechanisms of Development. 2004;121(9):1055–68.

FIGURE 1.16

Human embryo, six weeks. The black circle is the edge of the fundus of the eye. Visible here is the umbilical cord, a strand of tissue containing the two spiraling arteries that carry blood to the placenta (the organ embedded in the uterine wall that interfaces maternal and fetal circulations) plus one vein with return supply to the fetus.

Lennart Nilsson, TT/Science Photo Library

FIGURE 1.24

Human fetal legs at 16 weeks. The fetus can now grab and pull the long umbilical cord. The skeleton consists mainly of flexible cartilage, the soft precursor to bone.

Lennart Nilsson, TT/Science Photo Library

FIGURE 2.2

Origami skeleton: its shape and movement emerge as a consequence of its constraints – the dotted lines indicating where to fold the paper.

With thanks to Fergus Murray, the intrepid constructor

FIGURE 2.3

Myofascial cross-ply in body culture. A Dart's "double spiral arrangement" with regard to human anatomy and embryology was originally published in the Journal of the Institutes for the Achievement of Human Potential in 1967. B

Permissions

Dr Kurt Tittel's Muscle Slings in Sport, 1956. C Russian anatomist, Shaparenko, referred to the enantiomorphic (from enantios, or "opposite") arrangement of myofascial tubules circa 1980. D Askar's "aponeurotic expansions".41 E Scarr's schematic drawing of the cross-ply evident in the torso.

C, courtesy of the Kozyavkin Method. E, courtesy of Handspring Publishing

FIGURE 2.10

Compartmental arrangement of tubes typical of the limbs.

Courtesy of Handspring Publishing

FIGURE 2.12

Fibrillar, helical structure of muscle. The action of myosin "crawling" around the spiral staircase of actin inside muscle fibrils is an essentially spiral movement inside spiraling collagenous myofascial chains. Braids of tightly wrapped collagen filaments scale up in their bundles and form a seamless continuity with the contractile lengths that we call "muscle." Collagen itself is structurally helical.

Courtesy of Handspring Publishing

FIGURE 2.17

Poles apart: the cranial bones "fuse" along a fibrous joint that is not synovial, whereas the hip is a classic synovial joint with a host of densities to manage much different kinds of forces.

(Walker J. *Anatomy, Physiology and Hygiene.* Boston: Allyn and Bacon; 1900. p. 46)

FIGURE 2.36

Thoracolumbar continuities. (A) Posterior view of the back showing connections with the lattisimus dorsi, trapezius and gluteus maximus to the TLF and thoracolumbar composite (TLC). (B) Thoracolumbar fascia with gluteus maximus in situ.

A, with permission from the Willard/Carreiro Collection, University of New England. B, courtesy of Stecco C, Sharkey J, Schleip R. Fascia Net Plastination Project/von Hagens Plastinarium, 2018.

FIGURE 2.45

Space-making with the scapulohumeral rhythm: bringing awareness to drawing the humerus into the joint as it rotates will increase the sense of felt space as the movement progresses into greater complexity.

Image by Joanna Darlington with BSIP SA/Alamy Stock Photo. Demonstrated by Sarah Hatcher

FIGURE 2.46

Fourteen body segments of the fascial system. CP: Caput, CL: Collum, TH: Thorax, LU: Lumbar, PV: Pelvis, SC: Scapula, HU: Humerus, CU: Cubitus, CA: Carpus, DI: Digits, CX: Coxa, GE: Genu, TA: Tarsus, PE: Pes. Each segment comprises joint(s), portions of muscles that move the joint(s), and the fascia surrounding these muscle fibers. Latin terms are used to distinguish these segments from simple joints.

Redrawn with permission from Stecco C, Stecco AN. Fascial manipulation. 2012. https://www.researchgate.net/publication/288215443_Fascial_manipulation

FIGURE 3.8

Embryogenesis.

Image by Zephyris, labels modified by author. https://creativecommons.org/licenses/by-sa/3.0/deed.en

Permissions

FIGURE 3.9

The gut tube: perforation happens as the anus and mouth become apertures, and in humans, the mouth actually perforates first, at four weeks.

Walker J. *Anatomy, Physiology and Hygiene.* Boston: Allyn and Bacon; 1900. p. 46

FIGURE 3.16

Muscle fiber. Colored scanning electron micrograph of a freeze-fractured skeletal (or striated) muscle fiber. The fracturing of the fiber has revealed that it consists of a bundle of smaller fibers called myofibrils. The myofibrils are crossed by transverse tubules (horizontal lines), that mark the division of the myofibrils into contractile units (sarcomeres). (Magnification: x8000 when printed at 10 cm wide.)

Steve Gschmeissner/Science Photo Library

FIGURE 3.17

Classical systems anatomy.

https://www.canstockphoto.com/eula/

FIGURE 3.20

The Vedāntic version of the koshas from the *Taittirīya Upanisad*.

Artwork by Joanna Darlington

FIGURE 3.21

Illustration of the six chakras of Tantric yoga in Sanskrit and Hindi. One of eight colored plates, drawing explicit parallels between the yogic view of chakras etc., and the medical/anatomical view of the body. Svamihamsasvarupakrtam Satcakranirupanactiram: bhasyasamalamkrtam bhasatikopetan ca = Shatchakra niroopana chittra with bhashya and bhasha containing the pictures of the different nerves and plexuses of the human body with their full description showing the easiest method how to practice pranayam by the mental suspension of breath through meditation only.

Svami Hamsasvarupa. Sanskrit MS 391. Drawings by Shri Swami Hansa Swaroop. Wellcome Collection. https://creativecommons.org/licenses/by/4.0/

FIGURE 3.23

The Pancha Vayu (subtle srotamsi): udana, upward; apana, downward; samana, consolidating; prana, inward; vyana, expanding. Amy Hughes demonstrates the vayu in asana, with the body painted to draw awareness to vayu, "epistructural" routes (subtle srotamsi) of energy informing the felt sense of anatomy.

Illustration of The Pranic Body from: S. Saraswati. *Asana Pranayama Mudra Bandha.* Bihar Yoga Bharati; 1997

FIGURE 4.5

Classification of organismic and environmental constraints according its relatively faster or slower rate of change.

Adapted for yoga from Balagué et al.[16] https://sportsmedicine-open.springeropen.com/articles/10.1186/s40798-019-0178-z/ figures/3. https://creativecommons.org/licenses/by/4.0/

FIGURE 5.2

The diaphragm in continuity with the pericardial sac.

Courtesy of Stecco C, Sharkey J, S chleip R. Fascia Net Plastination Project/von Hagens Plastinarium, 2018

Permissions

FIGURE 5.3

Anatomical illustration by Arnauld-Eloi Gautier-Dagoty (1741–1771) for the Royal College of Medicine of Nancy in Lorraine, France. Dagoty elegantly depicted muscles of the human body as perceived by scientists in the 18th century with precise details. His illustrations offer us a glimpse of medical practice in the age of enlightenment.

The New York Public Library. Image public domain

FIGURE 5.4

A Dorsal view of a mouse brain stem–spinal cord preparation. B Oscillations of neural activity during inhalation and exhalation in the brain stem (top) and phrenic nerve (bottom) that innervates the diaphragm, illustrating the neural involvement in the cardiorespiratory rhythm.

(Reproduced from: Ausborn J, Koizumi H, Barnett WH, et al. Organization of the core respiratory network: insights from optogenetic and modeling studies. PLOS Computational Biology. 2018;14(4): e1006148. https://doi.org/10.1371/journal. pcbi.1006148. https://creativecommons.org/ publicdomain/zero/1.0/)

FIGURE 5.8

Basic anatomy of the eye showing visible light frequencies refracting through to the retina where light is transduced into neural information for higher processing in the brain. The meninges, connective tissue coverings of the brain and spinal cord, are continuous through the optic nerve and wrap around the eyes.

Christoph Burgstedt/Science Photo Library

FIGURE 5.14

Left: organismic, environmental, and task constraints as independently defined interacting entities. Right: organismic and environmental constraints as independently defined interacting entities, and task constraints as emergent properties of the organism–environment system.

Redrawn and adapted from Balagué N, Pol R, Torrents C, et al. On the relatedness and nestedness of constraints. Sports Medicine - Open. 2019;5:1. https://sportsmedicine-open. springeropen.com/articles/ 10.1186/s40798-019-0178-z/ figures/1. https://creativecommons.org/ licenses/by/4.0/

FIGURE A.3

Teaching yoga with biotensegrity principles in mind.

Photo by Charlene Lim

FIGURE A.4

Microvacuoles: the intersection of fibrils in three dimensions that form an irregular polyhedral unit of volume.

Image by Jean-Claude Guimberteau, courtesy of Handspring

FIGURE A.5

Image by clinical anatomist John Sharkey demonstrating the moist, fractal, multifibular, omnidirectional, chaotic nature of fascia.

Courtesy of John Sharkey

Permissions

FIGURE A.9

Fractal-like: bubbles on the polyhedral texture of your skin tell the story of how things continue into the deeper layers. In the bottom image, a saucer of hydrophilic chia seeds demonstrates the way round things coalesce geodesically in the most minimal-energy configurations.

Photo by Charlene Lim

FIGURE A.10

Soft matter: all things squishy, including you, me, and this modular presentation of gelatin.

Photo by Charlene Lim

FIGURE A.12

Strandbeest by the artist Theo Jansen. No muscles are contracting, and yet it moves!

Animaris Currens Ventosa Oostvoorne, 1993

FIGURE B.2

Open systems.

Image by Krauss. https://creativecommons.org/licenses/ by-sa/4.0/

TABLE A.2 Training or synergizing? Contrast of theoretical principles

Adapted for yoga from Pol R, Balagué N, Ric A, et al. Training or synergizing? Complex systems principles change the understanding of sport processes. Sports Med – Open. 2020;6:28. https://doi.org/10.1186/s40798-020-00256-9. https://creative-commons.org/licenses/by/4.0/

TABLE A.3 Training or synergizing? Contrast of methodological principles

Adapted for yoga from Pol R, Balagué N, Ric A, et al. Training or synergizing? Complex systems principles change the understanding of sport processes. Sports Med – Open. 2020;6:28. https://doi.org/10.1186/s40798-020-00256-9. https://creative-commons.org/licenses/by/4.0/

Index

A

Acharyas, 102
Akasha, 110
Amniotic fluid, 9
Anatomical position (AP), 20, 55
Andragogy, 147
Angular motion, 52
Anisotropy, 36e
Anna vaha srotas, 108
Anusara movement, 49
Apana vayu, 122–123, 126
Aponeurotic expansions, 40f
"Appropriate stiffness," 174
Archenteron, 101
Asana, 7
    Baddhakonasana, 152
    handstand filament, 60–62
    Janusirsasana A, 154
    Kounchasana, 153
    Marichyasana A, 155
    Marichyasana D, 156
    mayurasana, 61f
    Parighasana, 157
    Parivrtta Parsvakonasana, 150
    Prasarita Padottanasana C, 149
    suptavajrasana, 59
    trans, 7
    Urdhva Dhanurasana, 148
    Vriscikasana, 151
Ascending air, 123–124
Autonomic nervous system, 168
Auxetic materials, 169
Axial matrix filament, 65–73, 66f
    anatomical basis, 66–67
    flexion, 67–70
    inside and outside, 71–73
    twists, 70–71
Axial rotation, 53
Ayurveda, 93

B

Baddhakonasana, 152, 152f
Bandha, 172–174, 177
    breakdown, 174f
Basal tension, 200
Bilaminar disc, 9
Biological couplings, 41
Bioluminescence, 41
Biomechanical rhythms and couplings, 83
Biomotion, 41–43, 43f
Biopolymers, 12e, 44
Biorhythms, 8e
Biotensegrity, 16, 195
Biotensegrity, 40
Bipedal quadrupeds, 16
Blastopore, 97
Bone formation, 18
Bound water, 11
Breath, 119–128, 143–146, 161, 166–172, 177–179, 204, 206, 211

C

Central nervous system (CNS), 178
Chakorasana, 37e
Chakra, 118
Chirality, 12e, 16, 17
Chondrocytes, 9
Chordata, 8
Chronobiology, 141
Chronotype, 147
Circadian rhythms, 41, 141
Circulatory system, 10
Classical systems anatomy, 113f
Closed kinematic chains (CKC), 37, 40, 41, 43, 111
Collagen, 15e, 44
Comfort self-stress, 23
Complementarity, 164
"Conscious sleeving," 139

Index

Constraints, 16, 26, 37–39, 48–51, 81, 104, 114, 147, 183, 224–225
Continuum, 196
Cosmogony, 102
Coupled motion, 73–74
    handstand and footstand notes, 75–78
Coupling
    functions, 41
    kinematics of, 43–50
Cranial bones, 52
Craniofacial skeleton, 15
Crocodile pose, 21f
Cytoskeleton (CSK), 198

D
Deep fasciae, 79
"Deformation," 177
Dermatomes, 14, 14f
Dermomyotomes, 13
Derms, 15
Deuterostomes, 97
Dhatus, 107
Dorsolateral portion, of somite, 13
Doshas, 102
Double spiral arrangement, 40f
Downward dog position, 55f, 56
Dr Kurt Tittel's Muscle Slings, in Sport, 40f
Dvandva, 163–165
Dynamic reciprocity, 202

E
"Ecosystem," 197
Eighth week, of development, 20
Electromagnetic energy, 124
Electron transfer (ET), 41
Embryogenesis, 5, 99f
Embryo, in eighth week of development, 20
Embryology, 6–9
Enantiomorphic arrangement, 40f

Enantiomorphic pair, 14e
Endopelvic fasciae en route, 24
Enthesis organ, 140
Epaxial structures, 66, 66f
Erythrocytes, 198
Eumetazoans, 97
Extracellular matrix (ECM), 11, 14e

F
Fascia, 12, 162
Fasciatomes, 13
Fast breathing, 171
Ferns unfurl, 5e
Fibonacci, 10e
Fibrillar, 46f
Filament
    axial matrix, 65–73
    footstand, 63–65
    handstand, 60–62
    hip, 62–63
    shoulder, 58–59
Filamentous matter, 80
Filifusus filamentosus, 226f
Five filaments (5F), 37, 136, 146, 189
    general ideas about, 81–82
    logos of, 139
    rubric, 58–73, 81
        axial matrix filament, 65–73
        footstand filament, 63–65
        handstand filament, 60–62
        hip filament, 62–63
        shoulder filament, 58–59
    structural perspective of, 162
    for yoga, 50
Flexagons, 32e
Foot fingers, 26, 27
Footstand filament (FF), 63–65
Forearm supination and pronation, 54f

Index

G

Gastrulation, 7f, 8, 9
Geometric progression, 25e
Geometric series-powered logarithmic spirals, 28e
"Gesture of the pond, 176, 176f
Gheranda Samhita, 4
Gliding motions, 52
Golden ratio, 25e, 26e
Gomukhasana, 49f
Granthis, 119
Grounding footstand (GF), 64–65, 65f
Grounding handstand (GH), 60, 61f
Grounding handstand spiral, 150f
Grounding Hip Spiral (GHS), 63, 63f
Grounding Shoulder Spiral (GSS), 59, 59f
Ground reaction force (GRF), 28, 62, 171
Ground substance, 10
Gut tube, 100f

H

Hallux, 27
Handstand and footstand notes, 75–78
Handstand filament (HF), 60–62, 150f
    anatomical basis, 60–62
    grounding spiral, 60
    opening spiral, 60
Hasta, 28
Hatcher, Sarah, 147
Hatha Yoga Pradipika (HYP), 4
Heart rate variability (HRV), 112
Helical coupling, anatomy of, 47f
Helicoid pipe cleaner, 6f
Helix, 6
Heron pose, 153f
Hierarchy, 29
Hip
    filament, 62–63
    spirals, 68
    tissue, 52

Hoberman Sphere, 169f
Human embryo
    in development, 7f
    six weeks, 19f
Human fetal legs, at 16 weeks, 28f
Hypaxial structures, 66, 66f
Hyperboloid structures, 69f

I

Ida, 118
Ida and Pingala, 11e
Iliofemoral joint, 53
Iliotibial band (ITB), 70
Inchoate, 20
Interconnectedness, 205
Intermediate filaments (IFs), 199
Intrinsic stress, 198

J

Janusirsasana A, 154

K

Kapha, 102
Kha, 93
Khecara, 93
Kinematics, 43
Kinesiology, 51, 56
Klein bottle, 71
Knees, 15
Koshas, 112, 116, 116f
Kounchasana, 153, 153f
Krishnamacharya, 78
Kriyas, 4
Kumbhaka, 170
Kurmasana, 67f

L

Language, 135
Lateral (or external) rotation, 53
Law of Tripled motion, 51

Index

Lever model, 23

Levers, 5

    and loads, 5f

Levin and Martin's poles, of rotation, 50f

Light and Life, 164

Limb, 16–17

    an invitation, 23

    compartmental arrangement of tubes in, 44f

    development, 18

    limbs unfurling, 17–21

    symmetry, 23–28

    tuned into tension, 21–23

Linear (translational) motion, 42, 42f

Linkages, 45

Liquid crystal, 34e

Logarithmic spiral, 25e

Logos, 142

Long bones, rotation of, 54f

Lumbo-ilio-sacral matrix, 53

Lymphatic system, 10

M

Mahaswastikasana, 37f

Maitrayaniya Upanishad (Maitri), 165

Mamsa, 12, 111

    vaha srotas, 111f

Mayurasana, 61f

Mechanical forces, 141

Mechanotransduction, 12

Medial (or internal) rotation, 53

Meniscus, of knee, 83

Meridians, 114

Mesenchymal derivatives, 15

Mesenchyme, 10

Mesoderm, 10, 12

Mesokinetic organ, 48

Meso story, 9–12

Metameric array, 201

Microfilaments, 199

Microtubule system, 29e, 199

Microvacuoles, 194f

Mighty somites, 12–14

    head, shoulders, knees and toes, 15

Möbius strip, 71

Modularity, 200

Morphologic constraints of spirality, 147

Motion, defined, 41

Movement (intentional motion), 162

Movement, mapping, 38–41

    biomotion, 41–42

Mula bandha, 174f

Multipotent neural crest cells, 12

Multistability strategy, 222

Muscle fiber, 113f

Musculoskeletal movement, 22

Musculoskeletal system, 12

Myofascial cross-ply, in body culture, 40f

Myofascial system, 111

N

Nadis, 119t

Nagadi vayu, 121

Nakrasana, 21f

Nauli kriya, 123

"Nestedness," 147

Neural crest cells (NCC), 12

    in vertebrate embryos, 15

Neurulation, 8, 9f

Neutral, 29–31

Newtonian constraints, 48

Newtonian mechanics, 30t

Noise, 223

Nonlinearity, 218

Nonlinear pedagogy theory, 218

Non-proportionality, 219–220

Notochord, 6e, 8

O

Obstetric dilemma, 62

Ontological tree, 11f

Index

Opening footstand, 64, 64f
Opening handstand, 60, 60f
Opening hip spiral, 62–63, 63f
Opening shoulder spiral, 58, 59f
Open systems, 220f
Organismic constraints, 28e, 38
    and morphological constraints, 38
Origami, 26
Origami skeleton, 39f
Oscillating motion, 42, 42f

P
Pada bandha, 28
Padmasana, 181f
Pancha prana, 121
Pancha vayu, 122t, 125f
"Parametric controls", 222
Parastichies, 31e
Parivrtta Parsvakonasana, 150
Parsvakonasana, 60
Paryangasana, 82f
Pascal's triangle, 24e
Pelvic tilt, 180f
Pelvifemoral Rhythm, 62–63
    anatomical basis, 62–63
    grounding spiral, 62
    opening spiral, 62
Phyllotactic-type algorithm, 33e
Phyllotaxis, 30e, 31e
Phylogenic Tree, 96f
Pingala, 118
Pitta, 102
Poles of movement, 49
Pollex pedis, 27
Potent, 15
Prakrti, 102
Prana, 95, 105–106
Pranadi vayu, 121–122
Pranapana, 202, 205
Prana vaha srotas, 108

Prana vayu, 122, 126
Prestress, 21, 23
Primary bandhas, 174
Pronation, 55
Protein, 10
Protostomes, 97, 98
Pulmonary ventilation, 166
Purvottanasana, 177
Pythagorean Tree, 26e, 27e, 34e

Q
Quantum biology, 8e, 164
Quiet breathing, 171

R
Radioulnar joints, 76f
Rainbow pelvis, 129f
Raja yoga, 117
Rasayana, 115
Reciprocating motion, 42, 42f
"Regular polyhedra," 18e
Resonance, 41
Respiratory diaphragm, 166
Rhythm-with-movement, 172
Rotary (rotational) motion, 42, 42f
Rotational motions, 52
Rotational redux, 51–55

S
Sacroiliac joints (SIJ), 62
Samadhi, 117
Samana, 126
Samana vayu, 123
Samasthitih, 65, 144, 145f
Samkhya, 142
Sattva guna, 94
Scapular and hip rotation, 53
Scapulohumeral rhythm, 58–59, 78f
Schumann Resonances, 28e
Sclerotomes, 13

Index

Screw-home mechanism, 20
Secondary bandhas, 175
Segmental limb boundaries, 24
Shareera, 105
Shariram, 105
Shoulder, 15
    filament, 58–59
        anatomical basis, 58–59
        grounding spiral, 58
        opening spiral, 58
    spirals, 68
Siddhasana, 181f
Sierpiński Triangle, 70f
Single dorsal root ganglia, 14
Siva Samhita, 118
Slow (deep) breathing, 171
Somite, 11, 13
    dorsolateral portion of, 13
    role of, 14
    ventromedial portion of, 13
Somites, 6e
Somitogenesis, 13
Spatiotemporal sculpture, 21
Sphere-based vector space, 204
Spinal Engine theory, 73–74
Spinal nerve segmentation, anatomy of, 13f
Spiral mesogastrium, 102f
Spiral motion, in yoga, 56–58
Spiral movement, cross-ply patterns facilitating, 57
Spiral pipe cleaner, 6f
Spirals and movement, 78–82
Spira mirabilis, 25e
Sravanam, 105, 107
Sriyantra, 22e
Srotamsi, 11e, 107–110
Srotas-kinematics
    akasha, 110
    gastronomical, 101–103
    gross and subtle, 96–101
    hole in the middle, 93–95
    integration, 125–128
    mystery, 103–105
    prana, 105–106
    srotamsi, 107–110
    srotas, 111–115
    steady and comfortable, 92–93
    subtle body, spiral bound, 118–120
    vayu, 120–125
    weaving the threads, 115–118
Srotomaya, 107, 108
Sthira-suhkham, 92, 139, 162
Strandbeest of Theo Jansen, 208f
"Stretch," 138
Subacromial space, 94f
Sukha, 39, 92, 93
    dukha, 93, 93f
Sunflower seeds, 30e
Supination, 55
Suptavajrasana, 59
Sushumna, 11e, 118
Sushumna nadi, 93, 119
Svadhyaya, 142
Syndetome, 13, 14
"Synergetic," 204
Synovial joint classifications, 52f

T
Tadagi Mudra, 176
Talar mortise, 64
Tantra, 117
Tantric yoga, six chakras of, 117f
Teleology, 138
Tendinous tissues, 14
Tensegrity icosahedron (T-icosa), 20e
Tensegrity models, 12, 189, 195, 201
Tension and compression, 190f
Tetrahedron, 13e
Tetrahelix, 14e
Therapeutic modalities, 92

Index

Thixotropy, 127
Thoracolumbar fascia (TLF), 24f, 68, 70
Throupled motion, 43, 51, 73–75, 79, 165, 167, 202
Throupling, 169
T-icosa model, 192
Tissue formation, 12
Toes, 15
Toroflux, 114f
Torus, 98, 100–101, 100f
Traditional Chinese Medicine (TCM), 104
Trampoline, 167
Transanatomical, 7
"Transformation," 162
Tri-dosha theory, 18e
Trikonasana, 45, 45f
Tubification, 13
Tubular chiralities, 57
Tubular movement, 136
Turing patterns, 29e
Twists, 70–71. *See also* Axial matrix filament

U
Udana, 126
    vayu, 123–124
Uddiyana bandha, 123
Unicellular organism, 6
Upa pranas, 125
Upper and lower limbs
    allied parts in, 25t
    autopod in, 27f
Urdhvadanurasana with duhkha, 94f
Urdhva Dhanurasana, 145, 148, 148f

V
Vacuolar system, 193
Vajrasana, 182f
Variability, 140
Variation, 140
Vata, 102

Vayu, 11e, 105, 120–125
Ventral-dorsal rotation, 20f
Ventromedial portion, of somite, 13
Vertebrates, characteristics of, 16
Vesalius, 10f, 11
Vestibular sense, 29
Vinyasa, 57, 177
Virañchyasana, 53f
Virasana, 63, 64
VITAL tool, 140, 142
Volitional breathing, 170
Vriscikasana, 151
Vyana, 126
    vayu, 124–125

W
Warp and weft, 33e, 37e
Weaving, 39e
Windlass, 77f
Windlass mechanism, 28, 77

Y
Yoga, 15, 135
    deconstructed method, 140
    ekam, inhale, 79
    posture, chiral, 16
    practitioners, 135
    raja, 117
    as self-transformation, 127–128
    spiral motion in, 56–58
    sutras of Patanjali, 39
Yogic sitting
    Padmasana, 179
    Siddhasana, 179
    Sukhasana/Svastikasana, 179
    Vajrasana, 179

Z
"zero state" of equilibrium, 144